Treatment and Prog

General Pr

Philip Spencer.

Treatment and Prognosis
GENERAL PRACTICE

Edited by

Sir Michael Drury OBE, FRCP, FRCGP
and
Richard Hobbs, MB, ChB, FRCGP

Series editor
Richard Hawkins MMBS FRCS

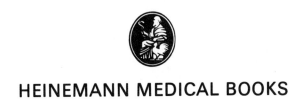

HEINEMANN MEDICAL BOOKS

Heinemann Medical Books
An imprint of Heinemann Professional Publishing Ltd
Halley Court, Jordan Hill, Oxford OX2 8EJ

OXFORD LONDON SINGAPORE NAIROBI IBADAN KINGSTON

First published 1990

British Library Cataloguing in Publication Data
General practice.
  1. Man. Diseases
  I. Drury, Michael   II. Hobbs, Richard
  IV. Series
  616

ISBN 0–433–00682–X

Typeset by Latimer Trend & Company Ltd, Plymouth
and printed in Great Britain

Contents

Foreword

When I began in General Practice (over 35 years ago!) our knowledge of therapeutics went little beyond an understanding of the actions of digitalis and the equipotent efficacy of the different forms in which it was available. Prescribing was, in the main, more an art than a science: compounding elegant formulae and masking unpleasant tastes (except where that effect was desired). Drug interactions were virtually unknown. Medical journals would regularly feature articles by general practitioners describing their *favourite* remedies.

Many of the medicines thought to be active were, in reality, little more than placebos. In fact, in those days we rarely admitted to prescribing a placebo.

Ointments were prepared individually for each patient and often compounded specially; so too, were some of the tablets and even suppositories. I remember writing prescriptions for my own 'cocktail' of ergot, aspirin and barbiturate for the treatment of migraine. Individual doses of the powder were poured by local pharmacists into empty capsules. (When I visited French pharmacies on behalf of the Nuffield Pharmacy Inquiry a few years ago, I was not as surprised as some of my colleagues were to see this practice still being carried out).

Medicines were labelled: 'The Medicine', 'The Capsules', 'The Ointment', and so on. In those days, we assumed, probably correctly, that our patients did not want to know what they were getting. Today every dispensed medicine is fully labelled, though in my part of London, a number of patients still speak of the 'blue tablets' rather than the name that is now always on the label.

Today, a knowledge of therapeutics is at least as important in general practice as it is in hospital practice. Until recently most of the textbooks in this field were written by hospital-based specialists with little or no experience of the practical every day problems of caring for people in the community. The arrival of an authoritative, well referenced textbook on treatment and prognosis written by general practitioners for general practitioners is, therefore, very welcome.

Stuart Carne, 1990

List of contributors

P E Bundred MD, DCH(SA), DCM (Cape Town)
Senior Lecturer in General Practice, Department of General Practice, Univeristy of Liverpool, New Medical School, Ashton Street, Liverpool

A J B Carson MB, ChB, BSc, MRCGP
Lecturer, Department of General Practice, Medical School, University of Birmingham, Vincent Drive, Birmingham

J Draper MD, MRCGP
Course Organiser, Vocational Training Scheme for General Practice, The Clinical School, Addenbrookes Hospital, Hills Road, Cambridge

V W M Drury OBE, FRCP, FRCGP, FRACGP
Professor and Head of Department of General Practice, Medical School, University of Birmingham, Vincent Drive, Birmingham

F D R Hobbs MB, ChB, FRCGP
Senior Lecturer, Department of General Practice, Medical School, University of Birmingham, Vincent Drive, Birmingham

R Hull MB, FRCGP
MacMillan Senior Lecturer in Palliative Care, Department of General Practice, Medical School, University of Birmingham, Vincent Drive, Birmingham

M D Jewell MA, MRCGP
Senior Lecturer, Department of General Practice, Bristol University, and Consultant, Epidemiology and Public Health Medicine, Canynge Hall, Whiteladies Road, Bristol

M H Kelly MBChB, MRCGP
Lecturer in General Practice, University of Glasgow, Woodside Health Centre, Barr Street, Glasgow

D R Morgan MBChB, FRCP, MRCGP, DCH, DRCOG
Senior Lecturer in General Practice, Department of General Practice, Medical School, University of Birmingham, Vincent Drive, Birmingham

B B Reiss OBE MRCP, FRCGP
Past Director of GP Studies, University of Cambridge, The Clinical School, Addenbrookes Hospital, Hills Road, Cambridge

J Southgate MB ChB, FRCGP, MClinSci
Senior Lecturer, Academic Department of General Practice and Primary Care, Medical Colleges of St Bartholomew's and London Hospitals, Charterhouse Square, London

D W Wall MB ChB(Hons), MRCP(UK), FRCGP
Associate Advisor in General Practice, University of Birmingham and General Practitioner, Sutton Coldfield

J H Walker and Members from the Division of Primary Care
Department of Family and Community Medicine Medical School, Framlington Place, Newcastle-upon-Tyne

J F Wilmot MBChB, FRCGP, DCH, DRCOG
Senior Lecturer in General Practice, School of Postgraduate Medical Education, University of Warwick, Coventry

Disease directory

10 Dermatology 235

1

The Female Genital Tract

L. J. Southgate

Premenstrual Syndrome

The premenstrual syndrome (PMS) is difficult to define as there are no generally agreed criteria; neither is the timing of the premenstrual phase consistently defined. Physical and emotional changes occur with such frequency in relation to the menstrual cycle that many women accept them as a normal aspect of life. However a proportion find the changes cause severe disruption to function and well-being. Drummond and Tonks[1] cite the work of Rees as an example of a 'middle-of-the-road' description of the syndrome. He reported the commonest complaints as tension and irritability (100% of sufferers), depression (80%), anxiety (77%), swelling of fingers or legs (74%) and painful swelling of the breasts (60%). Clare[2] found that 75% of women studied reported at least one premenstrual symptom. Women with a score on the General Health Questionnaire indicative of psychiatric morbidity were more likely to report symptoms relating to mood or behaviour, but were no more likely to report physical symptoms.

The prevalence of PMS is uncertain but it is much greater in those studies which use a questionnaire than in those using a daily diary to record changes[1]. It is likely that the syndrome represents the severe end of the normal spectrum of premenstrual changes and that up to 10% of women find these changes a problem. Particular difficulties are encountered by those women who not only have severe symptoms but who experience them throughout the luteal phase of the cycle[3].

There are many theories about the causes of the premenstrual syndrome such as abnormalities of the sex hormones (e.g. high ratio of oestrogen to progesterone, increased prolactin levels); water and sodium retention (e.g. increased aldosterone or antidiuretic hormone production), and psychological theories (e.g. adverse early experience of menstruation). There is at present no conclusive evidence to support any of these hypotheses. A recent theory[4] postulates a deficiency of essential fatty acids, particularly gamma-linolenic acid which is a precursor of prostaglandin E, which in turn attenuates the biological action of prolactin.

PROGNOSIS

- PMS is a difficult problem to help and sufferers often endure major disruption over several years.
- The condition often appears or worsens when women are in their 30s and 40s.
- The prognosis is improved when the patient is in the care of an understanding doctor who can negotiate with her the maze of unproven therapies to find the one which suits her best.

TREATMENT

1. The most important part of treatment is to allow the patient the opportunity to discuss her symptoms fully and the effect they are having on her daily activities and relationships. Many women already feel that their problems are not taken seriously by doctors and indeed it is deeply offensive to a woman to be told that a source of major disruption to her life is 'normal' or due to her 'hormones'[3].

2. Many women benefit from a self-help approach to PMS[4]. A menstrual diary in which symptoms and emotional changes can be recorded daily is a useful aid to understanding their timing and severity. This in turn enables the patient to anticipate the onset of difficulties and to plan her life accordingly.

3. Drug therapy in PMS is controversial as very few approaches have been shown to be effective when evaluated against placebo in a double-blind controlled trial[1]. Many women are helped by one of the following therapies but it is important to remember that studies of PMS have found a high placebo response; care should be taken to select the least intrusive therapy that is effective for the individual woman.

4. Pyridoxine 50–100 mg daily is given for depression, irritability and breast tenderness.

5. Natural progesterone may be given as a vaginal pessary, or the synthetic progesterone dydrogesterone may be given, 10 mg b.d. during the luteal phase.

Bromocriptine 2.5 mg daily may be given if breast pain is a major symptom. This drug is a prolactin antagonist, but is said to be effective in women with mastalgia in the absence of raised prolactin levels.

Some women benefit from a diuretic during the luteal phase despite the lack of reported evidence for premenstrual salt and water retention[1]. The aldosterone antagonist spironolactone can no longer be recommended in PMS due to worries of possible carcinogenesis in rodents[5].

  . Oil of evening primrose (gamma-linolenic acid) may be given as 500 mg capsules b.d. after food from 3 days before the onset of symptoms until the start of menstruation. The preparation is not available on prescription. This approach is currently the subject of research, but appears to be of benefit to some women in whom other treatments have failed.

  . Benzodiazepines are *inappropriate* therapy for PMS and cause more problems for the woman in terms of tiredness, depression and dependence.

FOLLOW-UP

Review of symptoms and medication depends on the therapeutic approach selected and its success. The practice nurse is an ideal person to conduct follow-up and may also convene a group for women who are experiencing major problems.

[1] Drummond L, Tonks C (1985) The premenstrual syndrome. In *Psychological Disorders in Obstetrics and Gynaecology* (Priest R ed.). London: Butterworths.
[2] Clare AW (1983) *Psychol. Med.* Monograph (**suppl. 4**): 1–58.
[3] Reid RL (1986) *Am. J. Obstet. Gynecol.*, **155**, 921–6.
[4] McPherson A (ed.) (1988) *Women's Problems in General Practice*. Oxford: Oxford University Press.
[5] Current Problems (1988) Committee on safety of medicines, **21**.

Menopausal Symptoms

The menopause is the consequence of the rapid decline in ovarian function which occurs at or around the age of 50. The mean life expectancy for women is now 83 years and postmenopausal women comprise 18% of the UK population[1], thus the problems they suffer are of major social and economic importance.

The menopause is experienced differently in different cultures and in some languages no word exists for it. In the western world 50–80% of women suffer hot flushes and night sweats; 12% of flushes are severe and accompanied by profuse sweating. The episodes are characterized by a reduction in core temperature, an increase in peripheral temperature by 5°C and tachycardia. Nocturnal flushes cause insomnia and some women are severely affected. Falling oestrogen levels also lead to atrophic vaginitis with dyspareunia, discharge and vaginal burning, while effects on the bladder trigone and urethra result in frequency, dysuria and urgency. Declining ovarian function leads to increased cholesterol and triglyceride levels, lower high-density lipoprotein and increased very low density lipoprotein.

While these changes are usually seen as detrimental, interpretation of clinical sequelae is much more difficult. Well conducted studies have shown that difficulty in making decisions, loss of confidence, difficulty in concentrating and low self-esteem reach peak prevalence just before the menopause, although adverse life events did not cluster around the climacteric[2].

A major consequence of the climacteric is osteoporosis which results from an increase in bone resorption. This is thought to be due to the fact that oestrogen regulates the secretion of calcitonin; the level of calcitonin declines in postmenopausal women. A 30% reduction in bone mass occurs by the age of 70 and 50% of women will have sustained one or more fractures of the wrist, vertebral bodies or femoral neck by the age of 75[2,3]. Small, thin, fair women, heavy smokers and those with a family history are at greatest risk. Women experiencing a premature menopause (before the age of 44) and women who have been castrated are particularly prone to severe problems during the climacteric.

PROGNOSIS

- Some 25% of women are asymptomatic and require no advice. There may however be 'rapid bone losers' in this group who are at greater risk of osteoporosis in later life.
- While oestrogen therapy does not reverse already established osteoporosis, studies have shown a reduction in the incidence of fractures in postmenopausal women on long-term hormone replacement therapy (HRT). The dilemma is to identify those women particularly at risk and to weigh up the risks and benefits for each patient in the light of present knowledge[4].
- Theoretically, oestrogen therapy should decrease the risk of ischaemic heart disease while progestogens may increase it. Treatment with combined preparations makes the outcome difficult to assess until current research clarifies the situation.

TREATMENT[5]

1. It is important for general practitioners to acknowledge the distress caused by the symptoms presented by many menopausal women. Time spent in talking about the effects on work, home and relationships with partners enables most women to cope better.
2. Contraception may pose problems; most authorities recommend continuing with contraception until 1 year after the last period in women over 40. A follicle-stimulating hormone level of >15 iu/l is in the menopausal range.
3. Women with distressing symptoms or those in the high-risk group for osteoporosis who have a uterus may be treated with continuous oral oestrogen with progestogen for 10 or more days in each cycle to avoid the risk of endometrial hyperplasia and subsequent endometrial carcinoma. Natural oestrogens have a more beneficial effect on the blood lipid profile than synthetic oestrogens and are to be preferred.
4. Several combined preparations are available, e.g. Prempak-C 0.625 or 1.25 mg. Women often have cyclical bleeding. Providing it is regular it is harmless and is often well tolerated by the patient as a small price to pay for relief of symptoms. Irregular bleeding must be fully investigated.
5. Women who have had a hysterectomy benefit from continuous treatment with unopposed oestrogen, e.g. Progynova 1 or 2 mg daily.
6. Occasionally implants may be used. Oestradiol 50 or 100 mg is inserted into the subcutaneous fat of the anterior abdominal wall under local anaesthesia. The procedure can conveniently be carried out in general practice. Subcutaneous therapy avoids the enterohepatic circulation, thereby producing a physiological ratio of oestradiol to oestrone[3]. The hormones are slowly absorbed over the following 6 months or more and the implant is repeated when symptoms return. Women with a uterus should also be given progesterone for at least 10 days each month.

   Women who are particularly affected by loss of libido and lethargy may benefit from an implant of testosterone 100 mg. This therapy is especially beneficial to women who have had surgical removal of both ovaries while young. This is because the ovary continues to produce androgens and some oestrogens in the postmenopausal period, making castration a particularly severe insult.
7. Vaginal cream (e.g. Premarin cream) is useful in treating vaginitis and bladder disturbances. The oestrogens are absorbed into the blood stream; vaginal cream must not be used in women with a contraindication to oestrogen therapy. Unlike oral preparations which are first metabolized in the liver, these hormones are absorbed direct and unchanged and are often effective in small doses. Continued sexual activity lessens the effects of vaginal atrophy and a lubricant such as KY jelly may be the only treatment necessary to deal with dyspareunia.
8. Skin patches which enable the direct absorption of oestrogen, avoiding the liver, are also available. Progestogens are indicated for women who have not had hysterectomies.
9. Oestrogens are contraindicated in women who have cancer of the breast, ovary, endometrium or malignant melanoma, or who have major thromboembolic disease, severe liver disease or severe diabetes[5].
10. Relative contraindications include irregular vaginal bleeding not yet diagnosed, gall bladder disease, untreated hypertension, smoking,

mild diabetes or the presence of increased risk factors for breast cancer.

. Beta-blockers may be of benefit for palpitations when heart disease has been excluded.

. Exercise and stopping smoking are important in minimizing osteoporosis.

All women presenting symptoms of the climacteric should receive advice regarding regular breast self-examination, cervical cytology, smoking, exercise and weight control as part of health education for women of this age. The history should include inquiry for irregular vaginal bleeding.

Women maintained on HRT require an annual pelvic examination to check on uterine size, blood pressure measurement and for breast examination. Fibroids may grow rapidly during oestrogen therapy. The duration of HRT will be decided during follow-up and depends on how long symptoms have lasted and the assessed vulnerability of the woman to osteoporosis.

[1] Whitehead MI (1985) The climacteric. In *Progress in Obstetrics and Gynaecology* (Studd J ed). London: Churchill Livingstone.
[2] Greene JG (1984) *The Social and Psychological Origins of the Climacteric Syndrome*. Gower. Aldershot, England.
[3] Savvas M et al. (1988) *Br. Med. J.*, **297**, 331–3.
[4] Heath D (1988) *Prescribers J.* Aug., 121.
[5] Coope J (1984) *Br. Med. J.*, **289**, 888–90.

Infertility

Up to 15% of all couples present to their general practitioner with involuntary infertility. The incidences of the various causes of infertility vary world-wide but in general the common causes are abnormalities of the fallopian tube, usually secondary to infection (20–30%), disordered spermatogenesis (15–25%), problems with ovulation (10–15%) and endometriosis (10%)[1]. Sexual difficulties are a cause in some cases. Infertility is associated with higher social class and increasing age of the woman; this combination is frequently seen in the UK as couples delay their first child for reasons of education and career. In couples where the woman is under 35 and where there is no obvious problem the more invasive investigations should be delayed until after 2 years as it is not until then that a couple can be said to be outside the normal range.

PROGNOSIS

● A total of 75% of couples who are not using contraception will achieve a pregnancy within 12 months and a further 5% will do so within the following year.

● The results from tubal microsurgery differ between centres. Term pregnancy has been reported in up to 25% of women after salpingostomy and up to 50% of women after salpingolysis. There is an increased risk of ectopic pregnancy after reconstructive surgery.

● In vitro fertilization leads to pregnancy rates of about one in ten per attempt with about 50% of women becoming pregnant after five attempts. Only 50–60% of the pregnancies result in live infants, amongst whom there is no increase in fetal abnormalities.

● Although 70% of women receiving clomiphene for anovulation appear to ovulate, only half become pregnant, usually within four treatment cycles.

● In 10% of couples infertility remains unexplained. Of these women, 50% become pregnant during the next 5 years, whether treated or not.

TREATMENT

1. Infertile couples are often under great strain and experience some relief when investigation

is begun. The process is, however, often lengthy and frustrating and the general practitioner can have a central role both in the initial assessment (which in itself is part of treatment) and in explaining and encouraging as the diagnostic process proceeds. The couple must be protected from doubtful therapies but ensured rapid and appropriate referral when it is warranted.

2. The initial assessment of the couple should include a joint interview with an exploration of the sexual relationship and any ambivalence or conflict within the couple regarding conception. The physical examination should concentrate on the genital and endocrine systems of both partners. The general practitioner should use the opportunity to build trust in case investigations and decisions become difficult later on. Preliminary investigations in general practice often clarify the situation sufficiently to enable an informed choice of specialist, whether for tubal surgery, treatment of ovulatory problems or male factors.

3. General practitioners can play a major role in the prevention of pelvic inflammatory disease (and hence tubal damage) by the proper diagnosis and adequate treatment of genital infections (see page 10).

4. In patients where tubal factors are thought to be responsible for infertility, function is assessed by hysterosalpingography and laparoscopy. These techniques only evaluate the anatomical status of the tubes; currently no methods are available to assess ovum pick-up and transport or the tubal environment for fertilization or the initial development of the embryo. While the hysterosalpingogram allows assessment of tubal patency, laparoscopy yields much more information as all the pelvic organs can be inspected and such conditions as endometriosis, extratubal adhesions, fibroids and ovarian abnormalities can be detected. Tubal microsurgery may restore tubal function but is best carried out in centres with special experience in the technique.

5. In vitro fertilization and embryo transfer techniques may be used when tubal blockage or dysfunction persists. In general the woman's ovaries are hyperstimulated and ova are retrieved using ultrasound or laparoscopy. The oocytes are inseminated 6 hours later and cultured under strictly controlled conditions. Transcervical embryo transfer is undertaken at 44–48 hours. The general practitioner should be available to discuss the ethical and emotional issues that such procedures may raise in the minds of the infertile couple.

6. a. Problems with ovulation may be revealed by the presence of amenorrhoea or irregular cycles. However 10% of women with regular cycles are not ovulating[1] and while dysmenorrhoea, premenstrual syndrome and mid-cycle pain or bleeding may suggest ovulation, the history itself is not an adequate assessment. Pointers within the clinical examination include low weight, lack of secondary sexual characteristics, galactorrhoea indicating hyperprolactinaemia, acne and hirsutism indicating polycystic ovarian disease or signs of thyroid dysfunction. Women who are menstruating regularly may be asked to keep a temperature chart as progesterone production by the corpus luteum may result in a rise in basal body temperature of 0.3°C in the second half of the cycle. A biphasic pattern certainly indicates ovulation but at least 20% of ovulatory women have a monophasic pattern. Three cycles are enough to provide useful information. The main use of a chart is to demonstrate the timing of ovulation, provide some guidance for the timing of intercourse and to monitor treatment.

b. The occurrence of ovulation is properly assessed by the measurement of serum progesterone levels in the mid luteal phase, which is 5–10 days before the onset of the next period. Levels of >30 nmol/l confirm ovulation, although assessment of the adequacy of corpus luteum function requires serial measurements.

c. Further investigation of women with absent or infrequent ovulation always includes measurement of serum follicle-stimulating hormone, luteinizing hormone, prolactin, thyroid function tests and an X-ray of the skull to examine the pituitary fossa for an adenoma in those women with hyperprolactinaemia.

d. Women with hirsutism or virilization should also have an androgen profile for polycystic ovary disease. Many of these investigations can be carried out by the general practitioner.

e. Anovulation is treated in most cases either by clomiphene or human menopausal gonadotrophin which contains a mixture of follicle-stimulating hormone and luteinizing hormone. The regimes need specialist monitoring to avoid hyperstimulation and multiple pregnancy.

7. a. Anovulation is affected by stress such as bereavement, family conflicts or a new job, and manifests with amenorrhoea. Low weight and strenuous exercise also affect ovulation and in all these situations the general practitioner can advise and encourage the patient in the knowledge that ovulatory cycles will resume when the underlying cause is dealt with.

b. Drugs which raise prolactin levels and hence inhibit ovulation include cimetidine and phenothiazines. About 1 in 500 women stopping oral contraceptives fail to start ovulating promptly; incidence is markedly increased in women with a history of previous menstrual irregularity[2]. Care should be taken before starting the pill in such women as about 12% of nulliparous women are still affected after 18 months[3].

8. a. A semen analysis may be arranged by the general practitioner. The sample is best provided by masturbation after 4 days' abstinence.

b. An abnormal sample has a volume <1 ml, sperm concentration of <20 million/ml, sperm motility $<40\%$ progressive motility and $<60\%$ normal oval forms. An abnormal result should be repeated on two further occasions before it is confirmed.

c. Men with oligospermia or azoospermia should be referred. Many men experience a severe reaction and loss of self-esteem which can lead to depression, aggressive behaviour or sexual difficulties.

d. Men with small testicles and grossly elevated follicle-stimulating hormone have primary testicular failure and no further investigations are necessary as the situation cannot be remedied[4].

e. A postcoital test can be performed in general practice and should be carried out on the day of ovulation. The woman can be examined in the morning after having intercourse the night before. Mucus is extracted from the cervical canal and immediately examined under the microscope. It should be clear and copious with a good Spinnbarkheit and in a positive test more than 10 motile sperm/hpf are seen. A positive result enables the general practitioner to reassure the couple that intercourse is adequate and that there is no cervical mucus hostility to sperm migration.

FOLLOW-UP

Many of these couples are investigated over a long period and often suffer many frustrations. The general practitioner should be available throughout and in particular must offer long-term support to those couples who have to accept that they are infertile and who have to deal with the painful emotional consequences that inevitably result.

[1] Pepperell R (1984) The investigation of infertility. In *Progress in Obstetrics and Gynaecology*, vol 4 (Studd J ed), pp. 272–89.
[2] Shaw RW (1984) Hypothalamic reproductive failure. In *Progress in Obstetrics and Gynaecology*, vol 4, pp. 279–89. London: Churchill Livingstone.
[3] Charnock M (1988) Problems with fertility. In *Women's Problems in General Practice* (McPherson A ed), pp. 285–313. Oxford: Oxford University Press.
[4] Pryor JP (1983) Treatment of male infertility. In *Progress in Obstetrics and Gynaecology*, vol 3 (Studd J ed), pp. 334–45. London: Churchill Livingstone.

Vaginitis

Vaginitis is a common problem in general practice; about 8% of women aged 16–45 present with a new episode each year[1]. It is usually caused by bacterial vaginosis, yeast infections (*Candida* spp.) or trichomoniasis. Rarer causes include an ulcerative vaginitis resulting from a forgotten tampon or cervical cap. In postmenopausal women, the vaginal epithelium becomes thin with oestrogen withdrawal, causing atrophic vaginitis which should be differentiated from the usual forms of infection.

Bacterial vaginosis

Bacterial vaginosis is present in 15–25% of women presenting in general practice and is characterized by an offensive vaginal discharge; the smell is particularly strong after intercourse. Many women are distressed and embarrassed by the odour and have difficulty talking about it. Clinical examination reveals a homogeneous, grey, uniformly adherent discharge. The vaginal pH is raised (5 or above) and addition of 10% potassium hydroxide to the discharge releases a fishy smell. Clue cells are present on the Gram-stained smear, and *Gardnerella vaginalis* and anaerobes (especially *Bacteroides* spp. and *Mobilluncus* spp.) are isolated[2].

PROGNOSIS

- The condition may recur after treatment. The reasons for this recurrence, the mode of transmission and complications such as increased risk of salpingitis are the subjects of current research.
- Women with an intrauterine contraceptive device (IUCD) in situ are four times more likely to have bacterial vaginosis.

TREATMENT

1. Metronidazole 400 mg b.d. for 7 days.
2. Acetic acid gel twice daily lowers the vaginal pH.
3. There is no evidence that the condition is sexually acquired.

FOLLOW-UP

Clinical examination, vaginal pH and potassium hydroxide test are adequate.

Candida albicans

Candida albicans is the commonest cause of vaginitis in general practice and may be the principal cause of vaginitis in 30% of new cases. The organism is harboured by many asymptomatic women, but when vaginitis is present, it is characterized by intense vulvovaginal itching, vulval oedema, external dysuria and thick white vaginal discharge. The diagnosis may be confirmed by wet mount or culture. The infection is commonly seen in pregnancy and may be the initial presentation of diabetes mellitus.

PROGNOSIS

- The mean late recolonization rate after treatment is 21% and is related to the past history of recurrence of vaginal candida in the patient.

TREATMENT (See p. 318)

FOLLOW-UP

Unnecessary for asymptomatic women.

Recurrent thrush must be confirmed by the presence of *Candida albicans*, as many of these women have other infections.

Treatment of the sexual partner with cream for his penis may improve the cure in refractory cases.

There is debate about the role of oral contraceptives. Susceptible women receiving antibiotics active against lactobacilli (penicillins, tetracyclines, cephalosporins) should however receive simultaneous antifungal therapy.

In intractable cases, monthly treatment with a single pessary of clotrimazole 500 mg between day 7 and 11 of menstrual cycle reduces recurences[3]. It is sometimes helpful to investigate these patients for low iron stores as correction of a low serum ferritin may lead to resolution of the infection. These women should have a random blood glucose taken to rule out diabetes.

Trichomonas vaginalis

Trichomonas vaginalis is a flagellated protozoan which is usually sexually transmitted and is often associated with gonorrhoea. Incidence figures vary widely, but the prevalence in general practice populations is about 5%. The age of peak incidence is 16–35 years with a high susceptibility in postmenopausal women. Symptoms and signs are very variable, but often include a profuse, frothy discharge and intense pruritis[4].

PROGNOSIS

- The infection may persist for years if untreated or if there is inadequate treatment of sexual partners.

TREATMENT (See p. 319)

FOLLOW-UP

Cultures should be taken after 7–10 days, as test of cure.

Atrophic vaginitis

Atrophic vaginitis results from changes in the vagina due to falling oestrogen levels at and after the menopause. The vaginal pH rises, allowing a change in the vaginal flora and sometimes leading to secondary infection.

PROGNOSIS

- If untreated these women develop a persistent bloody, purulent discharge. This situation must be differentiated from genital tract cancer.

TREATMENT

1. The health of the vaginal epithelium is maintained by regular intercourse.
2. The vaginal pH may be lowered by using acetic acid 0.92% in buffer as a gel to be inserted for 10 days.
3. Oestrogens are very helpful in restoring the vaginal epithelium. They also relieve the frequency and dysuria which often accompany atrophic vaginitis, due to similar changes within the bladder trigone. They may be given locally as a vaginal cream (e.g. dienoestrol cream) twice daily for 2 weeks as a short-term or intermittent treatment. HRT given as cyclical oestrogen/progesterone preparations is also most effective in this condition. For a fuller discussion of the use of oestrogens in postmenopausal women see page 4.

FOLLOW-UP

Women using acetic acid gel or a short course of vaginal cream need no follow-up except the usual 3-yearly cervical smear recommended for all women in the age group. They should be told to report any unusual genital symptom or recurrence of vaginitis.

Women on HRT require regular monitoring (see page 5).

[1] O'Dowd T, West R (1987) Clinical prediction of *Gardnerella vaginalis* in general practice. *J. R. Coll. G.P.*, **37**, 59–61.
[2] Amsel R *et al.* (1983) Nonspecific vaginitis: diagnostic criteria and microbial and epidemiological associations. *Am. J. Med.*, **74**, 14.
[3] Davidson F, Mould RF (1978) Recurrent genital candidosis in women and the effect of intermittent prophylactic treatment. *Br. J. Vener. Dis.*, **54**, 176.
[4] Rein M, Muller M (1984) *Trichomonas vaginalis*. In *Sexually Transmitted Diseases* (Holmes KK *et al.*, eds). New York: McGraw-Hill.

Cervicitis

Cervicitis is a common complaint and is often unrecognized as it may be asymptomatic. It is one of the causes of vaginal discharge, either alone or in association with vaginitis, and for this reason it may go untreated if the cervix is not inspected in women with vaginal discharge. Although *Candida albicans* and *Trichomonas vaginalis* can both cause exocervicitis, the major infectious causes of cervicitis are *Chlamydia trachomatis, Neisseria gonorrhoeae* and herpes simplex virus. *Frequently more than one of these causes is present in one patient.*

Chlamydial cervicitis

Chlamydia trachomatis is an obligate intracellular parasite which is always sexually acquired. The prevalence has been variously reported as 3–5% in asymptomatic women to 20% in women seen in sexually transmitted disease (STD) clinics. In one study of inner city general practice 8% of women seen for vaginal examination for any reason harboured the organism[1].

Chlamydial cervicitis is associated with a mucopurulent cervical discharge, cervical friability and hypertrophic ectopy (an area of ectopy which is oedematous)[1,2]. Clinical examination alone is unreliable for diagnosis, which should be confirmed by the methods locally available. In general, culture is difficult from general practice and most laboratories prefer a monoclonal antibody test such as MicroTrak or IDEA. If the infection is suspected for any reason and the expertise or facilities are not available for diagnosis the patient should be referred to the genitourinary medicine clinic.

PROGNOSIS

- Untreated infection leads to a chronic state which may persist for years.
- Some 8% of women with chlamydial cervicitis develop chlamydial salpingitis; 15% of these women are subsequently infertile.
- Untreated pregnant women have an increased risk of postpartum endometritis. Untreated women undergoing termination of pregnancy have a similarly increased risk.
- Perihepatitis is a rare but important complication. It is a more common cause of right upper quadrant pain in young sexually active women than cholecystitis.

- In the USA the incidence of chlamydial neonatal conjunctivitis is 18–25/1000 live births and the incidence of chlamydial pneumonia 5–10/1000 live births.

TREATMENT

1. Doxycycline 200 mg stat, then 100 mg for 10 days.
2. Erythromycin stearate 500 mg q.i.d. for 10 days.

FOLLOW-UP

Patients should be seen and retested for infection on completion of treatment. Sexual partners should be screened for infection; genitourinary clinics have the best facilities for investigation and treatment of male chlamydial urethritis. Discussion of the implications of chlamydial cervicitis should include information about its role in salpingitis and association with infertility and risk of ectopic pregnancy. This sensitive information must be imparted to enable the patient to modify her behaviour or that of her partner if she so wishes. The doctor should avoid appearing judgemental and should be aware of the potential damage to relationships that can occur when a sexually transmitted infection is diagnosed.

Gonococcal cervicitis

The endocervical canal is the primary site of gonococcal infection in women. Urethral colonization is present in 70–90%, rectal mucosal 30–50% and pharyngeal colonization in 10–20%

of patients. Infection of Bartholin's ducts and Skene's glands is common. The incubation period is about 10 days, although some women remain asymptomatic. Symptoms are those of lower genital tract infection and include vaginal discharge, intermenstrual bleeding, menorrhagia and dysuria. There may be a purulent cervical discharge and the cervix bleeds easily on contact. Diagnosis may not be made on clinical grounds alone as symptoms and signs are so variable, and other sexually transmitted infections (especially trichomonas and chlamydia) frequently coexist. Diagnosis is by culture and examination of stained smears; if these methods are not available to the practice the patient must be referred to the STD clinic.

PROGNOSIS, TREATMENT AND FOLLOW-UP

(See p. 320)

Herpes virus cervicitis (See also p. 323)

In the UK in 1979 genital herpes infections accounted for about 2% of all attendances at STD clinics. In 1977 8400 cases of herpes simplex virus (HSV) infections were seen in these clinics, but by 1983 the numbers had risen to about 18 000, an increase of 100% in 6 years[3]. Data from industrialized countries suggest that the disease is increasing in frequency, particularly amongst groups with a previously low prevalence. This appears to be the case for young middle and upper class adults although it is difficult to separate the effects of a greater awareness and reporting, and different diagnostic methods[3].

The first episode of genital herpes is characterized by multiple genital and extragenital sites, a prolonged period of viral shedding and generalized constitutional upset. Between 70 and 90% of women with a primary genital herpes infection have a herpetic cervicitis accompanying the painful lesions on the external genitalia. The mean duration of viral shedding from the cervical lesions is 11 days. Primary HSV cervicitis is characterized by diffuse or local areas of friability, or ulcerative lesions of the exocervix, or rarely an extensive necrotic cervicitis. In contrast to this picture, recurrent attacks are much milder, and only 15–30% of women with recurrent external genital lesions had HSV isolated from the cervix, which often appeared clinically normal.

PROGNOSIS

- Some 60–80% of women with primary HSV-2 infections develop recurrences, whereas the rate for infections due to HSV-1 is much lower[4].
- The median number of recurrences of genital herpes in a year has been reported as 5–8, but the pattern is very variable.
- Many studies have reported an association between HSV-2 cervicitis and cervical intraepithelial neoplasia, but the evidence for a causative role is not established.

TREATMENT

1. Patients with primary genital herpes infections often feel very unwell. Occasionally the pain of the external genital lesions is so severe that acute retention of urine occurs and the patient requires admission. General measures include rest and adequate analgesia.
2. The only effective treatment against the virus is *acyclovir*. Intravenous therapy is indicated in severe primary herpes; topical and oral preparations are available for use in the general practice setting. The drug does not eradicate the virus from the root ganglion and does not therefore prevent recurrent attacks.
3. Patients should abstain from sexual intercourse for 3 weeks after the primary attack to ensure that the virus is no longer being shed by cervical lesions.

FOLLOW-UP

Women with recurrent herpes need a sympathetic approach especially as there is no cure. The individual attacks are lessened by the use of oral acyclovir which must be started as soon as an attack begins. In patients with severe and frequent attacks long-term use may be justified and the drug may be given as 200 mg four times daily for up to 6 months. These patients should have an annual cervical smear. Some women are helped by contacting a self-help group.

[1] Southgate LJ, Treharne JD, Forsey T (1983) *Chlamydia trachomatis* and *Neisseria gonorrhoeae* infections in women attending inner city general practices. *Br Med J*, **287**, 879–81.

[2] Stamm WE, Holmes KK (1984) *Chlamydia trachomatis* infections of the adult. In *Sexually Transmitted Diseases* (Holmes KK *et al*. eds). New York: McGraw-Hill.

[3] Caul E, Roome A (1987) Genital herpes. In *Sexually Transmitted Diseases: A Rational Approach to their Diagnosis* (Jephcott A ed). London: Public Health Laboratory Services.

[4] Reeves WC *et al*. (1981) Risk of recurrence after first episodes of genital herpes. Relation to HSV type and antibody response. *N. Engl. J. Med.*, **305**, 315–19.

Uterovaginal Prolapse

Uterovaginal prolapse is a common condition which is a source of inconvenience and discomfort to many women and is the stated reason for 12% of hysterectomies carried out in the UK every year[1]. Prolapse of the upper vaginal wall involves the bladder (cystocele) and of the lower vaginal wall involves the urethra (urethrocele). Both commonly occur together and may be asymptomatic. A large cystocele may be associated with infected residual urine with frequency and dysuria and a sensation of a lump coming down. If the upper posterior vaginal wall is involved there is usually an associated herniation of the Pouch of Douglas which often contains a loop of bowel (enterocele). Prolapse of the lower posterior vaginal wall leads to a rectocele which is sometimes associated with difficulty with defecation.

Uterine prolapse is always accompanied by a degree of vaginal wall descent and has three degrees of severity:

1. The cervix remains within the vagina.
2. The cervix descends through the introitus when the woman is standing or straining.
3. The whole of the uterus prolapses outside the vulva.

The cause of prolapse is the failure of one or more of the vaginal or uterine supports and may be due to congenital weakness, trauma during childbirth and atrophy of the surrounding tissues at the time of the menopause. The condition may be familial and is exacerbated by obesity, chronic constipation and recurrent cough[2].

PROGNOSIS

Untreated

- An untreated uterine prolapse in which the cervix descends below the vulva leads to keratinization and thickening of the superficial epithelium. The cervix becomes elongated, oedematous and may ulcerate.
- Infection may follow leading to bleeding and discharge. Malignant change is very rare.
- Large amounts of residual urine within a cystocele may be chronically infected and eventually lead to pyelonephritis.
- A third-degree uterine prolapse may lead to chronic obstruction to the ureters with hydroureter and hydronephrosis.
- Some women have dyspareunia following surgery. This is particularly likely in older women in whom attempts to resume intercourse after

several months may be difficult due to post-menopausal vaginitis. Lubricants such as KY jelly and the use of oestrogen creams may be helpful in these circumstances.
- Some 75–90% of women who attempt conception after cervical amputation fail to become pregnant. Abortion and premature labour are increased in those who do succeed[2]. The procedure is not recommended for women who wish to have more children.

TREATMENT

1. Prevention: pushing during delivery should be avoided before the cervix is fully dilated, and a prolonged second stage is unadvisable. All lacerations and episiotomies should be carefully repaired in layers and the woman should be

encouraged towards early mobilization and regular pelvic floor exercises.

. Most parous women have a minor degree of prolapse for which no treatment is required unless there are symptoms.

. Surgical intervention is the treatment of choice, but only if the patient has symptoms or the prolapse is interfering with daily life. It may be left untreated if asymptomatic, provided there is no chronic urinary infection.

4. Vaginal prolapse may be treated by anterior and posterior repair respectively. If a utero-vaginal prolapse is present some surgeons advocate an anterior and posterior repair combined with amputation of the cervix and shortening of the transverse cervical ligaments (Manchester operation).

5. An alternative approach is a hysterectomy with approximation of the pedicles of the transverse cervical ligaments, the uterosacral ligaments and the broad ligaments.

6. All younger women undergoing repair with or without hysterectomy should have a full opportunity to discuss the implications for fertility and childbearing. Older women may be particularly reticent about discussing sexuality and the effects of the operation on intercourse. The general practitioner should ensure that they are enabled to do so should they wish.

7. Elderly women with complete prolapse (procidentia) are often admitted preoperatively for reduction of the prolapse and packing of the vagina with gauze impregnated with oestradiol cream. This promotes healing of cervical ulcers and improvement of vaginal tissues before operation.

8. Some women refuse or are too ill for surgery. Many benefit from a vaginal ring pessary which can be fitted and supervised by the general practitioner. The use of vaginal oestrogen creams is often helpful for older women using ring pessaries. For contraindications to the use of these preparations see p. 4.

FOLLOW-UP

Women using ring pessaries require review and a pessary change every 4 months. The vaginal vault should be inspected for trauma and the urine tested for infection.

Women who have undergone surgery should be followed up in general practice about 3 months postoperatively to ensure that symptoms are gone and a normal life, including sexual intercourse if desired, has been resumed.

[1] McPherson A (1988) *Women's Problems in General Practice*, 2nd edn, p. 113. Oxford: Oxford University Press.
[2] Tindall V (1987) *Jeffcoate's Principles of Gynaecology*, p. 260. London: Butterworth.

Cervical Cancer

Cervical cancer is the second commonest cancer in women, with an annual incidence rate of 24/100 000 women (including carcinoma in situ). It is extremely rare in women who have never had sexual intercourse and the risk increases with the number of sexual partners of the patient or her partner. The prevalence of cervical intraepithelial neoplasia (CIN) amongst patients in an STD clinic has been reported as 11.4%, compared with 6% amongst family planning clinic patients and 2% amongst American women[1]. Heavy smoking is an independent risk factor, whereas barrier methods of contraception are protective. More than one study has reported an increased risk with use of the combined oral contraceptive pill for over 5 years, but further evidence is awaited to confirm these findings[2].

The role of HSV-2 infections of the cervix as a co-factor for the development of CIN is not yet clear. Human papilloma virus-associated lesions are the most common abnormalities of the cervical epithelium in young women and in a significant proportion of cases are associated with CIN or even invasive cancer. The natural history of these lesions is presently unknown[3].

The spectrum of disease is continuous from CIN 1 through CIN 3 (carcinoma in situ) to the frankly invasive squamous cell carcinoma which comprises 90% of cases. Adenocarcinomata account for a further 5%.

CIN is asymptomatic and the cervix may be clinically normal—diagnosis is made by cytology—whereas invasive cancers usually present with offensive and coloured discharge. Vaginal bleeding is common and often postcoital. Advanced lesions are associated with abdominal pain, deep dyspareunia and low backache. Invasive tumours are seen easily on speculum vaginal examination.

PROGNOSIS

- Some 30–40% of women with CIN will develop true invasive carcinomas if left untreated.
- Although the lesions may remain superficial for up to 20 years, 5% of women with CIN develop invasive cancer within 3 years[4].
- Clinical staging of carcinoma of the cervix and 5-year survival rates are given below.
- There has been no recent improvement in survival for invasive cancer. Distant metastases are to liver, lungs and bone.

TREATMENT[4]

1. The management of all stages of the disease can vary with local facilities and expertise. The general practitioner should be aware of any differences which exist and refer the patient accordingly.
2. CIN 3, which includes severe dysplasia to carcinoma in situ, is often managed with laser surgery or cryotherapy which cures 70% of women. Those who are not so cured and others are treated with a therapeutic cone

Stage	Description	5-year survival
0	Carcinoma in situ: CIN3	100%
I	Confined to cervix	85–90%
II	Beyond cervix: not to pelvic wall Upper two-thirds of vagina may be involved	
IIa	No parametrial involvement	85–90%
IIb	Parametrial involvement	55%
III	Extension to pelvic sidewall and/or lower third vagina. Includes women with hydronephrosis or non-functioning kidney	15–35%
IV	Spread beyond pelvis, or involving mucosa of bladder or rectum	Very poor

biopsy which is curative and preserves reproduction. Occasionally, hysterectomy is carried out on older women.

3. *Invasive disease*
   a. Staging is done by clinical examination, colposcopy, curettage and initial investigation such as chest x-ray and intravenous urography.
   b. Stage I, IIa—Surgery and radiotherapy are equally effective. Surgery comprises a radical hysterectomy, including 2–3 cm vaginal cuff and pelvic lymphadenectomy. Bilateral oophorectomy is not mandatory as the tumour rarely spreads to the ovary. This factor is important in deciding best therapy. Surgery is preferred for adenocarcinomata. This operation gives best results in the hands of surgeons who regularly perform it and while early surgical morbidity is greater than radiotherapy, there are fewer late complications.
   c. Stage IIb–IV—Radiotherapy is the treatment of choice.

4. Chemotherapy has no place in the initial management of the disease, but does produce temporary remissions in women with advanced local or widespread disease.

5. Cervical cancer in pregnancy: the tumour occurs in 1 in 2500 pregnancies. Carcinoma in situ is monitored closely throughout pregnancy, whereas invasive disease in the first two trimesters is treated with radiotherapy which produces fetal death and inevitable abortion within 6 weeks. Unless there is grave risk to the mother's life from catastrophic haemorrhage, invasive disease during the last trimester is monitored until fetal viability is assured, when caesarean section is carried out. The general practitioner whose patient finds herself in these desperate circumstances should have a clear idea of the ethical as well as the emotional issues involved and be prepared to provide a forum where they can be broached.

6. The major role for the general practitioner is the early detection of CIN by cervical cytology. All general practices should provide this service for patients and have an obligation to ensure that adequate smears are taken and abnormal results are acted upon appropriately[5]. In view of the rapid changes within some tumours and the possible unreliability of a single smear, all sexually active women should have their first smear repeated after 1 year and then have the test at 3-yearly intervals.

FOLLOW-UP

All patients with CIN 1 and 2 must be closely monitored in consultation with the cytologist. Women with HSV or wart virus infection should have annual smears.

Women treated for CIN 3 and invasive disease should be followed up in consultation with the specialist unit. Late complications of radiotherapy include vesicovaginal or rectovaginal fistulae and vaginal stenosis.

Women with normal cervical smears should be warned not to ignore postcoital or irregular bleeding and discharge, as some tumours are very aggressive and can reach an incurable stage within 3 years. The rare adenocarcinoma is often not recognized by the cervical smear as it is high up within the cervical canal and is only detected with the onset of symptoms.

[1] Briggs RM *et al.* (1980) High prevalence of cervical dysplasia in STD clinics warrant routine cytolocic screening. *Am. J. Public Hlth*, **70**, 1212.
[2] Vessey M *et al.* (1983) Neoplasia of the cervix uteri and contraception: a possible adverse effect of the pill. *Lancet* **ii**, 930–4.
[3] Kaufman R *et al.* (1983) Statement of caution in the interpretation of papilloma-associated lesions of the epithelium of the uterine cervix. *Am. J. Ostet. Gynecol.*, **146**, 125.
[4] Souhami R, Tobias J (1986) *Cancer and its Management.* Oxford: Blackwell Scientific Publications.
[5] McPherson A (1985) *Cervical Screening: A Practical Guide.* Oxford: Oxford University Press.

Ovarian Cancer

Ovarian cancer is commoner in nulliparous and subfertile women, and causes the greatest mortality of all the gynaecological cancers. The incidence in the USA is six times that of Japan and evens out for Japanese women living in the USA within two generations. The incidence in the UK is 14/100 000[1].

Women with breast cancer have twice the standard risk of developing ovarian cancer. In some women there appears to be a familial factor and there has been an increase in the number of reports of familial ovarian cancer since the mid 1970s. Women who have used the combined contraceptive pill appear to be protected against ovarian cancer[2].

Symptoms are non-specific. Vague lower abdominal pain, bloating and pelvic 'discomfort' are common. Early diagnosis is of the utmost importance, particularly as the patients present late and only one-third have localized disease at the time of diagnosis. Two-thirds of all women with the malignancy die from the disease and the proportion of early diagnoses has not increased despite the widespread increase in pelvic examinations done at the time of cervical cytology. Early diagnosis may lie with pelvic ultrasound or the identification of chemical tumour markers specific for early-stage ovarian cancer: both are the subject of current research.

PROGNOSIS

- Depends on the type of ovarian tumour and the stage at which the patient presents.
- About 90% originate from the epithelial surface of the ovary; the degree of differentiation is of prognostic importance.

TREATMENT

1. In primary care the main contribution is to improve early diagnosis. Routine pelvic examination is likely to pick up only 1 in 10 000 ovarian cancers; the smallest ovarian mass that could be diagnosed in this way would be 1 cm², and then only with great difficulty. However 95% of tumours measure > 5 cm in diameter on diagnosis and the finding of a 5 cm or larger ovarian mass on pelvic examination, especially in a 40–60-year-old, requires further evaluation to determine malignancy.

2. All bilateral ovarian masses require immediate evaluation as they are much more likely to indicate malignancy.

3. A 5 cm cystic ovarian mass in a young menstruating woman may be functional and not malignant and is sometimes observed for two menstrual cycles. If it does not regress then it is suspected of malignancy[1].

4. Surgery is the bedrock of care and the initial

Table 1. FIGO (International Federation of Gynaecology and Obstetrics) staging cancer of the ovary: *figures for stage of presentation and 5-year survival rates*[3]

Stage	Definition	% of all women presenting	5-year survival
I	Growth limited to the ovaries	26%	61
Ia	Growth limited to one ovary		65
Ib	Growth limited to both ovaries		52
Ic	Ia or Ib plus ascites or positive peritoneal washings		52
II	Growth limited to the pelvis	21%	40
IIa	Spread to uterus and/or tubes		60
IIb	Extension to other pelvic tissues		38
III	Growth extending to abdominal cavity, including spread to small bowel or omentum	37%	5
IV	Distant metastases	16%	3

operation has greater bearing on the outcome than any subsequent therapy.

5. Treatment comprises a staging laparotomy with careful inspection of the whole of the abdominal cavity. Patients with stage I disease will have a total abdominal hysterectomy with bilateral salphingo-oophorectomy.

6. In patients with more advanced disease as much of the tumour is removed as possible. If this is not done at the initial laparotomy then a 'second look' procedure by an expert surgeon with tumour removal (debulking) is advocated. This has implications for the family doctor who should ensure where possible that the patient starts out under the care of a unit that is skilled in the management of this unpleasant tumour, thereby possibly avoiding an inadequate first operation.

7. Patients with stage II disease appear to benefit from postoperative pelvic irradiation; in contrast, those women with stage III and IV disease are given chemotherapy[3].

FOLLOW-UP

Women enduring these events need an open and continuing relationship with their family doctor. It is vital that the general practitioner ensures good communication between primary, secondary and tertiary care, and provides a safe place for the patient to explore her expectations, hopes and fears. A realistic but optimistic approach to the future should be adopted, with the aim of informing the patient and her family about prognosis. Timing and pacing of these discussions and co-ordination of explanations with those given by the specialist service are crucially important. For some patients the loss of fertility and a premature menopause may be particularly traumatic.

[1] Piver MS (1983) *Ovarian Malignancies: The Clinical Care of Adults and Adolescents.* London: Churchill Livingstone.
[2] Vessey MP, Muir G (eds) (1985) *Cancer Risks and Prevention.* Oxford: Oxford University Press.
[3] Souhami RL, Tobias JS (1986) *Cancer and its Management.* London: Blackwell Scientific Publications.

Fibroids

Fibroids are the most common benign tumours in women, and are present in 10–20% of women over 40. They comprise muscle and fibrous connective tissue and arise from the myometrium. They are slow-growing tumours which may be multiple and while the majority (70%) are interstitial they may also be subserous or submucosal; 1–2% are cervical. While most fibroids stop growing after the menopause 10% continue to enlarge. They are commoner in nulliparous women, may be familial and are associated with endometriosis. Black women appear particularly prone to develop fibroids.

Small tumours are often asymptomatic. Symptoms, when present, depend on the site and size of the fibroid. They include menorrhagia, pain due to torsion or degeneration, irregular bleeding from a pedunculated submucous fibroid and subfertility. The combined oral contraceptive pill, especially with a high progesterone content, may reduce the risk of developing fibroids[1].

PROGNOSIS

- Fibroids are benign and the prognosis after treatment is excellent.
- Sarcomatous change is found in 0.2% of tumours at operation.
- Some 20–25% of women having a myomectomy subsequently come to hysterectomy.
- In all, 40% of women who wish to conceive after myomectomy do so.
- Fibroids may grow rapidly and degenerate during pregnancy.

Although the majority do not affect the course of pregnancy distortion of the uterine cavity can lead to abortion, premature labour and malpresentation or position. A cervical fibroid may obstruct labour.

TREATMENT

1. Small, asymptomatic fibroids may be observed. A definitive diagnosis is essential to rule out ovarian and endometrial cancers.
2. If the uterus is more than 12/52 size, is growing rapidly or the tumour might complicate a future pregnancy then treatment is indicated.
3. *Medical treatment*
   a. Regression of uterine fibroids can be achieved with luteinizing hormone-releasing hormone analogues which suppress ovarian activity[2]. The drug is most effective given as a depot preparation monthly and causes amenorrhoea which may be useful in women who are iron-deficient as a result of menorrhagia. The fibroids grow again on cessation of treatment. This approach is still under evaluation and there are worries about the long-term effects on the mineral content of bone. It is best reserved for women approaching the menopause or as an adjunct to surgery.
   b. Menorrhagia may be temporarily controlled by norethisterone acetate or danazol.
4. *Surgical treatment*
   a. Myomectomy is the treatment of choice in women under 40 who wish to retain the option of childbearing.
   b. Hysterectomy is indicated if menorrhagia is not controlled by hormone therapy, if there are pressure symptoms or if the uterus is bigger than 14/52 and the patient wishes to have no further children.

FOLLOW-UP

No follow-up is necessary after hysterectomy for fibroids. Patients who are not treated should be examined annually to monitor the growth of the uterus and should be advised to seek advice sooner should symptoms such as menorrhagia occur.

---

[1] Ross R *et al.* (1986) *Br. Med. J.*, **293**, 359–62.
[2] Baird D (1988) *Br. Med. J.*, **296**, 1689.

Endometriosis

Endometriosis is the proliferation and functioning of endometrial tissue outside the uterine cavity. The commonest sites are the ovaries, the uterosacral ligaments and the pelvic peritoneum of the Pouch of Douglas[1]. The condition seldom occurs in extragenital sites without pelvic involvement, although cyclical symptoms anywhere in a woman's body should alert the clinician to the possibility of endometriosis.

The true incidence is unknown as it is an operative diagnosis and has been found in asymptomatic women undergoing surgery for unrelated reasons. The reported incidence amongst caucasian women undergoing laparoscopy is 10–25%[1]. It is commonest in the 35–45-year age group but can occur in adolescence when it is often associated with incapacitating dysmenorrhoea. It has been reported in postmenopausal women where it may be related to oestrogen replacement or to obesity resulting in extraglandular oestrogen production.

Principal presenting symptoms are dysmenorrhoea reaching a peak after the onset of menstruation, pelvic pain and deep dyspareunia. Tender nodules in the Pouch of Douglas, the uterine walls or the posterior aspect of the cervix with a fixed retroversion is highly suggestive. A definitive diagnosis should precede treatment.

Endometriosis is strongly associated wtih infertility but is not proven to be causal. The aetiology is unknown.

PROGNOSIS

- Cumulative recurrence rates 3 and 5 years after treatment have been reported as 13.5 and 40.3% respectively[2].
- Pregnancy does not prevent a recurrence but delays the onset. Persistent disease occurs more frequently than permanent cure after pregnancy.
- Infertile women undergoing conservative surgery have less chance of a subsequent successful pregnancy if they are older, have been infertile for more than 3 years or have had severe disease.
- The condition regresses with declining ovarian function.
- Malignant change has been reported but is rare.

TREATMENT

1. Treatment depends on the patient's age and wishes, the extent and severity of the disease, fertility hopes, and previous pelvic surgery. The treatment may be medical or surgical or frequently a combination of both.
2. Medical treatment aims to suppress ovarian function, ovulation and menstruation. It is preferred in young women who wish to conceive subsequently.

a. Low-dose oestrogen combined with a high-potency progestogen may be given continuously for 6–9 months. Some authorities prefer continuous progestogens alone, such as dydrogesterone or the injectable medroxyprogesterone acetate[3].

b. Danazol, which has complex actions on the reproductive system and is not just a selective antigonadotrophin as originally described[3], can be given in daily doses of 200–800 mg for at least 6 months. The side-effects of flushing, voice changes, breast atrophy, headache and depression make the drug unacceptable to some patients.

c. Medical oophorectomy can be achieved using luteinizing hormone-releasing hormone agonists and there is optimism for the beneficial effect for patients with endometriosis in the future.

3. Surgical treatment may be radical or conservative.

a. Conservative therapy comprises division of pelvic adhesions, laser treatment, diathermy or excision of local pelvic lesions, excision of ovarian endometriotic cysts, and ventrosuspension when indicated.

b. Radical surgery involves removing both ovaries and usually the uterus. This option is used for women near the menopause, or in severe disease where conservative treatment has failed.

FOLLOW-UP

Patients on hormone therapy require both regular monitoring of their symptoms and the usual supervision given to any woman on oestrogen/progestogen preparations.

As the definitive diagnosis of endometriosis is surgical the consultant gynaecologist will co-ordinate follow-up, at least in the short term. Repeat laparoscopy may be advised.

Family doctors will no doubt be asked to prescribe any recommended medication and can take the opportunity to remain in touch. This is especially important with the woman who is infertile who will need a lot of encouragement, particularly if she is encountering side-effects while taking danazol.

Patients who have had radical surgery and who are asymptomatic may be considered cured.

[1] O'Connor D (1987) Endometriosis. London: Churchill Livingstone.
[2] Wheeler JA, Malinak LR (1983) Recurrent endometriosis: incidence, management and prognosis. Am. J. Obstet. Gynecol., 146, 247–50.
[3] Tindall VR (1987) Jeffcoate's Principles of Gynaecology. Butterworths.

Salpingitis

Salpingitis is usually a complication of a sexually transmitted infection. It is a common problem, with an estimated incidence in industrialized countries of 10–14 cases/1000 women in the age group 15–45, and a peak incidence at age 15–24. Risk is associated with sexual activity and number of partners[1].

Most cases are caused by organisms which ascend from the lower genital tract, principally *Chlamydia trachomatis, Neisseria gonorrhoeae* and micro-organisms which are usually part of the normal vaginal, vulval or bowel flora and which may cause infections in tubes already damaged by STD agents. *Mycoplasma hominis* is also a possible cause of salpingitis. Rarely infection spreads from the appendix to the fallopian tubes (1% of cases).

The cervical mucus plug acts as a barrier to infection, and protection is lowered at the time of ovulation and menstruation. Hormonal changes affect the plug and hence progesterones and combined oral contraceptives are protective against infection[2].

Iatrogenic procedures which breach the barrier (IUCD) insertion, termination of pregnancy, dilation and curettage and insufflation of tubes) precede the onset of disease within 4 weeks in 12% of cases. The risk of salpingitis is 7–9 times greater for nulliparous women using an IUCD compared with non-users[3].

Diagnosis is difficult, as cultures from the lower genital tract do not establish with certainty the cause of the tubal infection. Presenting symptoms include lower abdominal pain, metrorrhagia, deep dyspareunia and purulent vaginal discharge. Some 5% of patients may have right upper quadrant abdominal pain due to chlamydial perihepatitis. Clinical signs include a temperature higher than 38.0°C, tender lower abdomen, cervical excitation, purulent discharge and tender fornices, with or without a palpable mass. The differential diagnosis includes ectopic pregnancy and appendicitis.

PROGNOSIS

One in five women have a repeat infection due to:

- Inadequate diagnosis and treatment of the initial attack.
- Lack of follow-up and treatment of partners.

- Postinfection damage leading to superimposed infection by endogenous flora.

Since the advent of antibiotics, death is rare in the acute attack and is inevitably due to a ruptured tubo-ovarian abscess, leading to peritonitis.

Late sequaelae include[1]:

- In 15% of women, chronic abdominal pain, more likely with repeated infections.
- A total of 17% of women become infertile due to tubal occlusion. The prognosis is better in younger women with gonococcal-associated salpingitis.
- Women who have had salpingitis have a 7- to 10-fold risk of ectopic pregnancy, compared with normal controls.

TREATMENT

1. In primary care, the first decision is about the severity of the illness. If there is severe constitutional upset, or the diagnosis is unclear, the patient should be referred urgently or admitted to hospital.
2. Women who are not in the above group require rest and antibiotics and should avoid coitus.
3. A full pelvic examination is mandatory, including adequate visualization of the cervix. Cervical swabs should be taken for *Neisseria gonorrhoeae* and *Chlamydia trachomatis*. If the facilities or expertise are not available, consideration should be given to referring the patient to the local genitourinary clinic for accurate diagnosis.
4. Usually antibiotics have to be started before the microbiological aetiology has been established; doxycycline 200 mg stat, then 100 mg daily and metronidazole 400 mg b.d. for 10–14 days is the preferred regime. Patients need encouragement to persevere with the treatment, as they often feel nauseated. They should avoid alcohol. Erythromycin stearate 500 mg q.i.d. is an adequate alternative to doxycycline.

Chlamydia trachomatis is *not* sensitive to amoxycillin/ampicillin, which is therefore an *inappropriate* treatment for salpingitis.
5. Sexual partners should be screened for STD and treated as appropriate.

If present, an IUCD should be removed once antibiotic cover is established, and the patient advised that it will from now on be an inappropriate form of contraception.

FOLLOW-UP

The woman should be examined after completion of antibiotic therapy and swabs repeated in the light of the original findings.

The general practitioner is ideally suited to advise the woman about limiting the number of sexual partners and avoiding the use of an IUCD. Tactful discussion of the possible effects on fertility and the risk of ectopic pregnancy should take place, to enable the patient to act appropriately, should she wish to become pregnant. Prompt treatment of recurrences should be stressed. Opportunities to share feelings of guilt or blame for the situation can be created within the consultation to help prevent future depression or relationship difficulties.

[1] Westrom L, Mardh P (1984) Salpingitis. In *Sexually Transmitted Diseases* (Holmes KK et al. eds). New York: McGraw-Hill.
[2] Westrom L et al. (1980) Incidence, prevalence and trends of acute pelvic inflammatory disease and its consequences in industrialized countries. *Am. J. Obstet. Gynecol.*, **138**, 880.
[3] Tatum H, Connell E (1986) A decade of intrauterine contraception: 1976–1986. *Fertil. Steril.*, **42**, 173–92.

Spontaneous Abortion

The World Health Organization recommends that the fetus shall be considered viable when the gestation is at 22 completed weeks or when it weighs more than 500 g. This is accepted in Australia and parts of the USA but not in the UK where the limit is 28 weeks and 1000 g. Pregnancies which end before this stage are deemed abortions; most occur in the first trimester. There is a large natural wastage of fertilized ova: of those which implant in the uterus, only 40–50% survive long enough to delay menstruation and lead to a recognized pregnancy. Over one-third of women become pregnant in one cycle of unprotected intercourse but only 55% of the conceptions progress to a clinically recognized pregnancy. Of all abortions, 90% occur without the knowledge of the woman. The risk of spontaneous abortion in a clinically recognized pregnancy is about 15%. Most fetuses die during weeks 2–8 although most abortions occur during weeks 7–13, hence intrauterine retention commonly follows fetal death[1,2].

Some 5% or more of all human conceptions have a significant chromosomal abnormality, but the selective effect of spontaneous abortion leads to a rate of 2.4% at 12 weeks and 0.6% at term[3]. Factors associated with early embryonic loss include failure to maintain the corpus luteum, the presence of a lethal gene and immunological factors, especially human leukocyte antigen compatibility between the couple.

Environmental factors such as smoking, diet, drugs and irradiation are likely but as yet unproven precipitants.

There is an association between colonization with *Mycoplasma hominis* and *Ureaplasma urealyticum* and recurrent and spontaneous abortion: the relationship of *Chlamydia trachomatis* infection to spontaneous abortion is also under scrutiny. Rubella infection is a cause of first-trimester abortion.

Later abortions are principally due to cervical incompetence which is present in 1 in 5 cases in the mid-trimester.

Uterine abnormalities such as a bicornuate uterus, a fixed retroversion or gross distortion of the cavity by uterine fibroids are rare causes.

PROGNOSIS

- In all, 60–80% of women who have a threatened abortion during the first half of pregnancy continue to term but they have double the risk of delivering a small-for-dates baby. The perinatal mortality rate is twice that of women who have never bled[4].

- Spontaneous abortion would occur relatively frequently even if the risk were the same for all couples, but research has demonstrated that some couples experience recurrent abortion more. The risk increases with the number of previous abortions and is greater in those women who previously aborted a fetus with a normal karyotype[5]. This implies that factors leading to recurrent abortion are not normally those leading to chromosomal abnormalities.

- Other factors associated with repeated abortion are abortion after the first trimester, a history of preterm births and a delay in conceiving after unprotected intercourse. Smoking and alcohol consumption are associated with an increased risk for chromosomally normal abortions and women experiencing recurrent abortion should be advised accordingly. The role of chronic endometrial infection in recurrent abortion is the subject of current research.

- There is a small increase in the proportion of chromosomal abnormalities in aborted fetuses after oral contraception use of more than 18 months; this is thought to be the result of a *lower* spontaneous abortion rate of normal fetuses amongst pill users.

- The rate of spontaneous abortion rises with age, but only after the mid 30s.

- A small proportion of couples do have abnormal chromosomes and referral for genetic counselling and chromosome studies is advisable after three abortions in the absence of other explanations.

The immunological processes which protect the fetoplacental unit are not initiated or are defective in some women with recurrent abortions. This is an area of research which may help many distressed couples and general practitioners must be aware of developments as they happen and refer patients accordingly[4].

TREATMENT

An abortion may be threatened, complete, incomplete or missed.

1. *Threatened* abortion (bleeding, slight pain and a closed cervix): rest for 5–7 days or while the bleeding remains bright red. There is no evidence that bedrest affects the outcome but it is sensible to restrict daily activities as the woman often feels unwell and insistence on full activity may lead to feelings of guilt should she later abort. Progesterone has not been shown to be of any value and should not be given.

2. *Complete* abortion: if the patient is seen at home and the abortion appears to be complete with no shock or heavy bleeding, a sterile vaginal examination should be carried out to inspect the cervix and if possible the material which has been passed should be examined. The patient may then be managed at home with careful observation; an ultrasound examination which confirms an empty uterus is of value. The Rhesus status of women cared for in general practice should be ascertained and anti-D gammaglobulin given where appropriate. The products of conception may be sent to the laboratory for further examination.

3. *Incomplete* abortion: the majority of these women present with severe, crampy pain and bleeding which may be very heavy: this situation can constitute a real emergency. While waiting for the ambulance pain relief can be achieved with pethidine 100 mg. A sterile vaginal examination should be made with a view to removing any placental tissue which may be distending the os causing shock; this may best be done with a finger. If the patient continues to bleed heavily ergometrine 0.5 mg i.m. may be given and on occasion it may be necessary to start an intravenous infusion. The uterus is evacuated by curettage after hospital admission.

4. *Missed* abortion: there is no urgency in treating missed abortion, although most women are very distressed if the situation is not resolved quickly. If the uterus size is under 12 weeks a dilation and curettage is performed; for gestations of more than 12 weeks vaginal or intravenous prostaglandins may be used.

5. Cervical incompetence is treated with a cervical suture at 14 weeks. In true cases of incompetence an 80–90% livebirth rate can be expected.

FOLLOW-UP

Abortion is always a significant and painful experience for a woman. For those women who were not pleased to be pregnant there may be a sense of relief coupled with guilt. If the pregnancy was planned most women feel angry and depressed and many are frightened and anxious about embarking on another pregnancy. Many women experience the loss as part of herself accompanied by a loss of self-esteem and a sense of failure as a woman. The primary need is to talk about the experience—this need is often denied by family and friends who find the subject embarrassing or painful. The general practitioner should be available to help during this difficult time and also to give support during the next pregnancy when lack of bonding and lack of confidence in her ability to carry the pregnancy to term may be a problem. The medical record should show the abortion as a significant life event as it may be an important factor in depression later in life.

Normally only moderate bleeding follows a dilation and curettage done to evacuate the uterus. Heavy or prolonged bleeding raises the possibility of an incomplete evacuation and the patient should be referred back to the gynaecologist for assessment.

Pyrexia, lower abdominal pain, and increased vaginal discharge indicate infection which must be promptly treated after cervical and high vaginal swabs have been taken. If the facilities to establish a microbiological diagnosis are not available or the patient is ill she should be referred for treatment. It is *inappropriate therapy* to give amoxycillin blind in these circumstances. Erythromycin and metronidazole may be commenced while the results of swabs are awaited.

Each woman should be seen about 4–6 weeks after the abortion for an examination and review of contraception if she wishes it. This consultation provides an opportunity to assess her psychological well-being and to arrange further follow-up if needed.

---

[1] Edmonds DK (1987) Early embryonic mortality. In *Spontaneous and Recurrent Abortion* (Bennett MJ, Edmonds DK eds). Oxford: Blackwell Scientific Publications.

[2] Miller JF *et al.* (1980) Fetal loss after implantation. *Lancet*, **ii**, 554.

[3] Hook EB (1981) Prevalence of chromosomal abnormalities during human gestation and implications for environmental mutagens. *Lancet*, **ii**, 169.

[4] Llewellyn-Jones D (1986) Fundamentals of obstetrics and gynaecology. London: Faber & Faber.

[5] Alberman E et al. (1975) Previous reproductive history in mothers presenting with spontaneous abortion. *Br. J. Obstet. Gynaecol.*, **82**, 366.

Ectopic Pregnancy

Ectopic pregnancy is an important cause of maternal and fetal mortality and morbidity and international data have shown an alarming increase in its incidence since the early 1970s. In England and Wales the rate per 1000 livebirths plus induced abortions was 3.7 in 1966 and 6.2 in 1976. Risk factors include increasing maternal age, a previous history of salpingitis, IUCD usage of increasing duration (including the first year after removal) and use of the low-dose progestogen only pill[1,2]. The vast majority of extrauterine pregnancies occur in the fallopian tubes but ovarian, abdominal and cervical pregnancies are rarely reported.

Presenting symptoms include abnormal vaginal bleeding and abdominal pain. Amenorrhoea may not occur in up to 45% of women although symptoms of early pregnancy may be present. Physical findings may be absent but pelvic and cervical tenderness are often present and a palpable adnexial mass has been reported in 30–75% of patients. The diagnosis is confirmed from clinical findings, accurate measurement of serum human chorionic gonadotrophin, ultrasound and diagnostic laparoscopy.

PROGNOSIS

- In general practice the prognosis for the individual woman is directly related to the doctor's level of suspicion and knowledge of risk factors, so that the diagnosis can be made before tubal abortion or rupture occur.
- Rupture leads to catastrophic bleeding and maternal death if prompt intervention does not follow. Mortality in the USA in 1980 was 0.8/1000 ectopic pregnancies. In the years 1970–1980 there was an overall decrease in the absolute number of deaths of only 35% despite a decline in the death/case rate[1] of 75%. The large rise in cases explains these contradictory figures.
- In 50% of women the opposite tube is normal at operation.
- In all, 70% will experience problems with becoming pregnant.
- Some 10–50% will have another tubal pregnancy[3].

TREATMENT

1. In women with a ruptured ectopic pregnancy salpingectomy is performed.
2. In patients diagnosed early, with a pregnancy in the mid or distal portion of the tube, conservative surgery is an option, especially if future fertility is important.

   Linear salpingostomy may be performed for ampullary ectopic pregnancy, and segmental resection and anastomosis using microsurgical techniques for pregnancies in the isthmus of the tube. Both procedures, carried out in women with only one tube remaining, have been reported as having been followed by successful intrauterine pregnancies[3].

FOLLOW-UP

Patients require careful advice about future pregnancies and contraception. They are at increased risk of another tubal pregnancy and should be dvised to consult their family doctor at once if they think they are pregnant or have unusual aginal bleeding or abdominal pain. Use of an UCD or minipill is contraindicated.

Frau L *et al.* (1986) Epidemiologic aspects of ectopic

pregnancy. In *Extrauterine Pregnancy* (Langer A, Iffy L eds). Littleton, Massachusetts: PSG.

[2] Westrom L (1980) Incidence, prevalence, and trends of acute pelvic inflammatory disease and its consequences in industrialized countries. *Am. J. Obstet. Gynecol.*, **138**, 848.

[3] Wingate M, Langer A. Surgical management of tubal pregnancy. In *Extrauterine Pregnancy* (Langer A, Iffy L eds). Littleton, Massachusetts: PSG.

Anaemia of Pregnancy

Healthy pregnancy involves changes in the circulating blood due principally to increase in blood volume and alteration in factors involved in haemostasis. The blood volume rises throughout pregnancy and peaks at the 32nd week. Plasma volume in a single uncomplicated pregnancy is about 40% greater than in the non-pregnant state[1]. Red cell mass increases by about 30%, but the disproportionate increase in the plasma volume leads to a fall in haemoglobin concentration in the first and second trimesters. Haemoglobin concentrations of <10.5 g/dl indicate anaemia.

Iron deficiency anaemia is the commonest haematological problem in pregnancy and is likely when a hypochromic, microcytic blood picture is seen. Serum ferritin levels correlate with the level of iron stores and levels of <35 µg/l[1] may indicate deficiency. Bone marrow examination is also a useful test, whereas the total iron binding capacity (TIBC) and serum iron are unreliable indicators of iron status in pregnancy[2].

The other common anaemia of pregnancy is the megaloblastic anaemia associated with folate deficiency, which is almost always due to poor diet, particularly a lack of green vegetables. The incidence in the UK is reported as 0.2–5.0% with many more women showing megaloblastic changes in their marrow[2]. An average mixed diet contains between 100 and 200 µg of folic acid which is normally sufficient. In pregnancy the demand increases by 50–100 µg daily; as a result pregnancy is associated with a negative folate balance which is reversed by folate supplements.

Phenytoin reduces folate absorption. The changes in the blood picture may be masked by iron deficiency and may only become apparent after iron therapy. A bone marrow examination may be required for definitive diagnosis as both serum and red cell folate levels in deficiency states overlap the normal ranges in pregnancy.

Iron deficiency anaemia

PROGNOSIS

- Iron deficiency is associated with poor nutrition, lower socioeconomic group, multiparity and poor antenatal care. It is difficult to assess its contribution to the poor pregnancy outcomes which result from these risk factors.

- Infants born to iron-deficient mothers are seldom iron-deficient at birth, but they have reduced iron stores demonstrated by low ferritin levels in cord blood. They are at risk for iron deficiency in infancy[1].

TREATMENT

1. *Prophylaxis: diet.* A normal mixed diet supplies about 15 mg iron daily, of which 1–2 mg is absorbed. The average daily requirement during pregnancy is 4–6 mg and although the absorption of dietary iron is enhanced during the last weeks of pregnancy, mobilization of iron stores is inevitable.

   The availability of iron in food varies, with the haem iron from animal haemoglobin and myoglobin in meats being much more efficiently absorbed than the non-haem iron in cereals, grains, fruits, eggs and dairy products.

Tea inhibits the absorption of iron whereas ascorbic acid enhances it.

2. *Prophylaxis: supplementation.* This is controversial. Some studies in the developed world have reported that 15–30% of women of childbearing age are iron-deficient and 84% of unsupplemented women are iron-deficient at term[1]. If pregnancies are well spaced and the diet is adequate then iron stores can be replenished, but many authors still recommend routine supplements containing 30–120 mg elemental iron daily. This is best taken after meals to ensure maximum absorption and minimum gastric irritation.

3. *Therapy:* oral iron is the best treatment for iron deficiency anaemia and patients should be encouraged to take it. A variety of preparations are available, often in combination with folic acid. Tolerance is improved by starting with a small dose (e.g. 60 mg daily) and gradually increasing over a few days.

The haematological response to parenteral iron therapy is not faster than to oral therapy and the injections are painful and may stain the skin. Intramuscular iron should rarely be needed if good antenatal care has encouraged the patient to persevere with oral medication. The use of a total dose infusion may result in fatal anaphylaxis and is seldom indicated.

Women presenting late in pregnancy may occasionally be transfused before labour if the haemoglobin level is < 8 g/dl.

FOLLOW-UP

These women require careful evaluation at postnatal examination and beyond. Advice about diet and spacing of pregnancies and contraceptive methods which reduce rather than increase the menstrual flow should be considered. Women who are breastfeeding may need continued supplementation.

Megaloblastic anaemia of folate deficiency

PROGNOSIS

● Extensive research has examined the possible association of folate deficiency with abortion, fetal abnormality, antepartum haemorrhage and prematurity. There is no evidence that folate deficiency during pregnancy is a cause of any of these, although preconception deficiency is possibly related to neural tube defects and harelip and cleft palate[3].

TREATMENT

Prophylaxis: diet
1. Folate is rapidly destroyed by cooking and while broccoli, spinach and brussels sprouts are very rich in folate, 90% of their content is lost during boiling or steaming. Bananas and mushrooms are also a good source.

Prophylaxis: supplementation
1. This is controversial. Dietary folate is inadequate to prevent megaloblastic changes in the bone marrow in about 25% of pregnant women. Women with a poor diet require a daily supplement of 200–300 μg daily[4]. The theoretical risk of harm to women with vitamin B_{12} deficiency from inappropriate folate therapy has never been substantiated by any case report of subacute combined degeneration of the spinal cord in any pregnant woman receiving folate[4].

Therapy
1. Megaloblastic anaemia due to folate deficiency is treated by oral folate 5 mg daily, to be continued for several weeks postpartum.
2. Parenteral folate may be used if there is no response.
3. Women with thalassaemia trait require oral folic acid 5 mg daily from early pregnancy.
4. Women with sickle cell anaemia or sickle cell trait require at least 5 mg folic acid daily during pregnancy.
5. Women on anticonvulsant therapy should be given oral folic acid 5 mg daily. The control of epilepsy may become more difficult[2].

FOLLOW-UP

These women require assessment after delivery. If the megaloblastic anaemia recurs when folate is stopped, causes other than poor diet and pregnancy must be excluded.

---

[1] Kelton J (1988) Hematologic disorders of pregnancy.

Medical Complications during Pregnancy (Burrow G, rris T eds). London: WB Saunders.

.etsky E (1987) Anaemia in obstetrics. In *Progress in ostetrics and Gynaecology*, vol 6 (Studd J ed). London: hurchill Livingstone.

[3] Smithells R *et al.* (1983) *Lancet*, **i**, 1027–31.

[4] Chanarin I (1985) Folate and cobalamin. *Clin. Haematol.*, **14**, 629.

Hyperemesis of Pregnancy

bout three-quarters of pregnant women experience nausea and vomiting between the xth and 16th week of pregnancy and in most no gastrointestinal lesion can be emonstrated. The cause of this common problem is unknown although the possibility of isordered upper gastrointestinal motility seems likely[1]. The nausea and vomiting are most evere during the morning. Uncommonly some women develop persistent and intractable omiting (hyperemesis gravidarum) leading to dehydration and electrolyte imbalance and arely to death. Patients with a hydatidiform mole or a twin pregnancy are more likely to uffer nausea and vomiting.

PROGNOSIS

- The condition is self-limiting for the vast majority of women.
- In severe cases hepatocellular jaundice and Wernicke's encephalopathy secondary to hyperemesis have been described.
- Extremely rarely the condition proves intractable and is fatal.

TREATMENT

1. The link between antiemetics and fetal abnormalities is unproven. It is best to avoid the use of all non-essential medication in early pregnancy and the majority of patients are pleased to avoid the use of drugs for this problem.

2. Most women have mild symptoms and can manage to cope by planning a daily routine which includes more rest and the avoidance of early morning rushing about. Rarely will drugs be needed, although metaclopramide is helpful in difficult cases.

3. Women with severe symptoms require hospital admission for rehydration and the restoration of electrolyte and calorie balance.

FOLLOW-UP

Women with troublesome vomiting should be seen more frequently in the antenatal clinic to give encouragement and to monitor the severity of symptoms. Distress from these symptoms can adversely affect the woman's feelings about the pregnancy and the child she is expecting.

[1] Connon J (1988) Gastrointestinal complications. In *Medical Complications During Pregnancy* (Burrow G ed). London: WB Saunders.

Pre-eclampsia

Although convulsions associated with pregnancy have been recorded since ancient times and the preceding triad of hypertension, proteinuria and (sometimes) oedema known since the late 1800s, a satisfactory definition of pre-eclampsia is still awaited. Nelson[1] proposed a definition in 1955 which has been widely accepted in the UK. More recently, MacGillivray has proposed a modification[2]:

1. Pregnancy hypertension: rise in blood pressure only in the second half of pregnancy.
2. Mild pre-eclampsia: hypertension (140/90 mmHg IVth phase or more) and proteinuria <2 g/l in 24 h.
3. Severe pre-eclampsia: hypertension and proteinuria >2 g/l in 24 h.

Epidemiological comparisons are beset with problems of vague definitions and varying standards of antenatal care. From 1968 to 1972 the incidence amongst Aberdeen primigravidae was 26% for pregnancy hypertension and 5% for proteinuric pre-eclampsia[2]. Risk is associated with first pregnancy, increasing age, family history (mothers or sisters), twin pregnancy and poorly controlled diabetes.

PROGNOSIS

- The death rate from pre-eclampsia per million maternities from 1973 to 1975 was 9.4 and for eclampsia was 10.9[3].
- Deaths from pre-eclampsia or eclampsia are from placental abruption, cerebral haemorrhage, acute renal failure and, more rarely, liver failure.
- True pre-eclampsia with hypertension and proteinuria is not associated with renal damage, hypertension or diabetes in later life[2]. If a woman does not have the immediate complications pre-eclampsia is completely reversible.
- The perinatal mortality rate amongst primigravidae with proteinuria and hypertension is more than double that of normotensive women. The rate is three to five times greater in women with pre-eclampsia who smoke more than 5 cigarettes a day[2].
- The risk of recurrence of pregnancy hypertension in a subsequent pregnancy is less than 5%.

TREATMENT

1. In general practice, management comprises planned observation to detect early evidence of onset. It is important therefore to follow up non-attenders for antenatal care and to ensure that practice organization and liaison with community midwives facilitate this.
2. A diastolic blood pressure of 90 mmHg or more in the second half of pregnancy, especially in a primigravida, requires a full assessment. If it returns to normal after 24 hours' rest, there is no proteinuria and other causes of hypertension have been ruled out, the patient may be managed at home with at least twice-weekly measurement of blood pressure and urine tests for protein.
3. If the blood pressure remains elevated urgent referral to an obstetrician is indicated.
4. All patients with proteineuria and hypertension (140/90 mmHg or more) require immediate assessment by an obstetrician.

FOLLOW-UP

All women should be normotensive with no proteinuria by the time of their postnatal examination. Those who are not require further investigation.

[1] Nelson TA (1955) Clinical study of pre-eclampsia. J. Obstet. Gynaec. Br. Empire, **62,** 48.
[2] MacGillivray I (1983) Pre-eclampsia: the hypertensive disease of pregnancy. London: WB Saunders.
[3] Report on Confidential Inquiries into Maternal Deaths in England and Wales (1979) London: DHSS.

2

Ear, Nose and Throat

J. F. Wilmot

Acute Otitis Media

Acute otitis media is one of the most common diagnoses made in children by primary care doctors in different countries. Inevitably diagnostic criteria vary between clinicians but there are two main varieties—suppurative and non-suppurative otitis media.

The typical episode of acute suppurative otitis comprises ear pain, initially with localized tympanic injection, which progresses to a bulging red or yellow eardrum[1]. Bacteria can be cultured from middle-ear fluid in 90% of such cases—most often *Haemophilus influenzae* (causing the majority of infections in children under 6 years) or *Streptococcus pneumoniae*[1]. In a minority of cases the drum will burst and discharge pus; in developed countries almost all such eardrums now heal. The annual consultation rate is 23.3 per 1000 patients[2]; peak age is 4–8 years[3].

Non-suppurative otitis media follows certain upper respiratory viruses. The chronic form is also known as otitis media with effusion or glue ear, but the clinical signs are similar. Deafness is likely to be a more prominent feature than ear pain. The eardrum is typically dull, may be retracted, and is pink, amber, grey-white or bluish[1]. The annual consultation rate is 16.6 per 1000[2]. Diagnostic difficulties arise from the presence of wax, or from the diffuse eardrum redness which can occur with upper respiratory infection, or even merely with crying or instrumentation in infants and toddlers[1]. Acute otitis media is therefore likely to be overdiagnosed[4].

PROGNOSIS

- The course of acute otitis media varies. About 50% of children (range 10–70%) have an effusion 10–14 days after diagnosis of acute suppurative otitis media, and 10% (range 8–25%) have such signs at 12 weeks[5].
- About 40% of children will suffer acute otitis media during childhood; about half will experience recurring attacks[3].

TREATMENT

1. The role of antibiotics is increasingly debated in ear as in throat infections. Acute otitis media is a milder disease in developed countries, and serious complications are rare.
2. A bulging or discharging eardrum is usually regarded as an indication for antibiotic therapy, which probably shortens the duration of ear pain or discharge[4]. Amoxycillin is preferable, especially in children under 6, to cover *Haemophilus influenzae*. Shorter antibiotic courses (e.g. 2–3 days amoxycillin 250 mg twice daily in children aged 3–10) seem as effective as longer more traditional courses[6]. Co-trimoxazole or cefaclor are slightly more toxic alternatives, while penicillin V and erythromycin penetrate poorly into middle ears[4,6].
3. A selective antibiotic policy is reasonable, and symptomatic treatment alone is entirely appropriate for a well child with a merely pink or diffusely red eardrum. The doctor must be prepared to review such children promptly in case of persisting symptoms; antibiotics may then be needed[4].
4. Adequate analgesia is necessary, especially when antibiotics are not used (paracetamol 60–120 mg for infants, 120–250 mg for 1–5-year-olds, 250–500 mg for 6–12-year-olds three or four times daily. Decongestants and antihistamines do not influence the course of otitis media[4,6].

FOLLOW-UP

Follow-up is not of proven benefit, but seems advisable in those with bilateral infections, previous middle ear problems, and chronic disease (especially Down's syndrome, cystic fibrosis and cleft palate, all of which predispose to effusion). Re-examination after 4–6 weeks would seem more rational than the usual 10–14-day period.

[1] Paradise J (1980) *Pediatrics*, **65**, 917–43.
[2] RCGP/OPCS/DHSS (1986) *Morbidity Statistics from*

General Practice: 1981–1982, third national study. London: HMSO.

[3] Fry J (1985) *Common Diseases: their nature, incidence and care*, 4th edn. Lancaster: MTP.

[4] Anonymous (1984) *Drug Ther. Bull.*, **22**, 53–5.

[5] Bluestone CD, Klein JO (1983) In *Pediatric Otorhinolaryngology*, vol II (Bluestone CD, Stool S eds). Philadelphia: Saunders.

[6] Bain J (1986) *Update*, **34**, 136–41.

Glue Ear

Otitis media with effusion (also known as secretory or serous otitis) is an inflammatory condition of the middle ear where fluid is present behind an intact drum; the chronic form is an episode persisting for 3 months or longer. 'Glue ear' describes the typically viscous quality of the secretions in children. The causes are unknown but may include chronic low-grade infection, Eustachian tube dysfunction, and allergy. Bacteria may be identified from up to 50% using special techniques[1]. The eardrum is typically dull, and may be pink, grey, white, amber or bluish[2]. Tympanometry is a technique for measuring reflected sound energy at differing levels of ear canal pressure, and abnormal patterns can be used to confirm the presence of effusions.

Otitis media with effusion typically results in a conductive hearing loss, either for low tones or across all frequencies, which can fluctuate in intensity.

Community typanometry surveys reveal a high point prevalence of middle ear effusions, e.g. 17–20% in 3-year-olds[3]. Screening detects less effusions among school-age children, but more in poor city children, in South Pacific and North American natives, and in caucasian as against Afrocaribbean groups[2].

Glue ear is most often treated surgically between the ages of 4 to 8.

PROGNOSIS

- Two-thirds of effusions detected at screening will resolve within 3 months. Spontaneous resolution is unlikely after this stage[3].

- In a group of severe bilateral cases in Ear, Nose and Throat (ENT) departments, 40% were unresolved after 3 years and 25% after 5[1]. Controlled prospective studies suggest that by school age children with a history of persistent glue ear have impaired articulation but no cognitive difficulties[4].

- Long-standing glue ear can be complicated by the development of a cholesteatoma, a keratin-forming cyst in a tympanic retraction pocket. This can erode bone and lead to serious septic complications[1,2]

TREATMENT

1. Middle ear effusions present in a matter of weeks. When recognized they are likely to resolve spontaneously and the reassurance of this information may be all the treatment required.

2. When an effusion follows an episode of acute suppurative otitis media, a single 7–10-day course of antibiotic (different from that used in the acute attack) may help to clear persistent effusion[2].

3. Antihistamines and decongestants are of no benefit in glue ear[5].

4. Inhaled bronchodilators and steroids, with nasal steroids, may benefit the effusions associated with rhinitis and asthma.

5. Surgical treatment is appropriately reserved for the cases where effusions persist for longer than 3 months, and where the hearing loss is causing poor speech development or impeding school progress.

   a. Adenoidectomy is likely to help preschool children with large adenoids[1,2,6].

   b. Myringotomy is a traditional procedure which does no lasting damage to the eardrum, but only provides temporary relief[5].

   c. Grommets are the commonest tympanostomy tube. They return hearing virtually to normal while in situ, but are extruded after 6–9 months, when the effusions may recur. Tympanosclerosis, not necessarily important, is a common late effect on the ear-drum[5].

d. Goode's T-tubes remain in situ for 2–3 years, during the age of maximum risk. They may require an anaesthetic for removal, and frequently leave dry perforations.

FOLLOW-UP

Those with definite glue ear are likely to require follow-up by an ENT department, possibly until the age of 8–10 years. Milder cases of short duration can appropriately be followed up in primary care, especially when hearing testing is available—in the practice, by the health visitor, or by audiologists.

[1] Maw R (1987) *Practitioner*, **231**, 1108–14.
[2] Bluestone CD, Klein JO (1983) Otitis media with effusion, atelectasis and Eustachian tube dysfunction. In *Pediatric Otorhinolaryngology*, vol II (Bluestone CD, Stool SE, eds). Philadelphia: Saunders.
[3] Fielau-Nikolajsen P (1983) *Ann. Otol. Rhinol. Laryngol*, **92**, 172–7.
[4] Hubbard TW *et al.* (1985) *N. Engl. J. Med.*, **312**, 1529–34.
[5] Cantekin E *et al.* (1983) *N. Engl. J. Med.*, **308**, 297–301.
[6] Anonymous (1986) *Drug Ther. Bull.*, **24**, 49–51.

Otitis Externa

In external otitis there is inflammation or desquamation of the external auditory meatus. General practitioners see 10[1]–12[2] patients/1000 population annually, with no age preponderance. Some 35% are deaf[2]. Risk factors include chronic suppurative otitis media, seborrhoeic or atopic eczema and local irritants[2,3]. Fungal infections are common in the tropics. Symptoms can include irritation, discharge or deafness; frank ear pain is more likely in children.

PROGNOSIS

● Some 60% of cases recur within 5 years[2]. Some individuals, especially with seborrhoeic tendencies, have many recurrent attacks.

TREATMENT

1. Treatment is through a combination of cleaning and local agents.
2. The condition is unlikely to subside without either removal of wax debris by syringing, which can cause increased bogginess, or aural toilet, which is preferable if skill and equipment are sufficient.
3. Especially after cleaning, local antimicrobials will help to settle the condition. These include Cicatrin powder or drops such as Sofradex (this is one occasion when combining an antibiotic and steroid is advisable, to avoid sensitization).

4. Marked oedema may suggest the need for packing with ribbon gauze soaked with drops. If external aural furunculosis is identified or suspected, systemic antibiotics such as flucloxacillin 250 mg qd daily for five days are indicated.

FOLLOW-UP

Follow-up is generally only required for recurrent symptoms.

[1] RCGP/OPCS/DHSS (1986) *Morbidity Statistics from General Practice: 1981–1982, Third National Study*. London: HMSO.
[2] Hodgkin KM (1985) *Towards Earlier Diagnosis*, 5th edn. Edinburgh: Churchill Livingstone.
[3] Hickish GW (1985) *Ear, Nose and Throat Disorders*. Edinburgh: Churchill Livingstone.

Wax in Ears

Each year 29 per 1000[1] of the population consult their doctor with external ear canal blockage due to wax. This is more likely in those with genetically determined (recessive) dry wax. Cotton buds and the ingress of water contribute to impaction. The problem becomes more likely with increasing age, and is more common in males (in a ratio of $2:1$)[2].

TREATMENT

1. Syringing is the method generally favoured in primary care, whether using the traditional Wood's syringe, the improved Shaw syringe, or the Bacon syringe incorporating rubber tubing to draw up water. Tap water may be used but must be near blood heat ($37.7°C$ is recommended[3]). This method is *contraindicated* where there is a history of perforation—a thinly headed scar may be ruptured.
2. Otitis externa may result from syringing; reactive tympanic hyperaemia may be difficult to distinguish from otitis media.
3. Wax-softening agents: clinical trials have not shown the superiority of proprietary preparations over sodium bicarbonate solution; this preparation, or alternatively glycerin or warm olive oil, is recommended for routine use for a few days before syringing[3,4].
4. Dry cleaning is preferred by otolaryngologists. A head mirror and lamp, or a head-worn lamp, should be used for illumination. The wax hook is used to remove cerumen; then the ear is cleaned using cotton wool pledgets on a probe.

FOLLOW-UP

Follow-up is normally only required for recurrent symptoms. Wax-softening drops used every few months by vulnerable individuals may help to avert the need for professional wax removal.

[1] RCGP/OPCS/DHSS (1986) *Morbidity Statistics from General Practice: 1981–1982 Third National Study.* London: HMSO.
[2] Hodgkin KM (1985) *Towards Earlier Diagnosis*, 5th edn. Edinburgh: Churchill Livingstone.
[3] Hickish GW (1985) *Ear, Nose and Throat Disorders.* Edinburgh: Churchill Livingstone.
[4] George CF *et al.* (1987) British National Formulary, no. 14. London: British Medical Association and Pharmaceutical Society.

Dizziness and Vertigo

Vertigo is a 'hallucination of movement' or 'disordered orientation in space', usually rotatory or rocking[1]. Dizziness may be the term used by patients for vertigo, lightheadedness, or unsteadiness ('like walking on cotton wool'). Dizziness arises from incompatibility of the neural information from the eyes, inner ears, and locomotor system[2]. Vertigo can arise from Ménière's disease, vestibular neuronitis, benign positional vertigo or occasionally from wax accumulation; the vertigo of brainstem disease (stroke, demyelination or tumour) is typically unremitting. Vertigo can also occur with strong lenses following cataract surgery, from toxic causes (e.g. acute alcohol intoxication), or from vertebrobasilar ischaemia, especially in combination with cervical spondylosis.

Unsteadiness typically arises from reduced input from peripheral receptors, and thus from any variety of lower limb peripheral neuropathy or in old age through multiple degenerative causes[2].

Lightheadedness is typically caused by decreased availability of oxygen within the brain, arising from ischaemia, cardiac disorder or hypoglycaemia. Postural hypotension is one variety[2]. Psychogenic dizziness is probably mediated by chronic low-grade hyperventilation, which can cause lightheadedness or true vertigo[3].

Dizziness from all causes results in 3.9 consultations per 1000 per year[4]. The consulting rate for females is $1\frac{1}{2}$ times that for males, and the rate increases steadily with increasing years (0.7/1000 aged 5–14 to 10/1000 in over 75-year-olds[4]).

PROGNOSIS

- Vertigo of peripheral origin will subside within 2–3 weeks as the eighth nerve is 'switched off'. Remorseless vertigo is thus more typical of brainstem lesions[1,2].

- Transient vertigo can be due to benign positional vertigo, typically when lying, or to vertebrobasilar ischaemia when the erect head is turned.

- Intermittent unsteadiness can arise from faulty brainstem adjustment from 'lost inputs', especially in old age.

- Arrhythmias cause an unknown number of such cases.

- Most other causes of dizziness may fluctuate but tend to worsen with increasing age (as suggested by the consultation rates).

TREATMENT

1. General examination, simple blood tests, and sometimes electrocardiography, including 24-hour recording, may help to differentiate the responsible causative disorders. Treatment of these may improve the symptoms.

2. Avoidance of sudden head movements may help dizziness due to positional vertigo or brainstem ischaemia; the latter may also benefit from the wearing of a collar.

3. Phenothiazines are best used for 3-week courses in labyrinthitis or Ménière's disease. When continued for long periods (perhaps because they relieve the anxiety, itself causing dizziness), extrapyramidal adverse effects are likely[5]. Prochlorperazine (Stemetil) 5 mg twice or thrice daily is appropriate.

4. Caution is advisable when using psychotropic, diuretic or other hypotensive agents in the elderly. These cause dizziness through postural hypotension and other mechanisms.

5. As dizziness is so often multifactorial in the elderly, a variety of generally simple measures may be helpful (improving ocular function, removal of wax, treatment of diabetes, control of rapid atrial fibrillation etc.). A walking stick may be particularly helpful in improving sensory input[2].

FOLLOW-UP

Review will be necessary, initially weekly, and then every few weeks, until symptoms have settled.

Laxton LM (1984) *Br. J. Hosp. Med.*, December, 315–21.

Wright A (1987) *Dizziness; A Guide to Disorders of Balance*. Beckenham: Croom Helm.

Lum C (1987) *J. R. Soc. Med.*, **80**, 229–31.

[4] RCGP/OPCS/DHSS (1986) *Morbidity Statistics from General Practice: 1981–1982 Third National Study*. London: HMSO.

[5] Pall MS, Williams AC (1987) *Br. Med. J.*, **295**, 30–1.

Labyrinthitis

The semicircular canals can be affected by bacterial infection, especially by direct spread from the middle ear in the presence of a cholesteatoma. The much more common disease is acute labyrinthitis of presumed viral origin (also known as vestibular neuronitis) or epidemic vertigo[1]. There is severe vertigo, nausea, vomiting, malaise and often fever. Reported incidence varies widely, from 0.18/1000 per year[2], to 2/1000 per year[3]. Some 28% are due to influenza A, and others may be caused by herpes[3,4]. Sudden vestibular failure can also arise from infarction, head injury, or diabetic neuropathy[1]. Nystagmus is present in at least half of the cases in the early stages[3]. Deafness and tinnitus do not occur.

PROGNOSIS

- Severe vertigo and nausea on movement, subsiding over 3–4 days, when patients can usually mobilize. Recovery takes about 3 weeks, but poor light and fatigue can produce symptoms for some weeks longer.

TREATMENT

1. Intramuscular sedation such as chlorpromazine 25 mg or prochlorperazine 12.5 mg is required, possibly repeatedly in the acute phase.
2. A 3-week course of oral labyrinthine sedatives (prochlorperazine 5 mg t.d.s., or cinnarizine 15 mg t.d.s.) will cover the likely duration of symptoms. Long-term phenothiazines should be avoided because of the risk of extrapyramidal side-effects.

FOLLOW-UP

Patients are likely to need review every few days in the acute phase, and then once or twice during the next few weeks.

[1] Hickish GW (1985) *Ear, Nose and Throat Disorders*. Edinburgh: Churchill Livingstone.
[2] Berzon DB (1983) *J. Laryngol. Otol.*, **97**, 817–24.
[3] Brill GC (1982) *J. R. Coll. Gen. Pract.*, **32**, 47–50.
[4] Anonymous (1984) *Lancet*, **ii**, 1439.

Meniére's Disease

This disorder comprises a triad of sudden and recurring episodes of vertigo (with nausea and vomiting), tinnitus, and fluctuating deafness. The mechanism is endolymphatic hydrops, and the cause is unknown. Suggested aetiologies include migraine, head injury, infection, allergy and hypothyroidism. Nystagmus usually accompanies the vertigo[1,2]. The true incidence is unknown, as milder cases may not be diagnosed, but 0.24/1000 per year is the rate reported from one practice[3]; such patients form half of all those seen by ENT surgeons with vertigo.

PROGNOSIS

- Overall prognosis is uncertain, but varies from those where the disease process arrests after a few attacks to those unfortunates who suffer frequent attacks and develop severe deafness[1].

TREATMENT

1. Acute vertigo, vomiting, and nystagmus call for phenothiazines, e.g. chlorpromazine 25 mg or prochlorperazine 12.5 mg i.m. Similar agents can be continued orally for 2–3 weeks (e.g. prochlorperazine 5 mg t.d.s. or cinnarizine 15 mg t.d.s.[1]).
2. Betahistine (Serc) 8 mg t.d.s. is an agent which may be helpful over a 6-week course.

3. Patients will need referral for confirmation of the diagnosis, and exclusion of other conditions, especially acoustic neuroma.

FOLLOW-UP

Review is likely on several occasions following an acute episode, and then as required for recurrent symptoms.

---

[1] Hickish G (1985) *Ear, Nose and Throat Disorders.* Edinburgh: Churchill Livingstone.
[2] Anonymous (1984) *Lancet,* **ii,** 1439.
[3] Berzon DB (1983) *J. Laryngol. Otol.,* **97,** 817–24.

Hearing Impairment

A socially significant hearing loss (i.e. with difficulty at conversational levels) occurs with a mean hearing loss of 30 decibels or more. Using this definition, 0.8% of males aged 15–24 years and 18% of males aged 75–79 have a significant problem[1]. Prevalence is lower in females at all ages, and higher in manual occupations or following noise exposure.

The causes of hearing impairment vary with age. In *infancy*, congenital causes are important; 1–2 infants per 1000 births are born with a severe hearing impairment[2]. The chief causes are infective (chiefly rubella in the UK in recent years), but include cytomegalovirus and neonatal meningitis, perinatal hypoxia or hyperbilirubinaemia, birth injury, and recessive inheritance. Later in *childhood* wax accumulation or otitis media with effusion commonly cause a conductive deafness; a sensorineural loss, often unilateral, may result from mumps infection. In *adult life* hereditary deafness may become apparent for the first time; Ménière's disease occurs. Otosclerosis is a progressive disorder of ossification of bony tissue in the ear, causing a bilateral conductive loss in middle life. In *old age* the degenerative condition of presbycusis, noise-induced damage, and wax accumulation are the important causes.

PROGNOSIS

- Sudden total hearing loss will be seen only a few times in a general practitioner's working life. Recovery is unlikely when the deafness has persisted more than 1 month, but is likely to occur in 90% of those treated within 1 week[2].

- Speech development is likely to be normal in congenitally deaf babies only when the problem is recognized early. Infants in most areas are tested by the distraction test at 6–9 months, but earlier recognition is preferable. This will be more likely if professionals pay attention to parents when they believe their baby is not hearing.

- Presbycusis appears to be more common in conditions of noise exposure. Hearing loss for high tones (4000–6000 Hz) increases by about 10 decibels for each decade of life[2].

- The prognosis for other causes will depend on the disease process responsible. Ménière's disease and otosclerosis will cause a progressive hearing loss. Toxic or infective sensorineural deafness will not improve, but most conductive losses will do so (i.e. wax can be removed, middle ear fluid is likely to resolve).

TREATMENT

1. The infant with marked hearing loss requires prompt referral for definitive diagnosis, amplification and special educational provision.

2. Sudden total hearing loss at any age requires prompt referral. Most cases are believed to arise from viral eighth nerve damage, and systemic steroids seem to improve prognosis[2].

3. Many causes of conductive hearing loss are amenable either to surgical treatment (e.g. glue ear, otosclerosis), or to simple measures like removal of wax.

4. Most patients with a bilateral hearing loss of 30 decibels or more at the speech frequencies (250–5000 Hz) are likely to benefit from hearing aids[3].

   a. Postaural aids are unobtrusive and suitable for most patients.

   b. Body-worn aids are prescribed for the severely deaf.

   c. Smaller aids which fit in the ear canal are commercially available and preferred by a few patients but only provide a lower level of amplification.

   d. Deafness is associated with stigma, and can result in isolation and psychiatric problems. In addition the adaptation required is more difficult at advanced ages when there are likely to be other difficulties. Thus patients should be referred when deafness is only moderate, and preferably before 65 years[3].

   e. Hearing therapists with a range of technical and educational skills are found in an increasing number of ENT departments[3].

5. Hearing dogs can be as useful for deaf individuals as the more familiar guide dogs are for blind persons[2,4].

[1] Rawson A (1973) *Deafness: Report of a Departmental Enquiry into the Promotion of Research*. Report on Health and Social Subjects no. 4. London: HMSO.
[2] Hickish G (1985) *Ear, Nose and Throat Disorders*. Edinburgh: Churchill Livingstone.
[3] Knight J (1987) *Practitioner*, **231**, 1121–6.
[4] Fogle B, Radcliffe A (1983) *Practitioner*, **227**, 1051–3.

FOLLOW-UP

Those with marked hearing impairment may well be reviewed at hospital, but subsequent primary care consultations can include checks on general functioning, including the use of hearing aids.

Tinnitus

An abnormal noise, typically ringing or buzzing, occurs spontaneously for short periods in one-third of adults. Tinnitus lasting 5 minutes occurs in 15% of the population: 2% are significantly bothered and 0.5–1% suffer serious effects on their lives as a result[1]. Hearing loss is generally associated, and the sound is believed to arise from damaged cochlear cells. The prevalence of tinnitus is highest in the 50–60-year age group[2] and is higher in manual workers and those who have suffered noise exposure. Different series reveal either an equal sex incidence or a slight male preponderance.

PROGNOSIS

● Tinnitus may remit spontaneously, especially when of short duration. Other patients adapt to the symptom.

TREATMENT

1. Reassurance must be based on an adequate assessment which defines the cause as far as possible. Accurate information may be very helpful to the patient in confirming that there is no intracranial tumour or other frightening disease.
2. Specific treatment for remediable causes may help (Ménière's disease, otosclerosis, acoustic neuroma[1]).
3. Masking therapy is the main treatment. An adapted hearing aid which produces white noise can reduce or abolish tinnitus, and the white noise will often persist for a number of hours after 2–3 hours' wear[1,2].
4. Psychologists may help by teaching relaxation, biofeedback and cognitive therapy[2].

5. Drug treatment has a limited place. Some patients have depressive disorders which can be specifically treated, while carbamazepine appears to help some patients (initially 100–200 mg daily, rising to 0.6–1 g daily, according to response; blood levels should be measured at higher doses). Night sedation may be useful, while daytime anxiolytics are best used for short periods only.

FOLLOW-UP

Severely affected patients may be followed up at specialist tinnitus clinics. The family doctor can help with sympathetic support for this distressing and chronic symptom; follow-up is as appropriate for the level of symptoms.

[1] Stephens DG (1987) *Practitioner*, **231**, 1115–18.
[2] Hazell JWP (1981) *Practitioner*, **225**, 1577–85.

Coryza

The common cold is of great economic importance—50% of sickness absence results from upper respiratory infections. The clinical significance is chiefly in immunosuppressed patients, or in those with severe asthma or heart failure. In all, 30–50% of colds are caused by the 100 serotypes of rhinovirus, 20–30% by two coronavirus serotypes, and the others by a variety of viruses[1]. Spread is both by droplet transmission and direct contact, especially via the hands after nose-blowing.

PROGNOSIS

- Symptoms can last from 2–10 days. Most illnesses are mild with nasal congestion and discharge. A minority (especially young children) may have malaise, fever and headache[1].
- When cold viruses are administered to volunteers, one-third to one-half will develop coryzal symptoms, one-third have subclinical infections, while the remainder are immune.
- As there is little cross-immunity between rhinoviruses, repeated infections are common, especially in youth. Infant schoolchildren suffer about 10 colds yearly (depending on definition of an episode), young adults 2–3 infections, and the middle-aged, 1 or less[1,2].
- Introverts and those with recent life events will have more severe infections for an equivalent viral exposure[1].

TREATMENT

1. Colds are self-limiting and practical therapy is presently entirely symptomatic. Hot drinks and steam inhalations may be comforting while simple analgesics will relieve headache or fever.
2. Decongestants are widely purchased over the counter for use during colds. Therapeutic considerations would be:
   a. Decongestant nasal drops such as ephedrine 0.5 or 1% can relieve nasal obstruction for several hours but may cause rebound effects if continued for more than 7 days[3].
   b. Systemic decongestants (e.g. pseudoephedrine 60 mg) do not cause the local effects, while being otherwise of doubtful value. Short-term use seems preferable, and as sympathomimetics they should be avoided in patients with hypertension, hyperthyroidism, coronary heart disease or diabetes. *Any* decongestants (local or systemic) may cause a hypertensive crisis in those taking monoamine oxidase inhibitors[3].
3. The dosage of inhaled bronchodilators and inhaled steroids may need to be increased in asthmatic patients. Likewise nasal steroid dosage should be increased in those with non-infective rhinitis.
4. The nasal administration of natural or recombinant interferon will avert the symptoms or prevent intrafamilial spread of rhinovirus infection. Unfortunately to date this is at the cost of a marked local inflammatory reaction.
5. General practitioners can usefully question patients about the reason for consulting, as well as about symptoms. Their answers may uncover relevant health beliefs, or various social or emotional problems. Any health education or other help and advice may then be more appropriately focused.
6. Many practices have adopted a non-prescribing policy for self-limiting illnesses such as colds, with a consequent reduction in their consultation rate[4,5].

FOLLOW-UP

Follow-up is not required for colds except when complications are present or suspected.

[1] Higgins PG (1987) *Update*, 98–104.
[2] Isaacs D (1987) In *Progress in Child Health*, vol 3 (Macfarlane A ed). Edinburgh: Churchill Livingstone.
[3] George CF *et al.* (1986) *British National Formulary*, no. 14. London: British Medical Association and Pharmaceutical Society.
[4] Marsh GN (1977) *Br. Med. J.*, **2**, 1267.
[5] Marsh GN (1981) *Br. Med. J.*, **281**, 1159.

Nasal Polyps

A nasal polyp is a shiny rounded opalescent structure which may fill the anterior nasal passage. It can easily be seen with a light and nasal speculum. Nasal polyps are detected in 2.3–3/1000 patients per year[1]. They are associated with non-infective rhinitis, especially the non-allergic or vasomotor variety. Hyper-reactivity of the mucosa and degranulated mast cells play a part in the pathogenesis of polyps[2]. They are chiefly found in later years, and in 30% of cases are associated with asthma, normally of late-onset 'intrinsic' type[2].

PROGNOSIS

- Nasal polyps are unlikely to disappear spontaneously, while recurrence is likely after surgical removal without other therapy.
- Long-standing polyps may occasionally destroy the nasal bones and result in widening of the nasal soft tissues[2].
- Asthma and polyps are likely to develop within 5 years of each other.

TREATMENT

1. Nasal polyps will require surgical removal for relief of symptoms.
2. Nasal steroids (e.g. beclomethasone) will relieve the rhinitis associated with polyps and may help to prevent recurrence.
3. The possibility of unrecognized asthma should be considered and treatment instituted with inhaled bronchodilators and steroids if appropriate.

FOLLOW-UP

One or two monthly reviews may be required, to assess response to nasal anti-allergic therapy which should be continued long-term. The patient should be warned of the possible later onset of wheezing or asthmatic symptoms. Re-examination of the nose may reveal recurrent polyps.

---

[1] Hodgkin K (1985) *Towards Earlier Diagnosis: A Guide to Primary Care*. Edinburgh: Churchill Livingstone.
[2] Drake-Lee A (1987) *Practitioner*, **231**, 1191–5.

Rhinitis

Non-infective rhinitis occurs in two forms—allergic (seasonal or perennial), and the vasomotor or non-allergic form. The latter is divided into eosinophilic and non-eosinophilic forms on the basis of nasal smear appearances; hyper-reactivity of the nasal mucosa is the underlying abnormality[1], in response to irritants or changes in temperature and humidity. About 10% of the population suffer from allergic disorders, which are becoming more common[2]. The consultation rate for hayfever is 19.7 per 1000, equal in both sexes and peaking in late adolescence[3]. Vasomotor rhinitis is less common, but occurs throughout adult life.

PROGNOSIS

- Hayfever (grass pollen allergy) causes most symptoms in May and June in northern Europe. Tree pollen causes symptoms earlier in spring, while mould spores and ragweed pollen (USA) cause symptoms in late summer[4].
- Hayfever symptoms tend to recur annually[2] for 5–15 years.
- Associated allergic conditions accompany hayfever; 30% of patients have asthma, 25% eczema and 5% urticaria.

TREATMENT

1. Antihistamines treat ocular as well as nasal allergic symptoms. Newer agents such as terfenadine (60 mg b.d.) or astemizole (10 mg daily) are both more effective and less sedating than other antihistamines. The latter is slow-acting, and more effective for obstruction rather than sneezing.
2. Nasal obstruction, due to allergic or non-allergic rhinitis, is best treated by intranasal steroids such as beclomethasone twice daily[1]. This can be combined with sodium cromoglycate eyedrops for ocular symptoms.
3. Nasal sympathomimetic drops and sprays are best avoided in non-allergic rhinitis because of the likelihood of nasal rebound symptoms[1]. Systemic agents such as pseudoephedrine

should be reserved for short-term use in exacerbations.
4. Systemic steroid treatments such as depot methylprednisolone 40–120 mg or triamcinolone 40 mg is highly effective in hayfever, but does not seem desirable on general grounds. Exceptional use for non-recurring demands (weddings, examinations) may be justified (but the patients may seek equally complete symptom relief in future years).
5. Desensitization for allergic rhinitis is associated infrequently with deaths from anaphylaxis. The Committee for the Safety of Medicines has advised against their use in the UK except when full rescuscitation facilities are available.

FOLLOW-UP

Review is needed chiefly to assess response to topical steroid or other prophylactic treatment, and to encourage compliance. It may be appropriate to encourage patients to attend before the start of the hayfever season, so that such advice can be reinforced.

[1] Jones AS, Lancer JM (1987) Br. Med. J., **294**, 1505.
[2] Fry J (1985) Common Diseases: Their Nature, Incidence and Care, 4th edn. Lancaster: MTP.
[3] Crombie D, Fleming (1987) Br. Med. J. 299, 279–83.
[4] Wood P (1986) Family Pract., **3**, 120–5.

Epistaxis

General practitioners will see bleeding from the nose at a rate of 3.6[1] to 5.8[2] per 1000 patients annually. It is less common in the middle years. In children and adolescents bleeding is usually from Little's area in the anterior septal mucosa, because of infective or non-infective rhinitis; in the elderly arteriosclerosis and hypertension are important, and bleeding is often more posterior. Anticoagulants, blood dyscrasias and trauma all may cause bleeding. Rarer causes are juvenile angiofibroma (males aged 10–20) and hereditary telangiectasia or Osler's disease (a mendelian dominant presenting in adult life)[3].

PROGNOSIS

- Recurrences are common although statistics are hard to find.
- At least 50% of elderly patients have recurrent bleeding after packing.

TREATMENT

1. The doctor may need to advise on first-aid management perhaps in the first instance over the telephone. Firm pressure on the fleshy part of the nose for 6–7 minutes (the clotting time) should be combined with ice packs or cold compresses.
2. Heavy or persistent bleeding calls for packing, using ribbon gauze soaked in 1:1000 adrenaline solution or bismuth iodoform and paraffin paste. A good light, angled forceps, a nasal speculum, and local anaesthetic spray are required. The nose is packed in layers from below upwards[3].
3. If the bleeding does not settle, hospital admission is indicated. Postnasal packing, balloon insertion, or even emergency surgery may be required.
4. Recurrences of bleeding from Little's area call for cauterization using silver nitrate sticks or trichloracetic acid after the application of a local anaesthetic spray.

FOLLOW-UP

Nasal packs will need removal after 24–48 hours. Review otherwise is as appropriate for the cause of epistaxis.

[1] RCGP/OPCS/DHSS (1986) *Morbidity Statistics from General Practice: 1981–1982, Third National Study*. London: HMSO.
[2] Hodgkin K (1985) *Towards Earlier Diagnosis: A Guide to Primary Care*, 5th edn. Edinburgh: Churchill Livingstone.
[3] Hickish G (1985) *Ear, Nose and Throat Disorders*. Edinburgh: Churchill Livingstone.

Sinusitis

An inflammation of the paranasal air sinuses is more often suspected from patients' symptoms than confirmed. The diagnosis strictly requires two of the following[1]: a purulent nasal or postnasal discharge; sinus tenderness, or deep facial pain aggravated by dependence of head; opacity of sinuses on x-ray or transillumination. The consultation rate is 14 per 1000 population; the condition is twice as common in females, and occurs mostly between the age of 25 and 65 years[2].

PROGNOSIS

- One-quarter of cases recur in 3 years[3]. Some of these develop chronic infections.
- Complications, especially of chronic sinusitis[4], are chiefly those of direct extension of infection. These include: cellulitis or osteitis; pyocele, or a frontal sinus mucocele; fistula to skin surface or mouth; intracranial spread from frontal or ethmoid infection; cavernous sinus thrombosis (rare).

TREATMENT

1. Steam inhalations, with short-term nasal or oral decongestants, may relieve congestion and aching of sinuses associated with upper respiratory infection, especially in those with vasomotor rhinitis.
2. Antibiotic treatment is indicated when there is fever, malaise or persistent pain. As the causative organism is likely to be *Pneumococcus* or *Haemophilus influenzae*, a broad-spectrum agent is indicated (tetracycline, ampicillin, amoxycillin, or co-trimoxazole).
3. Nasal steroids may be beneficial after acute episodes when an element of vasomotor rhinitis is suspected.
4. Those with chronic or troublesome recurrent infection, radiologically confirmed and unresponsive to the above conservative measures, may need ENT referral. Hospital management may include antral lavage for maxillary infection, surgery to correct a deviated nasal septum, or drainage procedures such as an intranasal antrostomy or the more radical Caldwell–Luc operation.

FOLLOW-UP

Acute episodes can be followed up according to the symptoms; definite or suspected chronic sinusitis will require review to arrange appropriate investigations and management.

[1] WONCA Classification Committee (1983) *ICHPPC-2 Defined (International Classification of Health Problems in Primary Care)*, 3rd edn. Oxford: Oxford University Press.
[2] RCGP/OPCS/DHSS (1986) *Morbidity Statistics from General Practice 1981–1982, Third National Study*. London: HMSO.
[3] Hodgkin K (1985) *Towards Earlier Diagnosis: A Guide to Primary Care*, 5th edn. Edinburgh: Churchill Livingstone.
[4] Hickish G (1985) *Ear, Nose and Throat Disorders*. Edinburgh: Churchill Livingstone.

Tonsillitis, Adenoiditis and Pharyngitis

The anatomically named forms of throat infection represent overlapping clinical clusters rather than strict entities, so are considered together. Tonsillitis is characterized by a sore throat, fever, red tonsils (often with pus), tonsillar and lymph node swelling (consultation rate 41.2 per 1000[1]. In adenoiditis—much less common—the adenoids are similarly affected; features include nasal speech, mouth breathing and halitosis. In pharyngitis there is a red throat, often without fever; this is about as common as tonsillitis[2]. Streptococci can be isolated from 30–50% of sore throats but up to half may be carriers[3]. Chronic tonsillar and adenoidal hypertrophy (1[1]–3.8[2] consultations per 1000) can cause snoring and sleep apnoea.

PROGNOSIS

- An acute throat infection lasts from 3 to 10 days.
- The peak incidence is in the first 2 years at school, but is common throughout childhood. There is a further peak in early adult life[4].
- Cervical adenitis often complicates throat infections (consultation rate 2.5[1]–17.5[2] per 1000).
- Peritonsillar abscess or quinsy may also occur (consultation rate 1.3 per 1000[2]).
- Scarlet fever occurs with certain strains of *Streptococcus pyogenes* (1.9 per 1000[1.2]).
- Rheumatic fever now has an annual incidence in developed countries of 0.6 per 100 000 children[5] or 1 per 30 000 of sore throats treated with penicillin as against 1 per 40 000 not so treated[5].
- Acute glomerulonephritis occurs in 1:13 000 treated sore throats, or 1:17 000 when untreated[6].

TREATMENT

1. The use of antibiotics in sore throats is controversial, although various surveys have shown that such treatment occurs in about 70% of cases seen by doctors[7].
2. Antibiotic therapy seems indicated for the ill or febrile patient with tonsillar redness, swelling, and exudate. Although these features predict the presence of streptococci fairly well, not all trials show a benefit from treatment even in this group.
3. The usefulness of throat cultures or rapid immunoassays for streptococci are limited by the high prevalence of streptococcal carriage.
4. Symptomatic treatment suitable for all cases would include aspirin gargles (in non-dyspeptic patients over 12) or paracetamol, combined with throat lozenges, ice for sucking and refraining from smoking.
5. If antibiotic treatment is thought appropriate, suitable guidelines would be as follows:
   a. Streptococci, overwhelmingly the bacterial throat pathogens, are invariably sensitive to penicillin. In patients who are markedly ill or vomiting, treatment can be commenced by intramuscular injection. (Penicillin G, 1 000 000 units for an adult, or combined with benethaquine and procaine penicillin in the long-acting Triplopen 2 ml.)
   b. Penicillin V (phenoxymethyl penicillin) is suitable for oral therapy; 500 mg 8-hourly, half an hour before food deviates slightly from British National Formulary guidelines but appears to be effective and acceptable[7].

   The optimum duration of a course is unknown but 5–7 days is likely to be sufficient[7].
   c. Erythromycin 500 mg t.d.s. is appropriate treatment in those allergic to penicillin; however, gastrointestinal side-effects occur commonly.
   d. Broad-spectrum antibiotics are not generally indicated for throat infections. Ampicillin and its derivatives are associated with greater toxicity, for instance the morbilliform rash which occurs in 90% of those with infectious mononucleosis. These agents are therefore particularly to be avoided for throat infections in adolescents and young adults. Cephalosporins, e.g. cephalexin, may have a place in those aller-

gic to penicillin (although 10% will react to these drugs also), especially in patients who develop gastric side-effects with erythromycin.

Apart from gross tonsillar and adenoidal hypertrophy, tonsillectomy is likely to benefit that restricted group of children who have several (e.g. five) throat infections in each of 2 successive years[4]. A month-long course of penicillin therapy may be a suitable first line of management in such cases.

Many children who suffer recurrent respiratory infections between the ages of 4 and 8 are catarrhal children, who react more strongly to ordinary pathogens[4]. Explanation and appropriate reassurance are an important part of management. The child may be presented when the problem is maternal anxiety or depression; the alert doctor will recognize this and direct attention appropriately.

FOLLOW-UP

Early review may be needed for persistent or severe throat symptoms; infectious mononucleosis will then need to be considered (and not only in adolescents). In recurrent cases, follow-up offers an opportunity to discuss longer-term management.

[1] RCGP/OPCS/DHSS (1986) *Morbidity, Statistics from General Practice: 1981–1982, Third National Study*. London: HMSO.
[2] Hodgkin K (1985) *Towards Earlier Diagnosis; A Guide to Primary Care*, 5th edn. Edinburgh: Churchill Livingstone.
[3] Foggo BA (1985) *Family Practice*, **2**, 101–7.
[4] Fry J (1985) *Common Diseases; Their Nature, Incidence and Care*, 4th edn. Lancaster: MTP Press.
[5] Howie JGR (1985) *J. R. Coll. Gen. Pract.*, **35**, 223–4.
[6] Taylor JL, Howie JGR (1983) *J. R. Coll. Gen. Pract.*, **33**, 783–6.
[7] George RM (1986) *Br. Med. J.*, **293**, 682.

Epiglottitis

Epiglottitis is an uncommon but dangerous infection, in which inflammatory oedema in and around the epiglottis may cause rapidly progressive respiratory obstruction. It is one of the invasive infections caused by *Haemophilus influenzae* type B, and the estimated annual incidence is 1 in 5000 children under 16, at least in inner city populations[1]. The child, typically aged 3–7 and an older singleton, will be found sitting up, toxic and anxious, dribbling saliva and with a harsh inspiratory stridor[2].

PROGNOSIS

- Few children now die in hospital, at least in major centres[1], but some still sustain respiratory arrest at home or during the journey to hospital[2].
- Epiglottitis also occurs in adults, and carries a mortality of around 7%[3].

TREATMENT

1. Immediate admission to hospital is required when the diagnosis is suspected. Attempts to inspect the epiglottis may provoke complete obstruction.
2. When a long journey to hospital is required, ampicillin or amoxycillin 250–500 mg should be given by i.m. or i.v. injection.
3. If the child sustains a respiratory arrest in transit, tracheostomy will be required to save life. The insertion of several wide-bore hypodermic needles between tracheal cartilages is recommended rather than a more formal surgical approach.
4. Opinions vary as regards ideal airway management in hospital, whether by tracheostomy or endotracheal inhalation. Prophylactic airway protection is combined with parenteral antibiotics; combination therapy including chloramphenicol or a third-generation cephalosporin will provide cover against ampicillin-resistant strains of *Haemophilus*[1,3].

Review is as indicated by the patient's condition after discharge from hospital.

[1] Dyas A, George RH (1986) *J. Infection*, **13**, 179–85.
[2] Drinkwater C (1982) *Medicine in Practice*, **1**, 369–73.
[3] Mayosmith MF *et al.* (1986) *N. Engl. J. Med.*, **314**, 1133–9.

Carcinoma of the Larynx

Carcinoma of the larynx represents 2% of all malignancies. It is the commonest cancer dealt with by ENT surgeons; more than 90% are squamous carcinomas[1]. The disease is almost confined to smokers, and is commoner in males but the incidence in women is increasing. There are three varieties—supraglottic, glottic and subglottic tumours. The chief symptom is hoarseness, especially as regards the glottic lesions.

PROGNOSIS

- Small tumours have a much better prognosis, especially if confined to the larynx. Survival is shorter when cervical lymph nodes are involved.
- The prognosis of anaplastic carcinomas is slightly worse.
- Some 10% later develop bronchial carcinoma[1].
- Cumulative five year survival[1]:

		Glottic	Supraglottic
Stage I	tumour	94%	91%
Stage II	tumour	85%	82%
Stage III	tumour	59%	49%
Stage IV	tumour	9%	9%

TREATMENT

1. Patients with hoarseness of more than 3 weeks' duration should be referred to ENT surgeons.
2. Radiotherapy is the treatment of choice for small tumours; 90% are cured with a return to normal voice.
3. Surgery is performed for failure to respond to radiotherapy (possibly conservative, leaving a reasonable voice). Radical laryngectomy will be required for failures of limited operations or for late tumours.
4. Rehabilitation is an important part of management.

    a. Laryngectomees will have a tracheostomy. Tracheal secretions, especially in chronic bronchitics, may call for suction apparatus which can be provided for community use. Tracheal crusting can cause obstruction and is best dealt with in hospital[2].

    b. Oesophageal voice is the usual communicative method, learnt by 65% of male laryngectomees[1].

    c. Speech aids are being developed; these include amplifiers for whispers and oesophageal speech, and electronic vibrators[2].

    d. A surgically created tracheo-oesophageal fistula can be used to recreate speech[5].

5. Prevention, either primary, by not smoking, or secondary and tertiary, by prompt hospital referral for hoarseness, offers the best long-term hope for these patients.

FOLLOW-UP

Laryngeal cancer patients will be followed up at hospital; as always, the support and help of the primary care team after discharge can be very helpful. Carcinoma of bronchus is common in these patients so the doctor should be alert for the development or worsening of chest symptoms.

[1] Harrison DFN (1986) In *Treatment and Prognosis; Surgery* (Hawkins R ed). London: Heinemann.
[2] Edwards N (1981) *Practitioner*, **225**, 1603–7.

3

The Respiratory System

J H Walker and Members from the Division of Primary Care, University of Newcastle

Chronic Bronchitis and Emphysema

Chronic bronchitis is defined as a cough producing sputum nearly every day for at least 3 months, in more than 2 successive years. Emphysema is defined as an increase in the acinus (the air space distal to the terminal bronchiole). This results in damage and, later, destruction of the walls. These conditions often occur together and can lead to permanent and generalized airways obstruction. The most important aetiological factor in both is cigarette smoking. Age, the environment, occupation, socioeconomic conditions, infection, and alpha[1] antitrypsin deficiency (present in 1/3000 of the population) are other aetiological factors, although less important. Males are more commonly affected than women and in the UK about 10% of men are sufferers. Over 30 000 working days each year are lost through chronic bronchitis and emphysema. During the winter acute exacerbations are common. The infections will most commonly be viral in the first place with superadded bacterial infection. In cities where there is high atmospheric pollution a clean air policy has undoubtedly reduced the incidence of chronic bronchitis, particularly in smokers.

PROGNOSIS

- In all 30 000 people die from these conditions each year in the UK—about one-quarter before the normal retirement age.
- Mortality increases greatly with age. Many young patients become severely disabled in middle age.
- Patients who continue to smoke cigarettes have a worse prognosis.
- Statistics show that smokers have a higher rate of hospital admission and absence from work than the normal population. They also have a higher mortality rate. A measurable predictable factor is forced expiratory volume in 1 second (FEV_1). When this is below the expected value prognosis is much poorer in those who continue to smoke[1].
- Five-year survival rate is about 30% in those with cor pulmonale, which may be the final stage in chronic bronchitis and emphysema[2].
- A poor socioeconomic status carries a worse prognosis. This may be due to poor nutrition and poor housing, together with living with other people who have similar habits of smoking and who easily pick up and pass on infections.
- Exposure to infection and high atmospheric pollution exacerbate these diseases.

TREATMENT

1. *Preventive*
   a. Stopping smoking is the most valuable measure in arresting the mild condition and possibly limiting those with more severe disease. Counselling by a doctor succeeds in about 10% of cases. Group therapy, psychotherapy, hypnosis and acupuncture have all claimed some success in smoking cessation.
   b. Work environments may provoke chronic bronchitis and emphysema, particularly where the atmosphere is dusty or contaminated by irritant gases. The Health and Safety at Work regulations make it obligatory for employer and employee to draw attention to these matters and have them dealt with appropriately.
   c. The weather may have an effect, particularly fog, and if this is predicted then the patient should stay indoors with the windows shut. Extremely cold weather may also aggravate bronchitis.

2. *Acute exacerbations*
   a. Broad-spectrum antibiotics are the first line of treatment, for example a 7-day course of ampicillin (250 mg four times a day) or tetracycline in the same dose. Other antibacterial drugs may have to be used if the infection proves resistant. Arranging sputum cultures is indicated in resistant cases. A coloured sputum usually indicates infection with *Pneumococcus* and/or *Haemophilus influenzae* but if the sputum is clear then antibiotics are unnecessary.
   b. Clearance of the sputum by coughing or physiotherapy is essential and should be ac-

tively encouraged; the services of a physiotherapist may be necessary. Expectorants and cough suppressants should not be used.

c. Mucolytics, such as bromhexine, are said to make the sputum more liquid; although it may be tried in a dose of 16 mg four times a day it is probably of little value. Dehydration should be prevented by the copious supply of oral fluids.

d. It is dangerous to give a sedative to patients with a serious respiratory complaint.

e. Bronchodilators such as beta-sympathomimetic (salbutamol or terbutaline), anticholinergic (ipratropium bromide), or xanthine (aminophylline or theophylline) drugs may help if there is reversible bronchial constriction. Drugs such as salbutamol should be tried first at home by inhaler or possibly by nebuliser.

f. When there is cyanosis and the partial pressure of oxygen is less than 70 mmHg, 24% oxygen should be administered. Too high an oxygen concentration will reduce the respiratory drive, leading to a higher carbon dioxide concentration and narcosis. The patient will of course be admitted to hospital.

Under these conditions physiotherapy is necessary in order to clear the bronchi of secretions and improve the airflow. For this the active co-operation of the patient is essential. When the patient is not fully alert due to hypercapnia, hypoxaemia and exhaustion, an intravenous injection of 2 ml nikethamide combined with intravenous aminophylline (250 mg) may produce enough stimulation and bronchodilation to allow the physiotherapy to be commenced.

3. *Long-term management*

a. Pre-winter vaccination against influenza is advisable, except in patients sensitive to eggs.

b. Prophylactic antibiotics to reduce acute exacerbations caused by bacteria may be advised, although drug resistance may develop. Choice includes ampicillin, amoxycillin, co-trimoxazole and tetracycline. These antibiotics may be given in short courses when the sputum becomes purulent or sometimes regularly throughout the winter.

c. If reversible bronchospasm is present then the use of bronchodilator drugs in aerosol inhalers may help.

d. Unless there is an asthmatic element corticosteroids either orally or by inhalation should not be used.

e. Oxygen used in the home can be beneficial if it is used continuously for over 15 hours a day. It will increase activity levels. The oxygen can be supplied in cylinders or in oxygen concentrators. Patients for oxygen therapy should be carefully chosen or the respiratory drive may be inhibited. Those with a partial pressure of oxygen of <55 mmHg are suitable. Short periods of oxygen convey no material benefit, except perhaps as a morale booster.

f. Mucolytics are of little use in reducing the viscosity of the sputum.

g. Diuretics (such as frusemide) are used in cor pulmonale and respiratory failure.

FOLLOW-UP

Many patients will benefit from long-term anticipatory care. Regular check-ups should include assessing the FEV_1 and arranging an annual chest X-ray. Obesity should be tackled. Patients should be encouraged to take light exercise such as walking, bowls or golf if they are able and the weather is fine. The doctor must be alert to depression.

[1] Fletcher C et al. (1976) *The Natural History of Chronic Bronchitis and Emphysema.* Oxford: Oxford University Press.
[2] Crofton J, Douglas A (1981) *Respiratory Diseases*, 3rd edn. Oxford: Blackwell.

Asthma

Asthma is a condition characterized by intermittent obstruction of the airways. The cardinal feature is wheeze but symptoms may be confined to shortness of breath or cough, which is often worse at night. Attacks may be preceded by upper respiratory tract infection or precipitated by exercise and may be described as recurrent colds or recurrent bronchitis. Pathologically there is production of intrabronchial mucus plugs, bronchial mucosal oedema, hypertrophy of bronchial or bronchiolar smooth muscle and hyperplasia or goblet cells and bronchospasm. These factors lead to airways trapping and the clinical feature of wheeze, cough and breathlessness. The underlying cause my be a bronchial hyperactivity to the chemical mediators of inflammation[1]. Such hyperactivity may be brought on by exposure to allergens, infectious agents such as viruses (especially respiratory syncytial virus), atmospheric pollutants, climatic changes, exercise, emotional factors or a combination of these factors. Asthma occurs in 5% of adults and 10–15% of children (i.e. about 100 patients in an average general practice of 2000 patients per doctor[2]. Occupational exposure to various chemicals can cause asthma (5% of adult-onset asthma).

In Children

Most asthmatic children present with recurrent cough, wheeze and breathlessness before 5 years of age, but only half are diagnosed by then[3]. The diagnosis of asthma is important as children labelled as wheezy are less likely to be treated appropriately[4,5]. (Wheezy bronchitis is not a diagnosis and should not be used.) It occurs in 10–15% of all children, although the incidence is difficult to gauge accurately because of the problems of applying the diagnostic criteria. Boys are affected twice as often as girls[6]. Many improve with age; by the time they are 20, 30–50% will be symptom-free. Common presentations include cough (especially nocturnal), exercise-induced cough or wheeze, difficulty in sleeping due to respiratory symptoms and prodromal itching. There is commonly a family history of atopy.

Counting the number of consultations for respiratory symptoms may help—more than twice a year is suspicious of asthma. Mentioning this possibility early to parents is helpful so that they understand and take appropriate action. Therapeutic trials may be necessary to confirm the diagnosis.

PROGNOSIS

● This depends upon the severity but can be graded as[7]:

Mild episodic—75% of childhood asthmatics, usually triggered by viral infections. Lung function is normal between attacks. Some 50% stop wheezing by 14 years; 15% have asthma as adults.

Frequent—20% of childhood asthmatics with multiple trigger factors. Between attacks 40% have decreased lung function. A total of 20% become asymptomatic but 25% have severe asthma as adults.

Chronic—5% of childhood asthmatics, all with persistently abnormal lung function. Only 5% become asymptomatic but 50% persist with severe asthma as adults.

● Asthma carries a significant mortality. In all, 40–50 children die of asthma annually in England and Wales, especially in the 10–14-year age group.

● Asthma has a significant mortality. In 1984 in the UK 39 children under 15 died of asthma[3].

● Respiratory syncytial virus bronchiolitis in infancy carries with it a significant problem of recurrent wheezing thereafter; the proportion varies from 42 to 51%[1].

● Some 50% of children suffer less severe symptoms as they become adolescent. However, even those without symptoms may have persistent airways obstruction and redevelop asthma later in life.

● The likelihood for asthma to improve is greater if the attacks are mild and the child is free of symptoms in between.

TREATMENT

General considerations

1. Education of the patient and family, perhaps using leaflets and written instructions about asthma and therapy, especially about when to seek medical help. The Asthma Society (300 Uppers Street, London N1 2XX) has useful information and patients may be encouraged to join.
2. Regular exercise and participation in sport should be encouraged. A feeling of disability should be strongly discouraged amongst asthmatics, their parents and teachers. Sodium chromoglycate (Intal) or an inhaled beta-agonist may be effective in preventing exercise-induced asthma.
3. Asthma may be prevented by noting and avoiding trigger factors, including the house-dust mite. Injections of desensitizing doses of allergen are not recommended.
4. Steam inhalations are effective in mild attacks.

Drug treatment

1. Infancy (up to 18 months): nebulized beta-agonists may be helpful but regular (daily) monitoring of an infant with wheeze is paramount. Hospital admission is required if feeding is impaired, if the infant is restless or obvious signs of respiratory difficulty occur, such as increasing respiratory rate.
2. Over the age of 2 children should be able to use a Nebuhaler. In those children who have occasional mild attacks, the use of a beta$_2$ agonist at the onset of an upper respiratory infection, continued for a week may be enough (terbutaline inhaler 0.25 mg per puff, 0.25–0.5 mg 3 or 4 times daily or salbutamol inhaler 100–200 µg puffs 3–4 times daily).
3. Over the age of 4, children are able to manage a tube-spacer delivering an aerosol or a Rotahaler delivering a powdered preparation.
4. Over the age of 8 children should be able to manage the metered aerosol without attachments.
5. Children who experience exercise-induced asthma may benefit from inhaled beta$_2$ agonists half an hour before exercise.
6. Those children who have frequent attacks (more than one a month) require prophylaxis. Oral theophyllines or inhaled sodium cromoglycate are alternatives.

a. *Oral theophyllines*: preparations such as Slo-Phyllin are useful. In children aged 2–6 years (10–20 kg) the dose is 60–120 mg twice daily. In 6–12-year-olds (20–35 kg) the dose is 125–250 mg twice daily, and in over 12-year-olds the dose is 250–500 mg twice daily.

This preparation may be released from its capsule; the time released pellets are placed on soft food to help swallowing. Initially the lowest dose is recommended. This may be increased gradually if optimal bronchodilator effects are are not achieved. If larger doses are used, blood theophylline levels should be checked.

b. *Sodium cromoglycate* may be delivered in aerosol or powder form. The usual dose of aerosol is 2 × 5 mg puffs four times daily, or 20 mg cromoglycate powder inhaled four times daily.

7. Failure to respond to the above measures necessitates the use of oral steroids.

a. Budesonide is available for use in a Nebuhaler, spacer or as a conventional metered dose aerosol and is given in a dose of 50–200 µg twice daily.

b. Beclomethasone dipropionate is available as a powder for use in a Rotahaler metered dose aerosol. Dosage is beclomethasone powder via Rotahaler 100 µg 2–4 times daily, or beclomethasone inhaler 50–100 µg 2–4 times daily.

Treatment of acute asthma

1. Severe attacks of asthma where there is cyanosis, drowsiness, pulsus paradoxus, a silent hyperinflated chest or restlessness should be treated in hospital.
2. Less severe attacks may be treated at the doctor's surgery with the use of nebulized salbutamol (2.5 mg) or terbutaline via a facemask. The child will be helped and reassured if he or she sits on the parent's lap while treatment is being given.

Dosage of terbutaline for average body weight 10 kg is 2 mg; for 15 kg 3 mg; 20 kg 4 mg; and 25 kg 5 mg. Improvement should be noted during treatment and the child should be monitored for signs of recurrence for an hour after treatment has finished.

Those children who have had nebulized

beta$_2$ agonists will require oral steroids to prevent another attack. Soluble prednisolone should be given in a dose of 1 mg/kg/day reducing over a week. Shorter courses of lower doses—2mg/kg on day 1, 1 mg/kg on day 2 and 0.5 mg/kg on day 3—are also effective[4]. Hospital admission should be considered where the peak flow rate after treatment is less than 75% of the expected value.

FOLLOW-UP

Follow-up involves regular assessment of symptoms including numbers of attacks of wheeze, days lost from school etc. and restrictions on normal activities, and measurement of the peak flow. Growth and weight gain should be measured and plotted on a centile chart. Assessment of inhaler techniques should also be performed regularly once the child has been taught to use the equipment. Techniques once learned can be forgotten and may be responsible for a worsening of symptoms.

If the child is able to use a peak flow meter, recordings three or four times a day will allow an assessment of the severity of the illness and whether there is variation throughout the day. Children with mild occasional attacks of asthma may be treated by the general practitioner. More severe cases should be referred to a paediatrician. Good liaison between the general practitioner and hospital consultant is vital to ensure optimum treatment.

In adults

Atypical presentations include chronic cough especially in non-smokers, chest tightness on exertion which may be confused with angina, and nocturnal breathlessness. The differential diagnosis in adults includes chronic bronchitis with emphysema, left ventricular failure, acute infective bronchitis, bronchiectasis and carcinoma of the lung. Trigger factors include anxiety infections, exercise, specific allergens, cold air, laughter and pets etc.

PROGNOSIS[10]

● Adult-onset asthma has a worse prognosis than childhood-onset asthma and episodic asthma

but a better prognosis than chronic continuous asthma.
● Some 2–3 deaths per 100 000 people are due to asthma and this mortality has been unaffected by modern therapy.
● Bronchitis adversely affects the prognosis.

TREATMENT

1. Education of patients in the aetiology and management of asthma. This includes appropriate use of inhalers and recognition of deterioration in their asthma. Written instructions may be helpful.
2. Treatment of attacks. Beta-agonists affect only the bronchospasm; steroids affect the inflammation (oedema and mucus).
3. Infrequent attacks:
   a. Use a beta-agonist inhaler as needed, even prophylactically if the trigger factor is known.
   b. Steam inhalations may also be helpful.
4. Frequent attacks:
   a. Continuous prophylaxis using a steroid inhaler 15 minutes after the use of a beta-agonist inhaler. If this stabilizes the patient's asthma, then regular inhaled steroid may be sufficient.
   b. If still inadequate, consider oral slow release aminophylline or theophylline (Phyllocontin Continus, Slo-Phyllin).
   c. If this fails or has too many side-effects, then short courses of prednisolone (orally) may be necessary. A high dose for a short period, such as prednisolone 30–40 mg daily, reducing when symptoms subside, is preferable to a low dose for a long time. Patients may be left with a spare course of prednisolone tablets so they can initiate a course early.
5. If the patient requires frequent (i.e. quarterly) courses of prednisolone then referral to a chest physician is advisable. This is to assess the patient's respiratory response to steroids and then gauge appropriate doses.
6. Severe attacks involving respiratory distress, tachycardia, tachypnoea, poor air entry and peak flow rate 50% less than predicted should be treated with a single dose of nebulized beta-agonist (although an ordinary inhaler used through a plastic cup[11] may be as effective) and

a course of oral prednisolone started. After 15–20 minutes, if there is no or little response, urgent admission to hospital for oxygen therapy is mandatory. If there is a response, seen clinically and by measurement of the peak flow rate, then the beta-agonist is repeated 4-hourly with review the next day.

FOLLOW-UP

Some practices find that a special asthmatic clinic may be useful to monitor their patients, using specific record cards. Others may rely on their repeat prescribing recall systems. The main aim is to enable patients to understand their own condition and choose the most appropriate therapy for their symptoms. Regular recording of the peak flow will assist management.

[1] Bierman CW, Pearlman DS (1983) Asthma. In *Disorders of the Respiratory Tract in Children* (Kendig EL, Chenick V eds) pp. 496–543. London: Saunders.
[2] Waine C (1987) *Asthma*. London: Royal College of General Practitioners.
[3] Levy M, Bell L (1984) *Br. Med. J.*, **289**, 1115–16.
[4] Anderson HR et al. (1981) *Lancet*, **ii**, 1030–2.
[5] Speight ANP (1978) *Br. Med. J.*, **2**, 381–2.
[6] Lee DA et al. (1983) *Br. Med. J.*, **288**, 1256–8.
[7] Martin AJ et al. (1980) *Br. Med. J.*, **280**, 1397.
[8] Anderson HR et al. (1983) Morbidity and school absence caused by asthma and wheezing illness. *Arch. Dis. Child.*, **58**, 777–84.
[9] Deshpande A, McKenzie SA (1988) Short course of steroids in home treatment of children with acute asthma. *Br. Med. J.*, **293**, 169–71.
[10] Campbell IA (1986) *Diseases of the Respiratory System* in *Treatment and Prognosis in Medicine* (Hawkins RL ed). London: Heinemann.
[11] Henry RL, Milner AD, Davies JG (1983) *Br. Med. J.*, **286**, 2021.

Lung Cancer

Carcinoma of the bronchus accounts for more than 50% of all male deaths from malignant disease in western countries. In the UK more than 30 000 men die of lung cancer each year. It is about four times more common in men than in women, and occurs most frequently between the ages of 50 and 75. Cigarette smoking is responsible for most cases. The number of deaths from lung cancer has steadily increased since the Second World War, directly in proportion with the increase in cigarette smoking.

PROGNOSIS

- Overall 5-year survival is 5%.
- Only 30% of the few patients with a resectable lesion survive 5 years.
- Unless surgery is practicable the average survival after diagnosis is less than 1 year.
- Early diagnosis provides slightly better results, but prognosis depends largely on histological cell type and presence of metastases.
- Weight loss, chest pain or a low serum protein confers a worse prognosis.
- Local extension of the tumour may cause vena caval obstruction or erosion of bone or blood vessel. Metastatic spread occurs early in the development of the disease, with the brain, liver and bone being the most commonly affected organs[1].

TREATMENT

1. All patients should be referred to a specialist for assessment and a treatment plan. Generally speaking this will be:
   a. Non small-cell tumours:
      i. surgical resection when practicable.
      ii. palliative radiotherapy for haemoptysis, bone pain or superior vena caval obstruction.
   b. Small-cell tumours: chemotherapy, with or without cranial irradiation.
2. Ideally full and frank discussion with the patient and family about the likely benefits and disadvantages of treatment is important. The general practitioner should obtain sufficient information from the hospital for this to occur.

3. Continuing support and care of the patient and family is of vital importance. It is important that the patient does not feel that he or she has been written off, especially if an attempt at cure is impossible.

   The role of the general practitioner in symptom control is often crucial[2].

4. *Pain*
   a. Mild analgesics such as aspirin, paracetamol, codeine or co-proxamol given regularly are used to begin with.
   b. Opiates usually become necessary. Morphine sulphate slow-release (MST Continus) 10–20 mg b.d. is useful initially. The patient and family require careful instruction on the use of opiates to ensure that an optimal dose is taken often enough to prevent the pain returning.
   c. Non-steroidal anti-inflammatory drugs, such as indomethacin 25 mg t.d.s. or 100 mg by suppositories, may be useful for the treatment of bony secondaries.
   d. Other causes of pain, such as constipation, arthritis, or postirradiation inflammation, must be excluded.

5. *Cough:* linctus codeine or methadone (Physeptone) are especially valuable at night.

6. *Anorexia:* prednisolone 10–20 mg daily in divided doses or dexamethasone 2–4 mg daily can stimulate appetite and produce a sense of well-being.

7. *Nausea:*
   a. Prochlorperazine (2.5–5.0 mg 4-hourly), metoclopramide or haloperidol may be required.
   b. The nausea caused by opiates usually abates in 2 or 3 days, when the anti-emetic may be ceased.
   c. Occasional vomiting may be preferable to the sedation caused by anti-emetics.

8. *Constipation:*
   a. Attention to the bowels is essential to prevent unnecessary discomfort and distress. Regular enemas may be necessary, though usually daily laxatives are sufficient.
   b. Patients on opioids must be given laxatives daily, such as Regulan, Normax, lactulose or Bisacodyl.

9. *Depression or anxiety:*
   a. Talking with the patient, seeking out fears and discussing them is a far better anxiolytic than the prescription of a benzodiazepine.
   b. Occasionally patients develop a true endogenous depression with biological features. This merits treatment with antidepressants such as amitriptylline 25–50 mg t.d.s. or single dose at night.
   c. Sleeplessness is best treated with short-term benzodiazepines. Chloral hydrate is a useful alternative.

10. *Dyspnoea:*
   a. This is a frequent symptom. The patient must be reassured that suffocation will not occur.
   b. Bronchodilators, diuretics, oxygen and antibiotics may have a place.

FOLLOW-UP

Early involvement of domiciliary nursing care with support or respite care from local hospice or community hospital is important. Scheduled regular visiting by the general practitioner should be carried out to anticipate and prevent crises in symptom development or morale of carers. Regular hospital follow-up is only necessary to prevent the patient feeling he or she has been written off. Short hospital admission for aspiration of pleural effusion or blood transfusion can be useful.

---

[1] Crofton J, Douglas A (1981) *Respiratory Diseases*, 3rd edn. Oxford: Blackwell.
[2] Taylor JH (1988) *Terminal Illness in Treatment* (Drury M, Beeley L ed). London: Kluwer.

Pulmonary Tuberculosis

In Europe and the USA pulmonary tuberculosis used to affect mainly young people, especially females, but there has been a major change in the age and sex incidence. Forty years ago 80% of patients were under 45 years of age, whereas now 60% are over that age and most are men. There is a much higher incidence among immigrants from the Indian subcontinent; these patients may present with the classical symptoms of cough, malaise, fever, weight loss and haemoptysis. Indigenous patients are more likely to be diagnosed inadvertently; haemoptysis is much more commonly associated with carcinoma of the lung.

PROGNOSIS[1]

- Adequate short-course chemotherapy has revolutionized treatment, and is curative in nearly 100% of patients.
- Residual lung damage is unusual unless the disease is advanced at the time of diagnosis.
- Mortality in the UK remains at 5%. Death occurs mainly among alcoholic and social drop-outs, and elderly patients, when presentation may be late and obscure. A high proportion of cases in the elderly are only discovered by post-mortem examination.
- Relapse is rare, except in patients who have had incomplete therapy. However, reactivation of pulmonary tuberculosis occurs in those middle-aged and elderly patients whose original infection was treated before the advent of chemotherapy in the 1950s.

TREATMENT

1. Treatment should be undertaken and supervised by a consultant who is familiar with the drugs and their side-effects.
2. Initially triple or quadruple chemotherapy is indicated for about 2 months, then followed by at least two drugs to which the mycobacterium is sensitive for a further 4–6 months. The drugs commonly used are rifampicin, ethambutol, streptomycin, isoniazid and pyrazinamide. All have toxic side-effects and treatment needs to be closely monitored.

3. Contact tracing is normally done by a health visitor or nurse attached to the chest clinic. Only close contacts need to be traced.
4. Patients whose sputum is negative on acid-fast staining are of low infectious risk, and should be so advised.
5. Smear-positive patients rapidly become non-infectious once treatment is commenced[1]. There is rarely any need to admit such patients to hospital, unless they are acutely ill.
6. Patients need to be counselled to counteract anxieties of social stigma and potential infectivity. Tuberculosis is still feared by many elderly people, who remember it as a scourge.
7. BCG confers protection for about 20 years in 70–80% of those vaccinated. Children of immigrant families are given BCG at birth in some areas.

FOLLOW-UP

No follow-up is required once an adequate treatment course has been completed. The number of patients treated by thoracoplasty in the pre-chemotherapy era is now dwindling. Many of those are still reviewed infrequently by chest physicians.

---

[1] Crofton J, Douglas A (1981) *Respiratory Diseases*, 3rd edn. Oxford: Blackwell.

Pneumonia

Pneumonia describes inflammation of the lung parenchyma accompanied by exudation into the alveoli. It is most commonly caused by viral or bacterial infections. Approximately 1% of people suffer pneumonia each year (usually in winter and early spring). The main predisposing factor is cigarette smoking. Immunosuppressed patients or those with chronic obstructive airways disease or alcoholics are also at increased risk. *Streptococcus pneumoniae* are the commonest cause in general practice, though in elderly patients *Haemophilus influenzae* must be considered. *Staph. pyogenes* causes 5% of cases (more in serious influenza epidemics), but the very serious *Klebsiella* only causes 1%. *Mycoplasma pneumoniae* represents 15% of hospital admissions for pneumonia, usually because they are resistant to the antibiotics commonly used in general practice.

PROGNOSIS

- Mortality rate is 5–10%.
- Mortality risk is increased if:
  1. Type 3 pneumococci, *Staph. pyogenes* or *Klebsiella* are involved.
  2. The patient already suffers from chronic bronchitis, carcinoma of the bronchus, or emphysema.
  3. The patient is immunosuppressed, particularly if suffering from acquired immune deficiency syndrome (AIDS).
  4. The patient is an infant or, more commonly, elderly.
  5. Where bacteraemia has occurred before treatment has commenced.
- Lung abscess (in 2%) and empyema (in 1%) may occur if treatment is inappropriate or inadequate. This worsens the prognosis.
- Persistent respiratory symptoms may follow lobar pneumonia, especially in cigarette smokers and those who live in poor conditions.

TREATMENT

1. In patients who are severely ill admission to hospital must be considered.
2. *Pneumococcal pneumonia:* in debilitated patients benzyl penicillin 1 Mu i.m. 6-hourly should be instituted. As the patient's condition responds phenoxymethyl penicillin 500 mg orally four times daily for up to 10 days is appropriate. Broad-spectrum antibiotics such as ampicillin 250–500 mg four times daily should not be used unless there is doubt as to the causative organism. Erythromycin 500 mg–1 g 6-hourly for 10 days is the best alternative in penicillin-sensitive patients.
3. *Staphylococcal pneumonia:* treatment of choice is flucloxacillin 250–500 mg four times daily for 2 weeks (sodium fusidate 500 mg three times daily for penicillin sensitivity). If *Staph. pneumonia* coexists with *Streptococcus pneumonia*, penicillin should be added.

   Lung abscesses are a relatively common complication of *Staph. pneumonia*. If they occur, postural drainage and prolonged chemotherapy are indicated.
4. *Haemophilus influenzae pneumonia:* more often affects elderly bronchitic people. Treatment of choice is ampicillin 500 mg four times daily or erythromycin.
5. *Klebsiella pneumonia:* most often involves the upper lobes and causes excavation or consolidation of one or more lobes. Sputum is frequently chocolate-coloured.

   The patient should always be admitted to hospital where a combination of chloramphenicol and gentamicin is the most appropriate treatment.
6. *Legionella pneumophila pneumonia (Legionnaires disease):* almost invariably affects smokers or ex-smokers, and is carried by ducted air systems. Erythromycin 500 mg–1 g orally in severe cases i.v. should be given four times daily for at least 2 weeks. If the patient does not respond then admission should be arranged for rifampicin.
7. *Mycoplasma pneumonia:* this is a pleomorphic bacterium capable of passing through a filter. Cold agglutinins can be demonstrated in most cases.

a. Pneumonia caused by anaerobes usually occurs in debilitated patients or where aspiration has occurred. Treatment is with metronidazole 400 mg three times daily by i.v. injection initially or orally if this is possible.

b. Rickettsial pneumonia (Q fever) is usually caused by contact with sheep or cattle. Treatment by erythromycin.

c. Chlamydia pneumonia (psittacosis or ornithosis) is usually caused by inhaling dust containing the faeces of infected birds, particularly parrots. Treated by erythromycin or oxytetracycline 250–500 g every 6 hours.

8. *Viral pneumonias:* there is no specific treatment, but bacterial superinfection is common (particularly with *Staph. pyogenes*).

9. Additional treatments might include:

a. 35% oxygen if cyanosis is present, administered preferably by double nasal cannulae or mask. Oral or intravenous fluids to counteract dehydration.

b. Analgesia if the infection has spread to the pleura.

10. *Fungal pneumonias*

a. Actinomycosis: benzyl penicillin up to 12 Mu daily is the most successful treatment. Phenoxymethyl penicillin may help in the later stages. Treatment has to be prolonged (for at least 6 months), but surgery is often essential.

b. Histoplasma pneumonia: treatment with amphotericin B by i.v. drip is usually successful, but it is toxic and can only be used under careful hospital supervision.

c. Nocardiosis: treatment of choice is sulphonamide or cephalosporin in hospital.

d. Other fungal pneumonias: i.v. amphotericin B in hospital.

11. In immunosuppressed patients immunocompetence should be restored if possible. In AIDS patients *Pneumocystis carinii*, a usually harmless organism, is life-threatening. Pentamidine is the treatment of choice; nebulized pentamidine may be prophylactic. Co-trimoxazole, 8 tablets twice daily, can also be used.

FOLLOW-UP

If the patient does not respond to treatment in 5 days, the treatment given should be changed. Chest X-ray at this time and 6–8 weeks later is appropriate. Sputum cytology is indicated if resolution is delayed.

---

[1] Campbell IA (1986) *Diseases of the Respiratory System in Treatment and Prognosis: Medicine* (Hawkins RL ed). Oxford: Heinemann.

[2] Crofton J, Douglas A (1981) *Respiratory Diseases*, 3rd edn. Oxford: Blackwell.

Pneumothorax

A pneumothorax exists when air is in the pleural cavity. A spontaneous pneumothorax occurs unexpectedly, and often suddenly, due to rupture of the pulmonary end of a pleural adhesion or of a subpleural emphysematous bulla. Occasionally rupture of a lung abscess or a tuberculous cavity can be the precipitating event. Traumatic pneumothorax occurs when rib fractures or wounds penetrate the chest wall or lungs, sometimes as part of medical procedures. Men (particularly young men of slim build) are five times more likely to suffer from this condition than women[1]. There are three types of pneumothorax: closed, when air enters the lungs from the pleura, but the entry route then closes over; open, when the fistula remains patent allowing air continually to enter the thorax; valvular (tension pneumothorax), where the communication between the lung and the pleural space acts in a non-return valve fashion, creating a build-up of pressure in the cavity.

PROGNOSIS

- In the case of a closed pneumothorax reabsorption of the air and the consequent re-expansion of the lungs take approximately 1–3 months.
- If respiratory function is already poor due to coexisting chronic lung disease, respiratory failure may occur.
- Tension pneumothorax, if untreated, will lead to complete lung collapse with mediastinal displacement interfering with the unaffected lung and eventually compressing the major blood vessels, leading to circulatory collapse and death.
- Some 30% of pneumothoraces will recur within 1 year. Without surgical intervention these recurrences increase in frequency.
- In case of trauma, the speed and effectiveness of the intervention decide the prognosis.

TREATMENT

1. If the pneumothorax is incomplete, and the patient is not seriously dyspnoeic, treatment is unnecessary, and observation over a week is desirable. The patient should be warned that recurrence is possible.
2. Where the patient is dyspnoeic, admission to hospital is essential. Initial treatment is by aspiration via a sealed intercostal tube. The classic position for insertion is through the second intercostal space in the mid clavicular line in men. In women, the fifth intercostal space or the axilla is more suitable. It usually takes from 24 to 48 hours for re-expansion to occur[2].
3. Valvular (tension) pneumothorax is an emergency. Immediate insertion of a wide-bore needle is essential before proceeding to other measures.
4. If a second pneumothorax occurs on the same side, tube drainage and intrapleural tetracycline are indicated. The tetracycline helps to create pleural adhesions.
5. A third episode of pneumothorax always indicates surgical treatment is necessary.
6. If the patient is very dyspnoeic oxygen should be used.

FOLLOW-UP

A chest X-ray after 48 hours and then at 3 months is advisable to confirm healing. The patient should be warned of the symptoms of recurrence, and recommended to return for treatment if this occurs.

[1] Crofton J, Douglas A (1981) *Respiratory Disease*, 3rd edn. Oxford: Blackwell.
[2] Campbell IA (1986) *Diseases of the Respiratory System in Treatment and Prognosis*: Medicine (Hawkins RL ed). Oxford: Heinemann.

Cystic Fibrosis

ystic fibrosis is a recessively inherited disorder which affects about 1 in 2000 livebirths. he disorder may present with intestinal obstruction due to meconium ileus in the neonatal eriod (10–15%) or more commonly later in childhood through failure to thrive associated ith recurrent lower respiratory tract infections and frequent pale bulky stools. The major linical features affect both digestive and respiratory tracts. In the pulmonary tree, viscoid ecretions lead to damage to the small airways producing obstruction, sputum retention nd overinflation. Chronic bronchial wall-thickening and micro abscess formation occur. rreversible pulmonary damage and bronchiectasis result. The common infecting organisms re *Staphylococcus aureus*, *Pseudomonas aeruginosa* and *Haemophilus influenzae*.

PROGNOSIS

- Cystic fibrosis has a variable prognosis, although the majority of patients now survive to adult life.
- Early referral to a specialist centre is indicated and has been shown to improve prognosis.

TREATMENT

1. The most important aspect of treatment is the clearing of sputum by postural draining and physiotherapy. Treatment must be carried out every day, preferably three times a day for a period of 10–15 minutes on each occasion. As the child grows, self-treatment may be sufficient, but does require careful monitoring.
2. Antibiotics, particularly flucloxacillin in childhood and gentamicin in adult life, may be indicated for prolonged periods if there is established infection, but should be used in high dosage for 2–3-week courses during intercurrent acute infection. Failure to respond to oral antibiotics should be an indication for hospital admission.
3. Wheeze in cystic fibrosis may be due to reversible airways disease and treatment with bronchodilators such as salbutamol may be useful. There is some evidence that these agents may also promote mucociliary clearance.
4. Mycolytic agents such as acetylcysteine are not generally recommended but may be worth a trial in patients with particularly viscid sputum.
5. Inhalation-moist therapy designed to deliver water to the lower respiratory tract is of great benefit to some patients.

FOLLOW-UP

Regular review by the general practitioner should aim to support the family and provide additional advice where required. This may include extra physiotherapy and advice on financial assistance as well as specialist review. Genetic counselling may also be indicated.

[1] Crofton J, Douglas A (1981) *Respiratory Diseases*, 3rd edn. Oxford: Blackwell.
[2] Doershuk CF, Boat TF (1987) In Nelson. Textbook of Paediatrics, 13th edn, pp. 926–35. London: Saunders.

Stridor

Stridor consists of noisy breathing heard on either inspiration or expiration and is due to obstruction of airflow, usually in the larynx or trachea. The degree of stridor varies with respiratory rate and degree of obstruction. Inspiratory stridor is usually associated with laryngeal obstruction, and expiratory stridor is more typical of tracheal narrowing below the vocal chords. Inhalation of foreign bodies is a frequent cause of stridor in infants and young children. There is often a history of acute onset of cough, choking or wheezing. Alternatively symptoms may develop gradually over hours or days. Diagnosis is based on an accurate history and careful physical examination. Most inhaled objects lodge in the bronchi, more often on the right than the left. Apart from the stridor, physical examination may reveal either diminished air entry or hyperinflation on the affected side. X-ray of the chest may be helpful. Bronchoscopy is essential if foreign body inhalation is suspected.

PROGNOSIS

- Ultimate outcome is excellent and depends upon the absence of residual collapse or chronic infection.
- Congenital stridor or laryngomalacia (due to indrawing of the largyngeal tissues during inspiration) is a benign self-limiting condition of the first few months of life.
- The prognosis is excellent and most children outgrow the problem by late infancy.

TREATMENT

1. Removal of the object by bronchoscopy must be followed by adequate physiotherapy and treatment of any secondary lung collapse or bacterial infection.

FOLLOW-UP

None is necessary.

Croup

Laryngotracheobronchitis or croup is due to an acute inflammation of the upper portion of the lower respiratory tract, usually due to the parainfluenza virus, the respiratory syncytial virus or rhinovirus. It commonly occurs in late infancy and early childhood with a peak incidence between the ages of 6 months and 4 years. The incidence is between 5 and 10 cases per general practitioner each year. It usually begins with upper respiratory symptoms of catarrh and congestion, followed by the development of hoarseness, a characteristic barking cough, and an inspiratory stridor. The development of intercostal and sternal recession indicates serious respiratory obstruction. In contrast to epiglottitis, the other major cause of stridor, croup progresses less rapidly and the child is less toxic. The possibility of respiratory obstruction nevertheless requires close monitoring.

PROGNOSIS

- Stridor may persist for up to 3 days. Many children retain a residual dry cough for 1–2 weeks.
- Recovery is the rule even in the small proportion (1–2%) of children who require intubation. Secondary infection must be anticipated but is comparatively rare.
- Recurrence of true infective croup is rare, although recurrent spasmodic croup associated with night cough and stridor, probably of atopic origin, occurs in some children. This usually responds to humidifying the atmosphere, as with infective croup, but treament with bronchodilators or cromoglycate may be necessary.

TREATMENT

1. Treatment at home is based on the fact that moist warm air may produce relief of symptoms. This can be achieved by placing the child in a hot bath or in a bathroom with the shower running or in the kitchen with kettles and pans boiling. Improvement may occur within 30 minutes to 1 hour.

2. Hydration should be maintained with warm drinks. Pulse, colour and rib recession should be carefully observed.

3. Signs of failure to improve or deterioration should lead to hospital admission. In that setting, the provision of warm, moist air may again be the only specific therapy, but confidence is induced by facilities for immediate intubation or tracheostomy.

4. Antibiotic treatment is not indicated and the use of steroids or bronchodilators remains controversial.

FOLLOW-UP

None is required, though the condition may recur and education of the parents is therefore necessary.

Tunnessen WWJ, Feinstein AR (1980) *J. Paed.*, **96**, 751.
Henry R (1983) *Arch. Dis. Child.*, **58**, 577.
Zach M *et al.* (1981) *Arch. Dis. Child.*, **56**, 336.

Acute Epiglottitis (See also p. 45)

Acute epiglottitis is an uncommon but life-threatening condition, of rapid onset. It may occur at any age from 6 months to 6 years, with a peak incidence in the second year of life. It is much more rare than croup, from which it must be distinguished, and may only be seen by a general practitioner once or twice in a lifetime. Infection with *Haemophilus influenzae* type B is the commonest cause although beta-haemolytic streptococci are occasionally incriminated.

Symptoms are due to acute infection with inflammatory oedema of the epiglottis and aryepiglottic folds, producing airways obstruction. Acute obstruction and respiratory arrest may occur at any time. The child presents with a rapid onset of sore throat and fever, followed by hoarseness, respiratory stridor and drooling. Toxicity is an important feature and in contrast to viral croup, the picture is one of rapid onset and progression in severity. The child may have an ashen grey appearance, suggestive of shock, and may be holding the head in extension in an attempt to relieve respiratory obstruction. The history and general findings should be sufficient to make the diagnosis. Examination of the mouth and throat are totally contraindicated as local intervention may exacerbate oedema and cause total respiratory obstruction.

PROGNOSIS

- Danger to life is maximal during the period before the child reaches hospital.
- With appropriate treatment, symptoms should resolve within 24–36 hours. Antibiotic treatment should nevertheless continue for 7 days.
- Recurrence is unusual.

TREATMENT

1. The child should be transferred to hospital immediately accompanied by the physician.
2. If acute respiratory obstruction should occur, a large-bore needle passed into the trachea below the cricoid cartilage may be life-saving.
3. In hospital, continuous cool moist oxygen may be required to correct anoxia, but the foundation of treatment will consist of the establishment of an adequate airway, preferably by nasotracheal intubation, but if necessary by tracheostomy. Intravenous antibiotic of choice is ampicillin 200 mg/kg per day, or if blood culture reveals a resistant haemophilus, chloramphenicol 50 mg/kg per day.

FOLLOW-UP

No follow-up is necessary.

4

The Cardiovascular System

P. E. Bundred

Hypertension

There is no absolute consensus on the level at which blood pressure readings are considered pathologically raised. The World Health Organization has set an arbitrary limit for 'normal blood pressure' at 160/90 mmHg on consecutive readings. Even at this level the risk of developing end organ damage is high—a 40% increase in risk of coronary artery disease with diastolic levels of 90 mmHg or more[1].

The aetiology of hypertension is unknown in 95% of cases. These patients have primary or essential hypertension. In the other 5% a cause can be found (secondary hypertension). These include chronic renal disease, renal artery stenosis, phaeochromocytoma, primary aldosteronism, Cushing's syndrome, corticosteroid therapy and the oral contraceptive pill.

Hypertension produces few symptoms. Some patients complain of general lassitude and occasionally, when the blood pressure is very high, they may complain of vague sensations in the head. It is the lack of symptoms in the majority of patients which makes hypertension such a difficult disease for the general practitioner to identify and treat.

PROGNOSIS

- The prognosis is dependent on a number of factors—the level of both systolic and diastolic pressures[2], the duration of disease and the effectiveness of therapy.

- Hypertension is uncommon under the age of 20. Adolescents who have a blood pressure in the upper range for age have a higher risk of developing hypertension in later life[3].

- Untreated hypertensives have a sevenfold increase in the incidence of stroke, a fourfold increase in the incidence of heart failure and a threefold increase in the incidence of coronary artery disease.

- A raised systolic blood pressure of over 148 mmHg in the absence of a raised diastolic blood pressure has been shown to increase the risk of coronary artery disease by a factor of two[4].

- All hypertensives below the age of 40 should be fully investigated, as many patients in this group have secondary hypertension.

- Adequate treatment of hypertension results in a fall in mortality and morbidity from stroke and renal disease. There is less evidence to suggest the same fall in mortality from coronary artery disease even in those patients who have had successful long-term management of hypertension[5].

- A number of studies have failed to show that elderly patients with mild to moderate increases in blood pressure in the range 160/95 mmHg gain any substantial benefit from lowering their blood pressure[6]. There is also a higher incidence of iatrogenic side-effects from treatment in this age group.

TREATMENT

1. The prime tasks of the general practitioner and practice team in the management of hypertension is the identification of all patients under their care with a raised blood pressure and to ensure that, once identified, they are well controlled. Routine measurement of blood pressure in all patients between 40 and 65 years should be undertaken at least every 3 years. This can be achieved in a number of ways:

   a. Systematic recall of all patients every 3 years for a health check.

   b. Opportunistic measurement of patients' blood pressure on visits to the surgery.

   c. Systematic screening of all high-risk patients using the practice nurse as a facilitator.

   Regular assessment of blood pressure monitoring in the practice should be carried out. The method described by the Oxford Heart and Stroke Group[7] can be adapted for use in most practices. Computerized age–sex registers can be of great assistance in the management of such an audit.

2. Non-medical management of hypertension is central to any treatment regimen.

a. Overweight patients should be encouraged to lose weight as this may produce a fall in blood pressure.

b. All patients should be encouraged to reduce alcohol intake to 2 units or less daily.

c. Patients should stop smoking. Although smoking is not associated with a rise in blood pressure, it is associated with an increased risk of developing coronary artery disease and stroke in patients with hypertension[8].

d. Regular daily exercise lowers blood pressure and patients should be encouraged to take some form of exercise[9].

e. A reduction in salt intake to 2 g/day will cause a fall in blood pressure in a small percentage of patients[10].

f. Stopping the oral contraceptive pill is essential in women with hypertension.

3. Where non-medical measures fail to reduce blood pressure to the expected range, a regimen using one or two hypotensive agents will reduce blood pressure in up to 90% of hypertensives. Where possible, a single daily dose of the drugs is more likely to lead to compliance than the use of more complicated dosage schedules.

4. Low-dose thiazide diuretics (bendrofluazide 2.5–5 mg daily) are the first line of treatment. However they are contraindicated in diabetes and they may cause hyperuricaemia. In elderly patients prolonged use may cause hypokalaemia. Impotence was reported in one study using a 10 mg dose of bendrofluazide[11].

5. If thiazide diuretics alone fail to reduce blood pressure, a beta-blocking agent should be added. Long-acting drugs such as atenolol (50–100 mg daily) or metoprolol (100–200 mg daily) are best in terms of compliance. Both thiazide diuretics and beta-blocking agents have a flat dose–response curve and once the patient has reached the optimal dose, further increases in dosage will not result in further fall in blood pressure. There is evidence that beta blockers may have fewer beneficial effects in hypertensives who smoke[11].

6. Nifedipine (40–60 mg daily) is an effective hypotensive agent as a third-line drug. Side-effects, including headache, palpitations, nausea and flushing, are lessened by the use of a slow-release preparation.

7. Angiotensin-converting enzyme inhibitors, such as captopril (25–150 mg daily) or enalapril (10–20 mg daily), should be used in non-responsive patients only. They are powerful agents and have some side-effects, although new varieties, such as lisinopril, are reported to have less. Side-effects tend to be dose-related and with captopril few occur when the daily dose is below 100 mg. Above this dose proteinuria, rashes and leukopenia can be a problem. In patients with renal impairment or in some patients on diuretic therapy, a precipitous fall in blood pressure may occur and admission to hospital for initiation of treatment is advised. All patients should be started on a low dose and the dosage gradually increased.

8. Vasodilator drugs such as hydralazine (100 mg daily in divided doses) or prazosin (0.5 mg gradually increasing to a maximum of 20 mg daily in divided doses), which is now believed to act more by an alpha blocking action, can be used. Side-effects include tachycardia, headache, nausea and postural hypotension. This last side-effect can often be overcome by starting treatment with a nighttime dose of the drug. Vasodilators should be regarded as third or fourth-line therapy.

9. Methyldopa has a place in the management of hypertension resistant to other treatment. A dose of 250 mg three times daily is recommended. This can be increased to a maximum daily dose of 3 g. Side-effects include dry mouth, depression, sedation, diarrhoea and ejaculatory disorders. Occasional liver damage occurs and regular monitoring of liver function tests is recommended. Since the other serious complication is an autoimmune haemolytic anaemia, all patients should have regular full blood counts and a direct Coomb's test at 6-monthly intervals.

10. The management of hypertension in pregnancy requires special consideration. Treatment should begin as soon as the diagnosis has been made. First the patient should be put to bed on a low-salt diet. If the blood pressure remains elevated hypotensive therapy should be commenced. The drug most suitable in pregnancy is methyldopa (750 mg–3 g daily). Beta blockers such as oxprenolol and atenolol can also be used and vasodilators such as hydralazine and prazosin are also effective

with few complications. It is important to remember that many pregnant hypertensive women will become normotensive after delivery and their treatment should then be stopped.

11. Patients who have recently had a stroke should be treated vigorously as control of blood pressure often prevents further episodes. The blood pressure should, however, be lowered slowly, particularly in elderly patients, as a rapid fall in pressure may cause an extension of the stroke.

FOLLOW-UP

All young hypertensive patients need close follow-up. Once blood pressure has stabilized they should be seen at least every 3 months by one of the practice team in order to ensure compliance. The older hypertensive needs less close monitoring and can be seen 6-monthly once blood pressure is controlled. Hypertensive clinics run by adequately trained practice nurses produce compliant, well controlled patients and should be considered in practices using a multidisciplinary team approach.

[1] Stamler J et al. (1984) Am. J. Med., 76, 13.
[2] Kannel WB (1977) In Hypertension, p. 888. New York: McGraw Hill.
[3] Sokolow M, McIlroy M (1986) In Clinical Cardiology, p. 218. Los Altos, California: Lange Medical Publications.
[4] Shaper A (1985) J. Epidemiol. Commun. Hlth, 39, 197.
[5] Hypertension Detection and Follow-up Group (1979) J.A.M.A., 242, 2562.
[6] Amery A et al. (1985) Lancet, ii, 1349.
[7] Oxford Heart and Stroke Prevention Group.
[8] Isles C et al. (1979) Br. Med. J., 1, 579.
[9] Wilcox R et al. (1982) Br. Med. J., 285, 767.
[10] McGregor G et al. (1982) Lancet, i, 351.
[11] MRC working party on mild to moderate hypertension (1977) Br. Med. J., 2, 1437.

Coronary Heart Disease

Each year nearly one hundred and fifty thousand people die from coronary heart disease (CHD) in England alone[1]. This represents 28% of all deaths. It is the largest cause of death in the UK, even exceeding malignancy.

The cause of CHD in almost all cases is occlusion of the coronary arteries by atheromatous plaque and this may present clinically as either an acute total occlusion (myocardial infarction) or partial occlusion (angina pectoris)[2].

The incidence of the disease increases with age, to peak in the 55–65 year group. The cause of CHD is multi-factorial and a number of risk factors have been described which contribute to the increased chance of an individual developing this condition. These include social class[3], sex, family history, a history of smoking, stress, hypercholesterolaemia, diabetes, hypertension and obesity.

PROGNOSIS

- The prognosis of CHD is influenced by the extent, nature and anatomical position of the coronary occlusion.
- Stable angina is associated with a mortality rate of between 0.3–8%, though this can be made worse by the presence of cardiac failure and hypertension.
- Following an acute myocardial infarction, prognosis depends on the age of the patient, the extent of myocardial damage and the efficiency of management. The overall mortality rate in the first month is 30% with most deaths occurring in the first 12 hours after infarction.
- Mild attacks with no complications have a much lower mortality rate (5%).
- Overall outcome depends on the severity of the lesion. The five year mortality of triple vessel disease is ten times greater than that of single vessel disease. Poor left ventricular function also adversely affects prognosis.

TREATMENT

The clinical management of myocardial infarction

nd angina are dealt with in their respective ections. This section will concentrate on the prevention of CHD.

General measures to prevent CHD

f coronary heart disease is to be prevented each ndividual should be made aware of the risk factors associated with it. The general practitioner is ideally placed to measure risk factors, since most of the information can be found in the patients records.

In order to verify the accuracy of his or her records, prior to starting a CHD preventive programme, the practitioner should carry out an audit. The method of audit described by the Oxford Prevention of Heart Attack and Stroke Project is recommended[5].

1. *Smoking.* Cigarette smoking is associated with an increased risk of developing coronary heart disease. Those who have never smoked are at a considerably lower risk than those who have given up, and risk seems to be related to the number of years of smoking rather than the number of cigarettes smoked each day[6].

2. *Raised blood pressure.* Patients who have a raised and untreated blood pressure are at greater risk from developing heart attacks than normotensive subjects. This risk is twice the norm in those with a blood pressure in the top 40% of all systolic readings and increases as the mean systolic level rises. A mean diastolic level greater than 95 mmHg is associated with a three-fold rise in risk.

3. *Serum total cholesterol.* As serum total cholesterol rises so does the risk of developing coronary disease. Figures from the Seven Countries Study indicate that mean serum total cholesterol levels in a community is the most accurate factor for the assessment of risk. At least 60% of British males have a serum total cholesterol in the range which increases their risk[7].

4. *Body mass index.* Increased body mass is associated with increased risk of developing raised blood pressure and raised serum total cholesterol. It should not be regarded as an independent variable in the calculation of risk. Body mass index is an easy screening procedure and as such should be used to identify individuals who require a full risk factor assessment.

5. *Previous history of coronary heart disease.* Patients who have had a myocardial infarction are at much greater risk of having a further episode than those with no history.

6. *Diabetes mellitus.* Patients who have diabetes have an increased risk of developing both peripheral vascular disease and coronary heart disease.

7. *Family history of CHD.* Although the mode of inheritance is not clear it has been shown that there is an increased risk in those individuals in whom a parent has died prematurely from the disease.

Calculation of risk factors

Shaper has suggested that General Practitioners use the following method for calculating risk factors:

Number of smoking years $\times$ 7.5 plus systolic blood pressure $\times$ 4.5 plus 260 if patient has CHD plus 150 if patient has diabetes plus 150 if patient has angina plus 80 if patient has history of parental death from CHD.

Using this scoring system it is possible for the practitioner to calculate the relative risk for each patient in his practice. These scores can then be compared with the standard percentiles of risk by age.

Age group	40–44	45–49	50–54	55–59
50th centile	755	820	900	935
80th centile	870	950	1935	1095

An individual with a score greater than the 50th centile for his age group has a more than 50% risk of developing CHD.

Strategies for Prevention

1. *Stopping smoking.* In the average list of 2000 patients approximately 700 will smoke, and 25% of these smokers will die prematurely. In a general practice setting a successful anti-smoking campaign will depend on three objectives.

   i Educating patients in the knowledge of the harmful effects of smoking.

   ii Effective counselling and support mechanisms for all those who wish to give up smoking.

   iii These practice based objectives should be

supported by effective media campaigns from central government.

2. *Dietary modification.* This has two goals.

   i The reduction of the patients weight to levels of the body mass index below 2.75.

   ii A reduction in the intake of fats so that less than 35% of daily energy requirements are obtained from this source. High risk patients should be encouraged to reduce their fat intake to less than 30% of energy requirements, with only 10% being made-up of saturated fats.

   In practical terms patients should be advised to reduce their intake of eggs to two per week; to use polyunsaturated margarines instead of butter; to reduce the consumption of dairy products and to use skimmed or semi-skimmed milk; to reduce the consumption of red meat as far as possible; and to increase their consumption of fish, poultry, and roughage.

3. *Increased physical exercise.* The reason why vigorous exercise prevents CHD is not known. Recent work has suggested that short bouts of aerobic exercise are more protective, as it is thought that this type of exercise may have a direct bearing on the levels of high density lipoprotein.

Practically, patients should be encouraged to take regular exercise on at least two occasions each week (children at least three occasions) for a period of at least 20 minutes. Where possible patients should be taught to monitor their own heart rate during and after periods of exercise.

FOLLOW UP

If general practitioners are to make an impact on coronary heart disease in their practices they need to identify and follow-up their high risk patients very closely. Routine assessment of risk factors and the use of nurse counselling services are very important. The screening of the children of coronary victims is mandatory.

[1] DHSS, Broken Hearts, (1987) London: HMSO.
[2] Sokolow M, McIlroy M. (1986) *Clinical Cardiology,* Los Altos, California. Lange Medical Publications.
[3] Pocock SJ et al. (1987), *Lancet* **2,** 197–201.
[4] Kouchoukos NT et al. (1974) *Circulation* **50,** 11–16.
[5] Fullard EM, Fowler GH, Gray JAM, (1987) *Br. Med. J.* **294,** 1080–82.
[6] Shaper AG, Pocock SJ, Phillips AN, Walker M, (1987) *Health Trends,* **19,** 37–39.
[7] Shaper AG, Pocock SJ, Walker M, Cohen NM, Wale CJ, Thomson AG, (1982) *Br. Med. J.,* **283,** 179–186.

Angina

Angina is a specific type of pain associated with myocardial ischaemia and is characterized by tightness and pressure in the praecordium which may radiate to the neck, lower jaw and left arm. The pain is induced by a decrease in blood supply to the myocardium and it is often relieved when oxygen demand falls. Stable angina can be precipitated by exercise, large meals, emotional stress, cold weather, tachycardia or a decrease in the oxygen content of the inspired air. In unstable angina there is pain following minimal effort or at rest, and with critical narrowing it may proceed to myocardial infarction. Angina is usually caused by atherosclerotic heart disease. It can be caused by aortitis, hyperthyroidism, anaemia, paroxysmal tachycardia, coronary arteritis, coronary spasm and syphilitic aortitis.

PROGNOSIS

● The annual mortality of patients with stable angina varies from 0.3 to 8%[1]; most deaths occur in the year following the onset of the angina.

● In one-third of new patients the symptoms will spontaneously remit.

● In stable angina the long-term prognosis is

related to the degree of cardiac damage. Multiple coronary vessel disease and poor left ventricular function carry an almost 100% 5-year mortality[2].

● The prognosis for unstable angina is worse than that for stable angina, and is related to the effectiveness of management.

● Poorly controlled hypertension and the presence of heart failure adversely affect the prognosis.

TREATMENT

1. *Nitrates*
Can be used to relieve acute pain or, preferably, for prophylaxis.
   a. *Relief of acute pain:* glyceryl trinitrate can be used as an oral spray (it has a long shelf-life) or taken as a 0.5 mg sublingual tablet (short shelf-life) for prophylaxis or when pain occurs. The dose can be increased and patients should be advised that the drug can be taken repeatedly without it becoming ineffective or producing dependence. Pain relief occurs within 2–3 minutes and lasts 30 minutes. Isosorbide dinitrate sublingual tablets (30–120 mg per day in divided doses) should be started. Onset of pain relief is within 45 minutes and lasts up to 2 hours. Side-effects include headache, dizziness, nausea, flushing and occasionally syncope or hypotension.
   b. Prophylaxis: isosorbide dinitrate sustained-release preparations should be used initially (40–80 mg 2–3 times daily). Isosorbide mononitrate (20–120 mg daily in two doses) has been shown to reduce the number of attacks of chest pain[3].

   A transdermal patch or ointment can be used as an adjunct to other treatment and should be applied daily to the lateral chest wall. These patches release 5–10 mg glyceryl trinatrate in 24 hours. Changing the site of the application will diminish the risk of hypersensitivity to the adhesive or ointment. Tolerance may develop to transdermal applications and this can be reduced by intermittent usage.

2. *Beta blockers*
Beta blockers reduce the myocardial oxygen needs by slowing heart rate, lowering systolic blood pressure and decreasing myocardial contractility. They are normally used in conjunction with nitrates as they are complementary in action. They should not be used in the presence of heart failure or when there is a history of bronchospasm. Beta blockers should be used with caution in diabetic patients and not used in patients suffering from peripheral vascular disease. Care should be taken to withdraw these drugs slowly because sudden cessation can precipitate acute angina or myocardial infarction.

Lipophilic beta blockers (propranolol and metoprolol) are absorbed well from the gut and broken down in the liver; they cross the blood–brain barrier and have a plasma half-life of about 6 hours.

Hydrophilic types (atenolol and nadolol) are not well absorbed and do not cross into the brain. They are excreted via the kidney and have a half-life of up to 24 hours.

Choice of drug and dosage will depend on individual needs. The hydrophilic types produce less fatigue and tend to be more cardio-selective, but care should be taken in patients with poor renal function.

Effective blood levels of beta blockers cause a sinus bradycardia. If the heart rate falls below 55 beats/min the drug should be discontinued.

3. *Calcium antagonist drugs*
Calcium antagonists are increasingly being used in chronic angina. They act by reducing coronary spasm. They also cause peripheral arteries to dilate, so reducing afterload. There are three calcium antagonists used in the management of angina—nifedipine (30–60 mg/day), verapamil (120–360 mg/day) and diltiazem (120–240 mg/day). Side-effects include postural hypotension, dizziness, nausea, headache, peripheral oedema and constipation (with verapamil).

4. *Surgical procedures*
   a. Percutaneous coronary angioplasty has transformed the management of angina in many patients. Dilatation of the coronary arteries using a balloon catheter (angioplasty) has a success rate of 60–80% with 5% morbidity and infarction, and mortality of 1%. Patients' symptoms are often greatly improved and they may be entirely pain-free. Re-stenosis is common but angioplasty can be repeated several times.
   b. Coronary artery bypass surgery using saphenous vein and internal mammary artery grafts has been used to relieve symptoms but the procedure does not affect the underlying atherosclerosis. There is evidence to show that prognosis is considerably improved in certain patients who have

severe ischaemia[4]. At 1 year 90% of patients are symptom-free; this reduces to 75% at 5 years.

as their control may vary from one visit to the next. Patients who continue with symptoms on therapy should be referred for investigation.

FOLLOW-UP

Young patients with angina need careful supervision and monitoring, and should be referred early for cardiological opinion. Those who have had angioplasty need to be seen at least every 3 months as re-stenosis is common. Those patients on drug therapy will need to be monitored closely

[1] Frank CW et al. (1973) Circulation, **47**, 509.
[2] Sheldon WC et al. (1975) Prog. Cardiovascular Dis., **18**, 237.
[3] Muller G (1983) Klin. Wochenschr., **61**, 409.
[4] European Coronary Surgery Study Group (1980) Lancet, **ii,** 491.

Myocardial Infarction

Acute myocardial infarction is caused by a sudden decrease in the coronary blood flow with resultant ischaemic damage to the myocardium. This may be due to a thrombus in a coronary artery, haemorrhage within or beneath an atheromotous plaque, coronary artery vasoconstriction or arrhythmias which decrease diastolic filling time. Other factors which can cause a decrease in coronary blood flow include shock, dehydration and blood loss. The extent of myocardial damage depends on the artery involved, the degree of occlusion and the existence of a collateral coronary circulation. Infarcts can involve the full thickness of the myocardium or may be only partial thickness. Most infarcts can be regarded as being uncomplicated in that the patient does not develop life-threatening arrhythmias, cardiac failure and shock.

Up to 30% of patients who develop an acute myocardial infarction have visited their general practitioner with prodromal symptoms within 2 weeks of the acute event[1]. These symptoms may include weakness, shortness of breath and vague chest pain.

Clinical features of an acute infarction include retrosternal chest pain often radiating to the neck and left arm, sweating, weakness, apprehension, dyspnoea and hypotension. In more severe cases the patient may be shocked, with pulmonary oedema and left ventricular failure.

PROGNOSIS

- The overall mortality rate during the first month following a myocardial infarction is 30%. Most of these deaths occur in the first 12 hours[2].
- Some 25% of all early deaths are due to arrhythmias—mostly ventricular fibrillation in the first 1–2 hours.
- Mild attacks have a low hospital mortality rate, in the region of 5%.
- Recurrent attacks have a reported mortality rate of 50% or more. However these figures are artificially low since many patients with recurrences die before reaching hospital.

- Early recurrence or extension of an existing infarct takes place in approximately 15% of all patients[3].
- Patients with triple-vessel disease demonstrated at cardiac catheterization have a much poorer prognosis than those with single-vessel disease. The prognosis is worse if there is poor left ventricular function or heart failure—in these cases there is an almost 100% 5-year mortality rate[4].
- Only one-third of patients who have an infarct will return to work[3]. Even fewer return to work among those who were unemployed prior to the infarct or those who suffer from depression after the attack.

TREATMENT

The control of pain is paramount, and is best achieved by the use of narcotic analgesia in the form of diamorphine 5–10 mg i.v.

Oxygen, given by nasal catheter, may limit the extent of myocardial damage by correcting hypoxaemia[5].

. Admission to a coronary care unit: in general, all young patients with infarcts should be admitted to a coronary care unit together with all those with an arrhythmia. Older patients who exhibit cardiogenic shock should also be admitted, but uncomplicated infarcts in elderly patients can be safely treated at home provided that there are adequate support services[6].

. The main cause of death after an acute myocardial infarction is a ventricular arrhythmia. If this is suspected, the patient should be given lignocaine 100 mg i.v. as a bolus. Patients suffering from epilepsy should not be treated with lignocaine as it may precipitate an attack. It is also contraindicated in patients on cimetidine[7].

. Bradycardia should be treated with atropine 0.6 mg i.v.

. Left ventricular failure should be treated with frusemide 40–120 mg i.v.

. The use of intravenous thrombolytic agents (like streptokinase 1.5 million units by i.v. infusion over 1 hour) has been shown significantly to reduce coronary mortality[8]. For this therapy to be effective the drug must be given within 4 hours of the infarct taking place. The general practitioner should therefore expedite the patient's admission to a unit using this form of treatment.

8. The management of postinfarction patients is often the responsibility of the general practitioner. There is evidence to suggest that the long-term use of beta-blocking agents, such as timolol maleate (10–20 mg daily) is effective in reducing mortality and morbidity[9].

9. Recent research has shown that the use of aspirin 300 mg daily protects against myocardial infarction[10]. Higher dosage is not recommended because it causes increased side-effects and is no more effective.

FOLLOW-UP

As patients with a history of previous myocardial infarction are at a much higher risk of developing further episodes, it is important for the practitioner to emphasize prevention. This is discussed in the section on coronary artery disease (p. 67).

The family members of those patients suffering from an infarct should be fully investigated to assess their risk factors.

Much of the follow-up of postinfarction patients can be carried out by a practice nurse. When older patients are confined to bed, the district nurse should be involved with their day-to-day nursing care.

[1] Kuller L et al. (1972) Arch. Intern. Med., 129, 714.
[2] Sokolow M, McIlroy M (1986) Clinical Cardiology, 4th edn, p. 189. California: Lange Medical Publications.
[3] Marmor A et al. (1981) Am. J. Cardiol., 48, 603.
[4] Sheldon W (1975) Prog. Cardiovasc. Med., 46, 237.
[5] Benotti J (1987) Conn's Curr. Ther., p. 228.
[6] Hill J et al. (1978) Lancet, i, 837.
[7] Duff H et al. (1983) Circulation, 67, 1124.
[8] AIMS Trial Study Group (1988) Lancet, i, 545.
[9] Chamberlain D (1983) Br. Heart J., 49, 105.
[10] Boerboom L et al. (1985) J. Am. Coll. Cardiol., 5, 505.

Heart Failure

Heart failure describes a continuum of symptoms from mild ankle oedema to acute left ventricular failure. It is a state in which cardiac output is reduced relative to the metabolic demands of the body.

The main causes of heart failure are myocardial diseases (coronary artery disease, cardiomyopathy and myocarditis), increased load on the heart (hypertension, aortic valvular disease and hypertrophic cardiomyopathy), and an increased stroke volume (aortic insufficiency and congenital left-to-right shunts). Lastly, high output failure occurs when the body has an increased demand as in thyrotoxicosis, anaemia and pregnancy. Children with congenital heart disease who go into heart failure may present as failure to thrive.

Heart failure can be precipitated by a number of events such as arrhythmias, respiratory failure, pulmonary embolism, thyrotoxicosis, anaemia, infection and rheumatic carditis.

PROGNOSIS

- In mild heart failure the prognosis depends on the underlying cause and the response to therapy. In severe heart failure the prognosis is less than 18 months[1] even with aggressive management.
- Modern drugs have improved the prognosis. Where treatment is delayed, the prognosis remains poor. Heart failure is commonly a sequel of late diagnosis of potentially preventable conditions such as hypertension, thyrotoxicosis and rheumatic valvular disease.
- Some 50% of patients with a diastolic pressure between 110 and 120 mmHg have hypertrophy of the left ventricle and have a poor prognosis[2].
- When aortic valvular disease is the underlying cause, the life expectancy is only 1–2 years after heart failure occurs[3]. The prognosis for heart failure in mitral valve disease is better. Valve surgery improves the prognosis in both aortic and mitral valve disease when heart failure is present.
- In cardiomyopathy the prognosis is very poor—1-year survival is only 50%.
- Prevention of heart failure should be sought by screening those at risk; early diagnosis and adequate control of hypertension are especially important.
- The prevention of coronary artery disease is an important measure in the prevention of heart failure, and is discussed in the section on coronary artery disease (p. 67).
- The admission of young patients with myocardial infarction to coronary intensive care wards has improved the prognosis, because early complications such as arrhythmias and acute left ventricular failure can be treated promptly[4].
- In the elderly, heart failure is often overdiagnosed. Ankle oedema should be accompanied by other signs, such as tachycardia, raised jugular venous pressure and cardiomegaly, before the diagnosis is made.
- Where there is doubt about the cause of heart failure patients should be referred for specialist opinion.

TREATMENT

1. The main objectives in the treatment of heart failure are:
   a. To determine, and, where possible remove, the underlying cause.
   b. To increase the force and efficiency of myocardial contraction.
   c. To decrease systemic vascular resistance.
   d. To reduce sodium retention if it occurs.
2. Where heart failure is precipitated by anaemia, chest infection, arrhythmias and thyrotoxicosis, these problems should be treated initially. Surgical correction of both rheumatic valvular disease and congenital heart disease often controls underlying heart failure.
3. A reduction in physical workload can produce considerable benefit. Occasionally complete bedrest is needed and this may necessitate admission to hospital. Where general practitioner beds are available, there is no reason why patients should not be admitted for management. The degree of rest required depends on the severity of the heart failure and the underlying cardiac disease.

Patients undergoing treatment for heart failure should avoid adding salt to food.

Obesity aggravates heart failure and counselling with regard to weight control should be given.

Diuretics remain the mainstay of therapy. Thiazides (bendrofluazide 2.5–5 mg) help in mild failure. In more severe failure loop diuretics such as frusemide (40–500 mg daily) and bumetanide (1–10 mg daily) often produce rapid improvement in symptoms. Care should be taken in their long-term use as they may cause hypokalaemia, and potassium replacement may be required.

Digoxin (0.25 mg daily or twice daily depending on age and body mass) is the treatment of choice in cardiac failure associated with rapid atrial fibrillation. There is some doubt as to the usefulness of digoxin in the long-term management of heart failure[5]. The limited positive inotropic effect has to be balanced against the potential toxicity. In elderly patients toxicity can occur with low dosage, especially in the presence of poor renal function, so serum digoxin levels should be monitored closely. When digoxin is used with diuretics, the serum potassium should also be monitored as hypokalaemia potentiates digoxin.

8. There is good evidence that angiotensin-converting enzyme inhibitors can reduce mortality and improve well-being. In one study of patients with severe heart failure, mortality fell from 52 to 36% at 1 year in a group with added angiotensin-converting enzyme inhibitors[6]. Profound hypotension and occasionally death can follow a first dose in 5–10% of patients. Treatment should be initiated in hospital on a low dose and care must be exercised when increasing the dose.

9. Severe heart failure with pulmonary oedema is a medical emergency usually requiring immediate admission. The patient's condition should be stabilized before transfer. Diamorphine 2.5–5 mg, depending on body mass, should be given by subcutaneous injection to allay fear and reduce catcholamine release. High concentrations of oxygen at 6–8 litres per minute should be commenced (although lower concentrations should be given to patients with chronic respiratory disease), and the patient should be given intravenous frusemide (40–80 mg).

10. The management of arrhythmias which occur concurrently or which may be the precipitating factor are discussed in the section on arrhythmias.

FOLLOW-UP

Patients with heart failure need close monitoring. Regular measurement of their serum electrolytes and urea should be carried out with serum digoxin levels if that drug is used. Joint management with a cardiologist will achieve the best results for those with severe failure.

[1] Romankiewicz J (1983) *Drugs*, **25**, 6.
[2] Sokolow M, McIlroy M (1986) *Clinical Cardiology*. California: Lange Medical Publications.
[3] Massel BF *et al.* (1966) *Circulation*, **34** (suppl. 2), 164.
[4] McEnay T *et al.* (1977) *Circulation*, **56**, 249.
[5] Guyatt G (1988) *Am. J. Cardiol.*, **61**, 371.
[6] The consensus trial study group (1987) *N. Engl. J. Med.*, **316**, 1429.

Valve Disease

Acute rheumatic fever has for many generations been responsible for most cases of valvular heart disease. With a general improvement in living conditions and the use of penicillin in the management of streptococcal pharyngitis the incidence of rheumatic fever has declined in the western world. However it is important to remember that rheumatic valvular disease is still the world's most common form of heart disease accounting for much disability and premature death in the third world.

Rheumatic valvular disease is still seen in this country, usually in middle aged patients who have a childhood history of acute rheumatism.

Other causes of valvular disease include congenital valve disease, post ischaemic valvular disease and functional valve disease due to dilatation of the ventricles in heart failure and cardiomyopathy.

PROGNOSIS

Mitral valve disease

- Mitral valve disease is usually caused by rheumatic fever, or damage to the cordae tendinae after a myocardial infarction. In childhood it is usually due to a congenital abnormality.
- Patients often present in the fourth and fifth decade of life with early heart failure manifesting as dyspnoea, orthopnoea and occasionally haemoptysis. Mitral incompetence is three times more common and mitral stenosis nine times more common in women[1].
- Congenital causes account for only 1% of cases of mitral valve disease in adult patients.
- Valve surgery has improved the prognosis from mitral valve disease. However the prognosis is dependent on early diagnosis preferably before the patient develops atrial fibrillation. The ten year survival after mitral valve replacement is approximately 50%, depending on the type and severity of the underlying cause[1].

Aortic valve disease

- Aortic incompetence and stenosis accounts for about 35% of patients with valve disease, the most common cause being rheumatic fever. Other important causes include congenital lesions, infective endocarditis, cardiomyopathy, hypertension with left ventricular hypertrophy and ankylosing spondylitis.
- Without surgery the prognosis for symptomatic aortic valve disease is poor. After valve replacement the prognosis is improved but depends on the preoperative state of the patient and the underlying pathology. The presence of heart failure has a poor prognosis.
- Mixed mitral and aortic valve disease accounts for 10% of all lesions and is usually caused by rheumatic carditis in childhood. Patients with a combined lesion tend to develop symptoms earlier than those with single valve disease.
- Where valve disease is caused by rheumatic carditis the severity of the lesion and the long-term prognosis will be improved by the prevention of further episodes of carditis[2].
- Pulmonary and tricuspid valve disease are usually congenital in origin though they can be as a result of an acutely dilated heart in acute heart failure or cardiomyopathy. Prognosis depends on the underlying pathology. Both valves can be replaced and the long-term prognosis after valve replacement is very good.
- The long-term prognosis following valve replacement is not known, however complications such as endocarditis and embolism reduce life expectancy.

TREATMENT

1. Early diagnosis and referral for a cardiological opinion are important in the early management of valve disease.
2. Symptomatic treatment is important, this includes:
   a) Treating heart failure which is discussed in the section on heart failure. (p. 72)
   b) Treating atrial fibrillation which is discussed in the section on arrhythmias. (p. 77)

All patients with valve disease require antibiotic prophylaxis for dental procedures to prevent infective endocarditis. In patients not allergic to penicillin, amoxycillin (3 g 1 hour beforehand) should be used. In patients with known hypersensitivity to penicillin, erythromycin (1.5 g 1 hour beforehand followed by 0.5 g 6 h later) should be used[3].

. In most patients with symptomatic valve disease valve surgery is indicated. Patients who are asymptomatic but who have left ventricular dysfunction should also be referred for surgery[4].

. All patients with artificial valves require anticoagulation to prevent thrombus formation. In spite of this the incidence of thromboembolism is 5% per patient year[1]. It is therefore essential for the general practitioner to monitor the prothombin index in these patients closely to ensure adequate anticoagulation.

. In patients who have valve disease as a result of rheumatic fever it is important to consider whether the patient requires long-term penicillin prophylaxis against the β haemolytic streptoccus. All children and adolescents should be placed on prophylaxis for at least five years, or at least till their twenty-fifth birthday. Prophylaxis is best achieved by the use of parenteral long-acting penicillin (1.2 million units intramuscular every 4 weeks). In patients who are allergic to penicillin, oral erythromycin (250 mg twice daily) should be used.

FOLLOW-UP

Close follow-up of patients is important. All patients with valve disease should be referred for cardiological opinion. Subsequently those with less severe disease need only be seen annually but those with more severe disease or who have had complications such as heart failure or an arrhythmia need to be seen every 3–6 months. Routine monitoring of anticoagula therapy is important and should be carried out in conjunction with the anticoagulant clinic.

[1] Sokolow M (1986) *Clinical Cardiology* Los Altos, California: Lange Medical Publications.
[2] Tompkins D (1972) *Circulation,* **45,** 543.
[3] Delaye E (1985) *Eur. Heart. J.* **6,** 826.
[4] Opie L (1987) *Drugs for the Heart* Orlando, Florida: Grune & Stratton.

Arrhythmias

Supraventricular ectopic beats

Ectopic beats can arise either from the atrium or from the junctional area of the atrioventricular node. They are usually benign, and are more common with increasing age. They are also associated with coronary artery disease, digitalis toxicity and may be found in patients with left atrial enlargement due to mitral stenosis. They may precede atrial fibrillation or initiate supraventricular tachycardia. The patient may notice a slight irregularity of the heart rate which is usually abolished by exercise.

PROGNOSIS

● Supraventricular beats do not result in sudden death.

● In the absence of heart disease the extrasystoles are benign.
● In the presence of heart disease the prognosis is that of the underlying heart condition.

TREATMENT

Drug therapy is rarely needed unless supraventricular tachycardia or atrial fibrillation supervene. Reassurance, if symptoms are noticed, is the only requirement.

FOLLOW-UP

This is only necessary if there is underlying heart disease.

Supraventricular tachycardia

Supraventricular tachycardia is an episode of atrial or junctional ectopic beats occurring at the rate of 150 beats or more per minute. It occurs in 1–2 adults/1000 population each year[1]. It may be associated with a known conduction disorder such as Wolff–Parkinson–White syndrome or established heart disease, but more commonly it may occur spontaneously for no known cause. Palpitations may be the only symptom. In the presence of underlying heart disease, or if the rate is very rapid, other symptoms may occur. These include dizziness, chest pain, transient loss of consciousness or heart failure. These symptoms are more common in older patients. The electrocardiogram (ECG) usually shows normal QRS complexes, preceded by an abnormal P wave, but this is not always the case.

Supraventricular tachycardia occurs more commonly in young women. Precipitating factors include exercise, stress and caffeine consumption.

PROGNOSIS

- This depends on the underlying aetiology and heart rate. If there is no underlying disease, patients can be completely reassured.

TREATMENT

Of the acute attack
1. Eyeball pressure, straining at stool, Valsalva's manoeuvre, breath-holding or squatting all increase vagal stimulation and can abort an attack.
2. Firm massage for half a minute of first the right carotid sinus and then the left will sometimes return the heart to sinus rhythm.
3. Other methods of control are best carried out in hospital and include:
   a. Rapid digitalization with i.m. or i.v. digoxin (0.75–1 mg).
   b. Direct current cardioversion to restore sinus rhythm is usually successful and can be done under sedation or general anaesthesia.
   c. Other anti-arrhythmic drugs such as verapamil (5–10 mg as an intravenous bolus), non-cardioselective beta blockers (propanolol 40–80 mg three times daily) or amiodarone (600–800 mg twice daily) may be used.

Long-term control
1. Digoxin (0.25 mg daily) is the drug of choice.
2. Non-cardioselective beta blockers (propanolol 40 mg three times daily) are also useful if there is no underlying heart failure. They can be used instead of or in conjunction with digoxin.
3. Other anti-arrhythmic drugs such as verapamil (5–10 mg daily) or amiodarone (200–400 mg daily) can be used when other therapy fails.

FOLLOW-UP

Patients should be assessed regularly for symptoms of palpitations. It may be necessary to use 24–hour ambulatory electrocardiography to assess the efficacy of treatment.

Ventricular extrasystoles

Ventricular extrasystoles or premature beats (VPBs) are the most common of all arrhythmias. They are usually of little importance in the absence of heart disease. In the presence of coronary artery disease they may lead to ventricular tachycardia and sudden death. When they occur during or after exercise they indicate the presence of underlying heart disease. If VPBs occur at rest and disappear on exercise, they are more likely to be due to escape beats caused by a slow resting heart rate and are of little significance. Most patients are asymptomatic, but sometimes the beat after a VPB is more forceful and the patient feels a thump in the chest. The incidence of patients complaining of VPBs is about 1/1000 each year[1].

PROGNOSIS

- If there is no underlying heart disease, the prognosis is usually benign.
- In the presence of ischaemic heart disease, there is a risk of ventricular tachycardia and sudden death.
- The risk of sudden death increases if there are more than 10 VPBs per 1000 beats[2].

TREATMENT

The main objective is to prevent ventricular tachycardia.
1. In patients with no underlying coronary artery disease, treatment is often unnecessary. Alco-

hol, tobacco and undue stress should be avoided. Drug therapy as a cause of the VPBs should be excluded. These include digoxin, aminophylline, phenothiazines and tricyclic antidepressants.

If VPBs are frequent (more than 5/min), multiform or occur close to the T wave of the previous complex, drug therapy should be used to try to suppress them since ventricular tachycardia may ensue. Drugs such as procainamide (250–500 mg four times daily), propanolol (80–320 mg daily in four doses), or verapamil (80–120 mg daily) may be used.

FOLLOW-UP

Patients with VPBs need only be followed up if they have an underlying heart condition. Those patients who have coronary artery disease should be followed closely and regular assessments made of their risk factors.

Ventricular tachycardia

Ventricular tachycardia is a rapid ventricular rhythm of 150–200 beats/min. The onset is abrupt and decreased ventricular filling and low cardiac output result in dyspnoea, angina, hypotension and syncope. It commonly occurs after acute myocardial infarction, occasionally in hypertrophic obstructive cardiomyopathy, and as a result of some drugs (especially digoxin).

PROGNOSIS

● Ventricular tachycardia following myocardial infarction is common, occurring in up to 40% of cases in the first 3 hours after the attack[3].

TREATMENT

1. Ventricular tachycardia represents a medical emergency and patients should be transferred to a cardiac intensive care ward immediately, preferably with the practitioner acting as an escort.
2. Lignocaine (100 mg intravenously) as a bolus should be given if there is no evidence of severe cardiac failure. The bolus should be followed

by a constant infusion at the rate of 1–4 mg/min.
3. Immediate direct current cardioversion is usually indicated, particularly if there is hypotension or in patients with myocardial infarction who are likely to develop ventricular fibrillation.
4. Disopyramide (300 mg as a single loading dose) or flecainide (1–2 mg per kg body weight as a single intravenous injection) can also be used.
5. Long-term treatment with flecainide (100–400 mg twice daily), disopyramide (100–200 mg 6-hourly) or amiodarone (200–400 mg daily) can be used to prevent recurrent attacks of ventricular tachycardia. All patients on long-term drug therapy need to have regular 24-hour electrocardiographic monitoring.

FOLLOW-UP

Patients should be seen at regular intervals to assess symptoms and 24-hour electrocardiographic monitoring should be done to measure the response to treatment.

Atrial fibrillation

Atrial fibrillation occurs when the normal sinoatrial conduction is lost and the atrioventricular node is bombarded by a multitude of atrial stimuli. Some are conducted into the ventricular node but this occurs in a random fashion, resulting in beats that are irregular in time and force. In addition, atrial contractility is lost and this may further reduce ventricular filling and precipitate cardiac failure. Atrial fibrillation occurs as part of a degenerative disease of cardiac conducting tissue, in thyrotoxicosis, and when there is atrial dilatation (ischaemic, hypertensive or rheumatic heart disease). It is also a common finding in patients with mitral stenosis. It is more common in older patients and the incidence of chronic atrial fibrillation increases at the rate of about 2% over 20 years[4]. Symptoms include rapid irregular palpitations and heart failure. Some patients have no symptoms and the diagnosis is made incidentally when it is noted that the pulse is slower than the heart rate.

PROGNOSIS

- This depends mainly on the underlying cause, and providing this is amenable to treatment, controlled atrial fibrillation should not worsen the prognosis.
- A total of 10% of patients with atrial fibrillation in the Framingham study went on to develop cerebral emboli[4].
- Stasis of blood in the atrium results in thrombus formation; this may result in systemic and pulmonary emboli. This is more common in mitral stenosis.

TREATMENT

1. If atrial fibrillation is of recent onset, it is beneficial to try and convert the patient back into sinus rhythm since this reduces heart failure and the risk of emboli.
2. Direct current cardioversion is the most effective method of returning the patient to sinus rhythm. This is more successful if the cause of the atrial fibrillation has also been treated (e.g. thyrotoxicosis, after mitral valve surgery or after acute myocardial infarction). Some patients will revert back to atrial fibrillation, especially those with cardiomegaly or a long history.
3. For these patients and those with longstanding atrial fibrillation, it is most important that the ventricular rate is controlled. This is best achieved with digoxin (0.25 mg daily) to produce a ventricular rate of 80 beats/min.
4. Non-cardioselective[5] beta-blocking drugs (propanolol 40–80 mg three times daily) may be used with digoxin to control ventricular rate. Care must be taken in the presence of heart failure.
5. Other drugs such as verapamil (80–120 mg three times daily) and amiodarone (200–400 mg daily) can be used in patients who are unable to take digoxin or who do not have heart failure.
6. Anticoagulants are used during cardioversion and sometimes in the long-term management of patients with underlying mitral valve disease, to prevent thrombus formation and embolization.

FOLLOW-UP

Frequency of follow-up will depend on the underlying heart disease. All patients on long-term digoxin need to have regular estimations of the serum level together with their serum electrolytes. Hypokalaemia potentiates digoxin toxicity. Many of these patients are receiving diuretics and care must be taken to ensure that the serum levels are not low.

Bradycardia

Bradycardia is defined as a heart rate of less than 50 beats/min. In sinus bradycardia the sinus node discharges at a slow rate, as in myxoedema, sick sinus syndrome or with some drugs (beta-blocking agents, opiates, tranquillizers and phenothiazines). Bradycardia may also be due to an atrioventricular conduction defect (complete heart block) and with digitalis toxicity or following a myocardial infarction. It can present as tiredness, dizziness, transient loss of consciousness (Stokes–Adams attack) or heart failure. Occasionally it might be associated with ectopic beats causing palpitations.

PROGNOSIS

- This depends on the underlying cause. It is generally worse if the bradycardia is due to myocardial infarction, sick sinus syndrome or complete heart block.

TREATMENT

1. This depends on the cause and on the severity of the symptoms. Drug-related bradycardia should be treated by discontinuing the drug. Conditions such as myxoedema should be treated with appropriate medication.
2. If the symptoms are significant, a transvenous, demand cardiac pacemaker should be considered, even in the elderly, as the quality of life is much improved.
3. Patients with Stokes–Adams attacks should be admitted to hospital immediately for insertion of a pacemaker, as any episode of extreme bradycardia can prove fatal.

Patients should be seen at regular intervals to assess symptoms. They should be asked to report any episodes of syncope immediately. To assess heart rate 24-hour electrocardiographic monitoring may be necessary. Patients with pacemakers need periodic checks of pacemaker function. The patient and family members should learn to check heart rate and report any abnormality immediately.

[1] Hodgkin K (1976) *Towards Earlier Diagnosis*. London: Churchill Livingstone.
[2] Hinkle LE (1969) *Am. J. Cardiol.*, **24**, 629.
[3] Sokolow M (1986) *Clinical Cardiology*. Los Altos, California: Lange Medical Publications.
[4] Kannel WB (1982) *N. Engl. J. Med.*, **306**, 1018.
[5] Opie LH (1987) *Drugs for the Heart*. Orlando, Florida: Grune & Stratton.

Peripheral Vascular Disease

Peripheral vascular disease can present in a number of ways which include intermittent claudication, peripheral gangrene, aortic aneurysm and Buerger's disease. Factors predisposing to the development of these conditions including cigarette smoking, a raised serum cholesterol, hypertension, polycythaemia, obesity, diabetes and a family history of vascular disease. The aetiology of most of these conditions is associated with the accumulation of a fibrolipid plaque beneath the endothelium of large and medium-sized arteries, leading to narrowing of the arterial lumen. This causes a reduction of blood flow and ischaemia to the limb distal to lesion. The formation of plaque is not uniform and most commonly occurs at the bifurcation or at the branches of the vessel. The major complications include distal embolization with gangrene, and the formation of aneurysms with ultimate rupture of the artery. Buerger's disease is an uncommon condition affecting men aged 25–40; the aetiology is unknown.

PROGNOSIS

- Intermittent claudication is a progressive disease, and 5% of cases will need an amputation within 5 years of diagnosis[1].
- Some improvement can occur early in the course of the disease as collateral vessels develop.
- Some 75% of cases of acute arterial occlusion in the presence of peripheral vascular disease are due to emboli during atrial fibrillation or following acute myocardial infarction[2]. The high mortality of 10–20% is due mainly to the associated cardiac condition[3].
- Gangrene, the result of acute untreated vascular occlusion, has a high mortality especially when major vessels are occluded. The hospital mortality following above-knee amputation is 30%[3]. A total of 60% of all bilateral above-knee amputees will be dead within 5 years[4]. The prognosis following below-knee amputation is

better, with a 10% hospital mortality and many more of the patients becoming mobile again[5].
- Abdominal atheromatous aneurysms get progressively larger over the years and there is a 50% mortality if they rupture[6]. The operative mortality for elective surgery is less than 5%[7], therefore early referral is important even in asymptomatic patients. Following surgery for abdominal aneurysm, the 5-year survival is 65%[8]. Aneurysms in peripheral vessels rarely rupture but may be the nidus for a thrombus which may cause a distal embolus.
- The prognosis in Buerger's disease is directly related to the patient's smoking habits. Failure to stop smoking results in severe ischaemia. In all, 30% of patients develop peripheral gangrene with amputation of the limb[9].

TREATMENT

1. The general measures to reduce risk from

atheromatous vascular disease are discussed in the section on coronary artery disease. These include mandatory cessation of smoking, control of raised blood pressure, reduction of raised cholesterol, control of diabetes, reducing body mass and taking regular exercise.

2. Intermittent claudication can be improved in a number of ways.

   a. The most important medical treatment in the control of this condition is to encourage the patient to give up smoking.

   b. The use of vasodilator drugs has little effect.

   c. A number of surgical procedures can be carried out to relieve symptoms. Transluminal balloon angioplasty can be used to treat short segments of diseased vessel, especially in the aortoiliac region[10].

   d. Bypass surgery using a dacron graft has good results in the aorta, iliac and femoral arteries. The success rate is high, with an 85% 5-year patency. There is a 2–3% operative mortality[2].

   e. The surgical treatment of femoral occlusion is the femoropopliteal or femorotibial bypass using saphenous vein autograft. The success rate from this operation is not as high as dacron grafts in the aorta and iliac arteries. The 5-year overall survival in these patients is only 50%[2].

3. Pain at rest or early gangrene should be managed as a surgical emergency and patients should be admitted for urgent investigation. Arteriography will show the sites of occlusion and where necessary constructive surgery can be carried out in an attempt to save the limb.

4. Extensive gangrene requires amputation. Below-knee amputation gives better postoperative mobility, but may not heal as well as an amputation carried out above the knee. Where a *Clostridium* infection is suspected the patient should be treated with large doses of penicillin and hyperbaric oxygen.

5. Abdominal aneurysms require surgery unless they are small (less than 4 cm diameter). The operation most commonly carried out is the dacron tube graft. Ruptured abdominal aneurysm is a surgical emergency requiring urgent treatment in a specialized surgical unit.

FOLLOW-UP

Patients with peripheral vascular disease require careful long-term follow-up. In the early years of disease, support and encouragement with regard to lifestyle, especially smoking habits, can improve prognosis. After surgery it is important to ensure that the patient's recovery is monitored. Support from welfare organizations for amputees should be used where necessary. Patients should have regular chiropody, and those with underlying conditions such as diabetes need to be closely monitored.

[1] Taylor GW *et al.* (1962) *Br. Med. J.*, **i**, 507.

[2] Ward AS *et al.* (1985) *Medicine*, **2**, 861–5.

[3] Tracey GD *et al.* (1982) *Surg. Gynecol. Obstet.*, **155**, 377.

[4] Van de Ven CMC (1982) *Br. Med. J.*, **ii**, 707.

[5] De Cossart I *et al.* (1983) *Ann. R. Coll. Surg. Engl.*, **65**, 230.

[6] Soreide O *et al.* (1982) *Surgery*, **91**, 188.

[7] Walker FM *et al.* (1983) *Ann. R. Coll. Surg. Engl.*, **65**, 311.

[8] Fielding JWL *et al.* (1981) *Br. Med. J.*, **ii**, 355.

[9] Jones S (1985) *Medicine*, **2**, 818–19.

[10] Mosley VG *et al.* (1985) *Ann. R. Coll. Surg. Engl.*, **67**, 83.

Hyperlipidaemia

The risk of developing coronary artery disease is proportionally related to the serum levels of cholesterol and inversely related to the levels of high density lipoproteins[1]. Hyperlipidaemia leads to atherosclerosis and the aim of treatment of raised serum cholesterol is to reduce the risk of coronary artery disease[2,3]. A raised total serum cholesterol is also associated with increased risk of developing peripheral vascular disease, stroke and hypertension. Atherosclerosis is associated with a number of neurological conditions such as Parkinson's disease and pre-senile dementia. Raised triglyceride levels are associated with attacks of acute pancreatitis. Most cases of hyperlipidaemia are due to dietary indiscretion or to the effects of an underlying medical condition, such as hypothyroidism, nephrotic syndrome and alcohol abuse. A small percentage of patients (1 in 500–1000) have a genetic abnormality leading to the increase in blood lipids.

PROGNOSIS

- National morbidity and mortality figures for coronary artery disease are related to the mean level of cholesterol in the community. The higher the mean level of cholesterol, the more the population is at risk[4].
- In a study of 11 000 British men, two-thirds were found to have cholesterol levels exceeding 5 mmol/l[5]. The incidence of coronary artery disease is twice as great in patients with a cholesterol level of 6.5 mmol/l as in those with levels of 5 mmol/l[6,7].
- Cholesterol levels rise with age[4]. In general practice the following four categories of total serum cholesterol give the practitioner a guide to the level of risk: <5.2 mmol/l, not at risk; 5.2–6.5 mmol/l, increased risk; 6.5–8.0 mmol/l, moderate risk; >8.0 mmol/l, high risk.
- The incidence of myocardial infarction has been shown to decrease in patients with hyperlipidaemia who have a fall in their cholesterol level[8].
- Low levels of HDL cholesterol also appear to be a risk factor for coronary artery disease. Patients with HDL levels below 0.7 mmol/l are eight times more likely to develop coronary artery disease than those with levels of 1.7 mmol/l or above[9].
- Risk factors for coronary artery disease are multiplitive. The patient with an isolated elevated cholesterol with no other risk factors is probably at marginal increased risk.

TREATMENT

1. In general practice the main objectives in the management of the hyperlipidaemia are:
   a. The identification of those individuals who are at moderate to high risk.
   b. The lowering of total cholesterol to levels which reduce the risk of developing coronary artery disease.
   c. The treatment of underlying medical conditions which may increase lipid levels (hydrothyroidism, nephrotic syndrome and alcohol abuse).
   d. The reduction of other risk factors for coronary artery disease, in particular, smoking and hypertension.
2. Screening for hyperlipidaemia: the study group of the European Heart Society[10] have recommended three ways of identifying patients at risk:
   a. Selective case-finding in patients who on clinical grounds may be at risk (strong family history of coronary artery disease, obesity, clinical signs such as premature corneal arcus, xanthomas, obesity or diabetes). This method is probably the most effective in general practice[4].
   b. Opportunistic screening in specific population groups.
   c. General population screening is probably not effective as it puts too much stress on the available facilities.
3. Lowering of increased levels. Dietary measures

are the first line of treatment, especially when coupled with cessation of smoking, weight reduction, exercise and the control of hypertension and diabetes.

   a. The European Study Group[10] recommends that less than 30% of energy in the diet should be derived from fat, and less than 10% from saturated fat. The intake of complex carbohydrates and fruit and vegetable-derived fibre should be augmented, with increased use of polyunsaturated and monounsaturated fats. Intake of starch should be reduced and moderation in alcohol is advised.

   b. Lipid-lowering drugs may be required when dietary and lifestyle modifications fail after a sufficient period of trial (at least 6 months). All these drugs are associated with quite severe side-effects and should therefore be used with caution.

4. Bile acid sequestrants such as cholestyramine (16–24 g daily to a maximum 36 g daily) or colestipol (20–25 g daily in two doses) should be used as the first choice for the reduction of raised serum cholesterol. The major side-effects of these agents include constipation, heartburn and occasionally steatorrhoea. They may cause an increase in the serum triglyceride and should not be used when this level is already increased.

5. Nicotinic acid (1–2 g three times daily) reduces the secretion of lipoproteins from the liver and is used to reduce serum cholesterol. The major side-effects from these high doses include flushing, dizziness, palpitations, impaired glucose tolerance and occasional liver dysfunction. Flushing, which can be quite severe, can be reduced by using low-dose aspirin.

6. Fibric acid derivatives activate plasma lipoprotein lipase and should be used to lower serum cholesterol when there is a raised serum triglyceride. Clofibrate (500 mg 2–3 times daily) causes a number of side-effects including warfarin potentiation, cholesterol gallstones, abdominal discomfort and muscle pain. Bezafibrate (200 mg 2–3 times daily) and gemfibrozil (600 mg twice daily) have fewer side-effects but both potentiate warfarin and should not be used in patients on this drug.

7. Probucol (500 mg twice daily) is used to reduce hypercholesterolaemia. As it does not distinguish between low and high density lipoprotein it should be used with caution in patients with already low levels of HDL. It is also contraindicated in pregnancy and patients should not become pregnant within 6 months of stopping the drug.

8. Many drugs may increase serum lipids and should therefore be used with caution in patients with already raised levels. Non-cardioselective beta blockers should not be used in high-risk patients and should be replaced by cardioselective beta blockers and calcium channel blocking agents in the management of angina. Diuretic dose should be kept low in patients with hyperlipidaemia. Oral contraceptive agents should not be used in patients with coronary artery disease or with increased risk as they may cause an increase in serum lipids.

FOLLOW-UP

Patients with hyperlipidaemia and their families need careful long-term follow-up. It is important to remember that a raised serum cholesterol may take many months to fall and routine blood tests should not be carried out too frequently. As lipids tend to rise in the elderly, and as dietary fats often make up an important source of calories in this group, the long-term control of hyperlipidaemia in the elderly is questionable.

[1] Lipid Research Clinics Program (1984) *JAMA*, **251**, 351.
[2] Blackburn H *et al.* (1979) *Prev. Med.*, **8**, 609.
[3] Mann J (1987) *Lipid Rev.*, **1**, 25.
[4] Mann J *et al.* (1988) *Br. Med. J.*, **296**, 1702.
[5] Lewis B *et al.* (1986) *Proceedings of the Conference on the Current Views on the Diagnosis and Treatment of Hyperlipidaemia*, p. 7. London: Royal Society of Medicine.
[6] Lewis B (1986) *Lancet*, **i**, 956.
[7] Martin M *et al.* (1986) *Lancet*, **ii**, 933.
[8] Brensike J (1984) *Circulation*, **69**, 313.
[9] Gordon A *et al.* (1977) *Am. J. Med.*, **62**, 707.
[10] Study group of the European Heart Society (1987) *Eur. Heart J.*, **8**, 77.

Thrombophlebitis

Thrombophlebitis is the term used for a thrombosis occurring in a superficial vein, secondary in most cases to an inflammatory change in the wall of the vein[1]. The main causes of thrombophlebitis are external trauma to the vein, either from a blow or pressure from a bandage; internal trauma to the endothelium, usually by the introduction of an intravenous needle or cannula[2]; the result of local irritation, in the form of infection or malignancy, or occasionally recurrent episodes of thrombophlebitis, due to a primary abnormality of the vein wall fibrinolytic activity[3]. Superficial thrombophlebitis can be associated with varicose veins[4], pregnancy[5], thromboangitis obliterans (Buerger's disease[6]) and in association with occult malignancy.

PROGNOSIS

- Most cases of superficial thrombophlebitis are either self-limiting or disappear when the underlying cause is treated.
- When there is an underlying malignancy the prognosis is decided by the underlying disease.

TREATMENT

1. Infusion thrombophlebitis is best treated by stopping the infusion, or by varying the site of the infusion and by using a non-irritant cannula. The symptoms are best relieved by analgesia and a firm compression bandage.
2. Thrombophlebitis occurring in a varicose vein should be treated with compression bandages and brisk walking. Mild analgesia can be used (paracetamol 1000 mg 4-hourly) or if the thrombophlebitis is severe, a non-steroidal anti-inflammatory drug can be used (indomethacin 50 mg three times daily).
3. If the thrombophlebitis becomes infected ligation of the vein or venotomy may be required to prevent the infected clot acting as a source of infected emboli.

4. When the cause of the thrombophlebitis is shown to be a defect in the vein wall fibrinolytic activator, the use of a fibrinolytic activator should be contemplated (stanozolol 10 mg daily).

FOLLOW-UP

Most cases of thrombophlebitis need only be followed for a short period of time, usually during the acute episode. Where there is an underlying cause for the thrombophlebitis, or when there are recurrences, the patient may need to be followed until the cause has been found. Underlying problems such as varicose veins will need to be treated in the usual way.

[1] Browse NL et al. (1988) Superficial thrombophlebitis. In Diseases of the Veins. London: Edward Arnold.
[2] Brown GA (1970) Br. J. Clin. Pract., 24, 197.
[3] Browse NL et al. (1977) Br. Med. J., i, 478.
[4] Hushi EA et al. (1982) Surgery, 91, 70.
[5] Aaro LA et al. (1967) Am J. Obstet. Gynecol., 97, 514.
[6] Buerger L (1909) Int. Clin., 3, 84.

Deep Vein Thrombosis

Deep vein thromboses (DVTs) form in the veins beneath the deep fascia of the leg or in the pelvic or abdominal veins. The condition develops most frequently in the immediate postoperative period. The estimated incidence of DVT in this group varies from 5 to 15%[1], though for some surgical procedures the incidence is considerably higher. The main presenting features are calf pain, swelling of the lower leg, skin discoloration over the site of the DVT and occasionally venous gangrene. A DVT may also present as pyrexia of unknown origin or as pulmonary embolism with no symptoms of venous thrombosis.

Certain factors increase the risk of developing a thrombosis, including increased age[2], the type and length of operation[3], local trauma, prolonged immobility, a history of previous thrombosis, malignancy, obesity and oral contraceptive use[4].

PROGNOSIS

- The most common complication of this condition is pulmonary embolism which is said to occur in 10% of patients with DVT[5]. The mortality from untreated pulmonary embolism is 30%[6].
- Calf pump failure syndrome (the postphlebetic leg) occurs in approximately 20% of patients with a previous history of DVT[7].

TREATMENT

1. Patients who develop the condition at home should be admitted to hospital where the aims of treatment are: the prevention of fatal pulmonary embolism, the reduction in severity of calf pump failure and the reduction in severity of presenting symptoms.
2. The use of intravenous anticoagulants such as heparin (5000 units intravenously as a loading dose followed by 20 000–40 000 units daily) is the first line in treatment. Its use can often reduce mortality from pulmonary embolism and the long-term morbidity associated with DVT. Treatment should be started as soon as possible after the diagnosis has been made and should continue for 10 days. If there is to be a delay in admitting the patient to hospital, the loading dose can be given at home.
3. Long-term anticoagulation involves using warfarin (30 mg daily) initially and then a dose to maintain the prothrombin time at 2–3 times higher than normal. This should be continued for at least 3–6 months following the DVT.
4. Surgical removal of the thrombus using a balloon catheter can be carried out. The complication rate is high[8], and the operation should only be carried out as a life-saving procedure[9].
5. Thrombolysis using agents such as streptokinase (250 000 units initially then 100 000 units hourly for 3–5 days), urokinase (4000 units/kg initially then 4000 units/kg/h) can produce a marked decrease in the size of the thrombus. Unfortunately their use is associated with a number of complications (haemorrhage and allergic reactions) and there is some doubt as to their effectiveness[8]. Tissue plasminogen activator is a newer fibrinolytic agent and may have fewer complications and a higher rate of success.
6. Patients who have had a DVT are at risk from a further episode if they have an operation or severe trauma. The use of prophylactic anticoagulation in these patients reduces the risk of further DVT formation from an 83% chance to a 14% chance[10]. The general practitioner will need to inform the hospital of subsequent admission about a patient's history of this condition.
7. A past history of DVT is an absolute contraindication for the use of the contraceptive pill.
8. The long-term management of patients who have had a DVT is discussed in the section on varicose veins (p. 85).

FOLLOW-UP

In the short-term the general practitioner may be required to supervise the patient's anticoagulation. A prothrombin time of 2–3 times normal is acceptable. It is important to remember that a number of classes of drugs can affect anticoagulants. These include some antibiotics, non-steroidal anti-inflammatory drugs, diuretics, alcohol and tricyclic antidepressants. A full list can be found in the British National Formulary. The long-term follow-up is aimed at reducing disability and complications. Patients should be encouraged to use elasticated stockings and to walk regularly. If the patient begins to develop signs of the calf pump failure syndrome (postthrombotic leg) they should be referred to a vascular unit.

[1] Browse NL et al. (1988) Aetiology of deep vein thrombosis. In Diseases of Veins, Pathology, Diagnosis and Treatment. London: Edward Arnold.
[2] Short DS (1952) Br. Med. J., i, 790.
[3] Berqvist D (1983) Postoperative Thromboembolism. Berlin: Springer.
[4] Vessey M et al. (1986) Br. Med. J., 292, 526.
[5] Kakkar VV et al. (1969) Lancet, ii, 230.
[6] Barritt DW et al. (1960) Lancet, i, 1309.
[7] Browse NL et al. (1974) Br. Med. J., ii, 468.
[8] Kakkar V et al. (1985) Am. J. Surg., 150, 54.
[9] Browse NL et al. (1988) Deep vein thrombosis: treatment. In Diseases of Veins, Pathology, Diagnosis and Treatment. London: Edward Arnold.
[10] Sevitt S et al. (1959) Lancet, ii, 981.

Varicose Veins

Varicose veins are dilated tortuous veins found usually in the superficial tissues of the legs or occasionally in the skin of the abdominal wall. The incidence in the community varies from 21% to 68%[1]. The incidence and severity increase with age[2]. Varicose veins can be classified into large vein (including the long and short saphenous with perforator incompetence) and small vein varices (involving the superficial veins of the long and short saphenous systems with or without venous flaring).

Primary varicose veins occur with no underlying aetiology and are said to be associated with an erect posture, chronic constipation, a congenital abnormality of the vein wall and/or absence of the venous valves. The aetiology of the secondary varicose veins includes incompetence of the venous valves due to previous deep vein thrombosis, the presence of a large intra-abdominal mass (including the pregnant uterus, ovarian cysts and malignancy), compression and obstruction to the venous return from the leg and in the case of abdominal varices, portal hypertension.

PROGNOSIS

- The prognosis depends on the initial classification and on the severity of the lesions.
- Varicose veins are typically progressive over a number of years but can remain asymptomatic for a long time.
- Primary varicose veins in the calf rarely give rise to complications[2] though they may be associated with aching legs or a 'bursting' feeling.
- Secondary varicose veins can cause ankle oedema, varicose eczema, induration, inflammation and pigmentation of the skin and ulceration.
- Venous haemorrhage is a rare, but sometimes fatal complication of a varicose ulcer.
- Long-standing varicose ulcers may become malignant (Majolin's ulcer).

TREATMENT

1. Non-surgical
   a. The patient should lose weight and take regular exercise. Compression hosiery can stop progression, relieve symptoms and prevent ulceration. Class I hosiery is used for superficial or early varicose veins and those occurring in pregnancy, Class II for those of more severity and Class III where there is gross oedema, for ulcer treatment or for gross varices[3].
   b. Pain is best treated with elevation of the legs, and support stockings. The pain may be disproportionate to the size of the veins.
   c. Varicosities secondary to DVT should be treated wtih Class II hosiery. In conjunction with ligation of the ankle perforating veins this may prevent ulceration.

d. Lipo-dermatosclerosis or ulceration should be treated with compression bandaging and local dressings. Many are available and the principles are to prevent infection and to minimize 'sticking'. Secondary allergy to antibiotic agents and other chemicals is common and should be watched for. Dressings will need to be changed at a frequency to suit the ulcer but often it is helpful to leave them covered for several days or weeks. Practice or community nurses are best qualified to manage these problems. Those who are fit enough may require surgery to prevent recurrence.

e. Occasionally a short course of hydrocortisone 1% may be needed for eczematous lesions.

2. *Surgical*

a. Oestrogen-containing oral contraceptives should be stopped for 4–6 weeks before surgery and not restarted until 2 weeks after the patient is fully mobile.

b. Sclerotherapy with compression is best for minor varices and residual small branches after surgery. It has no value for major veins or veins in the upper thigh. Patients usually need help with their bandaging and must be encouraged to walk three miles (5 km) daily after injection.

c. Patients with major valvular incompetence of the long or short saphenous vein should be treated with surgical ligation and stripping. One-third of patients develop new varices and may require further treatment.

FOLLOW-UP

As varicose veins occur in a large proportion of the adult population the general practitioner can only follow up those with problems. All patients should be encouraged to control their weight. Postoperatively patients should be followed up to check for recurrences, which are extremely common. The main area of general practitioner involvement is in the long-term management of patients with varicose ulcers. Active management can result in complete resolution of the problem. Those patients who wear elasticated stockings should be encouraged to change them regularly as they lose their elasticity.

[1] de Silva *et al.* (1974) *Vasa*, **3**, 118.
[2] Hoare MC *et al.* (1982) *Surgery*, **92**, 450.
[3] *Drug Ther. Bull.* (1989) **27**, 7–8.
[4] Negus D *et al.* (1983) *Br. J. Surg.*, **55**, 777.
[5] Guillebaud J (1985) *Br. Med. J.*, **ii**, 498–9.
[6] Lofgren KA (1978) In *Venous Problems* (Bergan JJ, Yao JST eds). Chicago: Year Book.

Raynaud's Disease and Phenomenon

Raynaud's disease and phenomenon are characterized by attacks of pallor and cyanosis in the fingers (rarely the toes) precipitated by cold and emotional upset. The process is reversed by warming the extremities. During the warming process there may be intense flushing of the skin with some oedema and pain.

Raynaud's disease is a condition seen primarily in women, usually starting in the late teens[1]. It is progressive with symmetrical involvement of the fingers of both hands. The fingers can go into prolonged spasm which is very painful.

Raynaud's phenomenon is always associated with regional or systemic disease, the most common are systemic sclerosis, Sjögren's syndrome, systemic lupus erythematosus and other connective tissue diseases. Occasionally Raynaud's phenomenon is associated with the thoracic outlet syndrome or with the prolonged use of vibrating tools. Early attacks of Raynaud's phenomenon may only involve one or two fingers; however, as the disease progresses more fingers become involved and sometimes the palm of the hand is as well.

PROGNOSIS

- Raynaud's disease has a good prognosis. The condition is not associated with digital gangrene[1] and the pain which occurs at warming is usually short-lived.
- Raynaud's phenomenon has a poorer prognosis depending on the underlying condition. As the disease progresses there may be atrophy of the terminal fat pads in the fingers and gangrenous ulcers may appear on the fingertips[1].

TREATMENT

1. General measures include avoiding cold conditions and wearing protective clothing such as well insulated or heated gloves[2]. Patients with Raynaud's disease should not work with vibrating tools and those who develop vibration white finger should change their job.
2. Some improvement may be gained by stopping smoking.
3. Vasodilator drugs may improve the symptoms in some patients. Bamethan sulphate (25 mg four times daily) or cinnarizine (75 mg three times daily) may be used. Topical glyceryl trinitrate in the form of a slow-release patch (25 mg patch applied every 24 hours) may improve the pain and discomfort associated with warming.
4. Sympathectomy may be indicated if attacks are frequent. However after an initial period of improvement there is often marked deterioration. Sympathectomy is of little value when there is advanced disease of the digital arteries with gangrene.
5. When the underlying cause is a cervical rib, its removal may give a complete cure[3].

FOLLOW-UP

Mild cases need only be seen intermittently. However when there is an underlying collagen disease the patient will require close supervision and regular assessment in hospital.

---

[1] Erskine JM et al. (1987) Blood vessels and lymphatics. In Current Medical Diagnosis and Treatment (Krupp MA ed). Los Altos, California: Appleton & Lange.
[2] Kempson GE et al. (1983) Br. Med. J., ii, 268.
[3] Anonymous (1972) Br Med. J., ii, 782.

Pulmonary Embolism

Pulmonary embolism occurs when material—usually from a deep vein thrombosis—is carried to and impacts in the pulmonary circulation. This represents a medical emergency requiring urgent admission to hospital. A number of factors are associated with pulmonary embolism: surgical procedures (especially abdominal; pelvic and hip surgery); childbirth or prolonged bedrest; oestrogen-containing contraceptive pills; neoplastic disease, and lower limb venous compression (such as during long aeroplane flights). The clinical presentation depends on the severity of the embolus. Many small pulmonary emboli are silent or are associated with pleuritic pain and haemoptysis. Larger emboli can present with sudden onset of chest pain, dyspnoea and haemoptysis; however, only when approximately 50% of the pulmonary vascular tree is involved is there any adverse haemodynamic effect[1]. Progressive dyspnoea, exercise intolerance and syncope are associated with chronic thromboembolic pulmonary hypertension.

PROGNOSIS

- The prognosis from pulmonary embolism depends on a number of factors: the size and severity of the embolism; the duration of symptoms, and the presence of pre-existing cardiorespiratory disease.
- The true incidence is unknown but it has been estimated that 21 000 patients die each year from pulmonary embolism in England and Wales[2].
- The mortality rate from massive pulmonary embolism is in the region of 30%[2]. Most deaths (60%) occur in the first hour following the acute episode[3].
- Prompt admission to hospital with immediate treatment reduces the mortality to approximately 8%[4].
- Most patients who survive the first day have almost complete clinical recovery; however lung scans show that in most patients there is still evidence of residual occlusion at 1 year[4].
- Recurrent pulmonary embolism occurs in 5–10% of patients[5].
- The development of chronic thromboembolic pulmonary hypertension is very rare; it occurs in less than 5% of affected patients[5].

TREATMENT

1. Prevention of embolism is vital. Patients in bed at home should be encouraged to move their limbs and early mobilization should be aimed for.
2. In acute minor embolism (those patients with pleuritic symptoms and signs and/or a small haemoptysis) it is probably wise to admit the patient to hospital for anticoagulation as a more serious embolus may be prevented. When signs have been present for a week or more before the patient is seen, analgesia only is required unless an obvious deep vein thrombosis is present.
3. In all other patients the most important element is early diagnosis and prompt referral. Morphine and oxygen may be required for travel.
4. Patients with severe symptoms or who may have collapsed need to be moved to hospital immediately. They should be started on opiate analgesia at once (morphine 10–15 mg i.m.) and given oxygen (35–60% by nasal catheter or mask). An intravenous line should be set up for the administration of drugs but extreme care should be taken with the quantity of fluid given as right ventricular dilatation and pulmonary oedema can be a problem[1]. Some studies have shown that an intravenous infusion of dextran 70 improves the prognosis[6].
5. An immediate intravenous injection of heparin (15 000 units) has been shown to improve prognosis[7].
6. Surgical embolectomy can be a life-saving operation. It normally takes place under cardiopulmonary bypass and is used in those patients whose prognosis is very poor. In most series the mortality is approximately 26%[1].
7. Thrombolysis using streptokinase (250 000 units i.v. initially followed by 1 000 000 units/hour by slow infusion for 24–48 hours) pro-

duces a more rapid and complete resolution of the embolus[8].

8. The long-term management of acute pulmonary embolism involves the use of the oral anticoagulants. Warfarin (10 mg as a loading dose) should be given on the third day and the subsequent dose should be calculated to keep the prothrombin index between two and three times higher than normal. Patients should be maintained on anticoagulants for at least 3 months.

9. The prevention of deep vein thrombosis and subsequent development of pulmonary embolism is an important part of the postoperative management of patients.

   a. Patients should mobilize early; even before they are out of bed they should have passive exercise to the calf muscles. The use of intermittently inflated air bags on the calf muscle has been shown to reduce the incidence of deep vein thrombosis by half[9].

   b. Adequate fluids and the avoidance of hypovolaemia are important.

   c. Low-dose heparin (5000–8000 units by subcutaneous injection every 8–12 hours) has been shown to reduce the incidence of deep vein thrombosis[10].

   d. The use of low-dose aspirin has been advocated as a means of reducing platelet stickiness and thus the incidence of deep vein thrombosis. However the evidence for a reduction in the incidence is poor and since gastrointestinal complications are a problem, this method of prophylaxis is not recommended[11].

FOLLOW-UP

Most patients who survive the initial thrombosis make a complete recovery, though this may take many months. If they are due to have further surgery they should reduce their weight to an acceptable level and stop smoking. Supervision of anticoagulant treatment is important (see section on deep vein thrombosis) and patients should be advised about problems with this type of treatment. Care should be taken when prescribing other drugs which may interfere with the anticoagulants. Female patients who have had a previous deep vein thrombosis should not be put on oral contraceptive pills. Patients should be encouraged to wear elasticated stockings and to take regular exercise.

[1] Miller G (1988) Pulmonary embolus. In *Diseases of Veins, Pathology, Diagnosis and Treatment* (Browse NL *et al.* eds). London: Edward Arnold.

[2] Barritt DW *et al.* (1960) *Lancet*, **i**, 1309.

[3] Dalen JE *et al.* (1975) *Prog. Cardiovasc. Dis.*, **17**, 259.

[4] Urokinase Pulmonary Embolism Trial (1973) *Circulation*, **47** (suppl II), 1.

[5] Sutton GC *et al.* (1977) *Br. Heart J.*, **39**, 1135.

[6] Skine A *et al.* (1975) *Br Med. J.*, **ii**, 109.

[7] Bergqvist D *et al.* (1979) *Acta Chir. Scand.*, **145**, 213.

[8] Greenfield JL *et al.* (1981) *Arch. Surg.*, **116**, 1451.

[9] Browse NL *et al.* (1976) *Br. Med. J.*, **ii**, 1281.

[10] Bergqvist D (1983) *Postoperative Thromboembolism*, p. 98. Berlin: Springer-Verlag.

[11] Browse NL (1988) Deep vein thrombosis: prevention. In *Diseases of Veins, Pathology, Diagnosis and Treatment.* (Browse NL *et al.* ed). London: Edward Arnold.

5

The Gastrointestinal Tract and Liver

M. H. Kelly

Glossitis

Glossitis is characterized by excessive redness, atrophy of the lingual epithelium, shrinkage of the tongue and fissuring. It is more common in elderly, debilitated or dehydrated patients and gives rise to symptoms of soreness especially after spicy or salted foods. Dysphagia and weight loss may occur in some cases. It is associated with a deficiency of vitamin B_7 (nicotinic acid), vitamin B_2 (riboflavin), vitamin B_{12} (hydroxycobalamin) and folic acid[1] and is therefore a feature of pernicious anaemia, gastrectomy, blind loop syndrome or coeliac disease, Crohn's disease, alcohol abuse, carcinoid syndrome and Paterson–Kelly syndrome[2]. It may also be due to irritation from drugs, or sharp teeth and ill-fitting dentures.

PROGNOSIS

- Most cases improve with treatment of the underlying deficiency or cause.
- The complaint of sore tongue is common and even after full investigation no cause may be found.
- Coeliac patients do not respond to haematinics but to withdrawal of gluten from the diet[3].

TREATMENT

1. Treat underlying deficiency, e.g. with folic acid or mixed vitamin B preparations.
2. Give advice on avoiding spices and flavourings in diet.

FOLLOW-UP

No routine follow-up is required, after investigations to exclude underlying diseases have been carried out.

[1] Read AE, Harvey RF, Naish JM (1981) *Basic Gastroenterology*. Bristol: John Wright.
[2] Bouchier IAD *et al.* (1984) *Textbook of Gastroenterology*. London: Baillière Tindall.
[3] Wray D *et al.* (1975) Recurrent aphthae: treatment with vitamin B_{12}, folic acid and iron. *Br. Med. J.*, **ii**, 490–3.

Gingivitis

Gingivitis is common in those with a poor bite or dental gaps, especially if the diet is mainly bread and soft foods[1]. It is also associated with diseases such as Crohn's disease, coeliac disease, scurvy and kwashiorkor[2]. Symptoms include painful bleeding gums. Acute ulcerative (Vincent's) gingivitis is caused by an overwhelming proliferation of an anaerobic complex of spirochaetes and fusobacteria but is not contagious. It is common in young adults who have neglected their mouths and smoke heavily. If untreated, the infection can rapidly destroy the gingival margins and underlying base.

TREATMENT

1. Replace any underlying deficiency.
2. Dental plaque should be removed and instruction given on correct dental care.
3. Gingivectomy may be necessary.
4. If very severe, affected teeth may be extracted and prostheses fitted.
5. In acute ulcerative gingivitis the administration of metronidazole as well as attention to oral hygiene may hasten resolution.

FOLLOW-UP

No routine follow-up is required.

[1] Read AE, Harvey RF, Naish JM (1981) *Basic Gastroenterology*. Bristol: John Wright.
[2] Bouchier IAD *et al.* (1984) *Textbook of Gastroenterology*. London: Baillière Tindall.

Aphthous ulcer

Aphthous ulcers form in the mucosa of the cheeks, lower lip and underside of the tongue. They may be isolated as a result of trauma or dental treatment but more commonly occur in crops of three or four[1]. Predisposing factors include trauma, stress, nutritional deficiency and/or hormonal imbalance. A family history is found in 25–50% of patients and it is suggested that there is an increased frequency of human leukocyte antigen (HLA)A1, B_{12} and -AW29 in patients with recurrent oral ulcerations[2].

Minor ulcers occur singly and account for 80% of all recurrent aphthous ulcers. Major ulcers are larger in size and number and last for up to 30 days, causing severe pain.

Oral ulceration can occur with systemic diseases such as Behcet's syndrome, Crohn's disease, ulcerative colitis, yersinia infection, coeliac disease and vasculitis. Therefore, the diagnosis of idiopathic recurrent oral ulceration should only be made after a careful clinical examination.

PROGNOSIS

- Usually self-limiting; ulcers resolve from 4–20 days.
- Major ulcers recur more frequently.
- More than 60% of major ulcers heal with fibrosis and scar formation.

TREATMENT

1. *Prodromal stage:* topical steroids such as 0.1% triamcinolone in Orabase or 2.5 mg tablets of hydrocortisone sodium succinate used 3–4 times daily.
2. *Herpetiform ulcers:* tetracycline 250 mg q.i.d.
3. *Symptomatic relief*
   a. local anaesthetic lozenges.
   b. The immunostimulant drug levamisole has been tried but remains to be fully evaluated.
   c. Attempts to suppress ovulation in women have not been successful.
   d. Idiopathic recurrent aphthous ulceration

does not respond to prolonged treatment with iron, vitamin B_{12} or other members of the vitamin B group[3].

FOLLOW-UP

Any ulcer persisting for more than three weeks should be referred for specialist opinion for biopsy.

[1] Read AE, Harvey RF, Naish JM (1981) *Basic Gastroenterology*. Bristol: John Wright.
[2] Bouchier IAD *et al.* (1984) *Textbook of Gastroenterology*. London: Baillière Tindall.
[3] Wray D *et al.* (1975) Recurrent aphthae: treatment with vitamin B_{12}, folic acid and iron. *Br. Med. J.*, **ii,** 490–3.

Oral Thrush

Oral thrush is caused by *Candida albicans*. The mucosa of the upper alimentary tract is infected with resulting destructive changes. Main symptoms include oropharyngeal discomfort and dysphagia. White lesions which mimic lichen planus may be seen in the mouth[1].

Predisposing factors include underlying malignancy, diabetes mellitus, immunological disorders, treatment with antibiotics, steroids or immunosuppressive agents.

PROGNOSIS

- May be acute or chronic and can be associated with a disseminated and life-threatening candidal infection.
- May subside spontaneously if immunosuppression, steroids or antibiotics are discontinued.

TREATMENT

1. Correct underlying predisposing factors.
2. Ingestion of nystatin in viscous solution—1 ml q.i.d.s. The suspension should be in contact with the affected areas for as long as possible.
3. Daktarin gel, 5–10 ml q.d.s., is a useful alterna-

tive if the suspension cannot remain in contact long enough.
4. In severe cases amphotericin B has been successful.

FOLLOW-UP

Most patients with oral thrush do not need specific follow-up. If predisposing factors (e.g. antibiotics) cannot be avoided, prophylactic treatment may need to be considered.

[1] Bouchier IAD *et al.* (1984) *Textbook of Gastroenterology*. London: Baillière Tindall.

Oesophagitis

Oesophagitis is common, especially in obese and elderly people, with or without hiatus hernia. Pain is the most common symptom and may be indistinguishable from angina, especially the atypical (Prinzmetal) variety. Both may be relieved by nitrates, be worse after food and occur at night. Some 35% of patients with oesophageal mucosal pain due to reflux have no demonstrable oesophageal pathological abnormality. Other causes of oesophagitis include infection (e.g. *Candida*, herpes simplex), postirradiation, drug-induced (e.g. tetracycline, ferrous sulphate) and corrosive oesophagitis[1]. Complications of gastro-oesophageal stricture include oesophageal columnar epithelium (Barrett's oesophagus[2]), haemorrhage, stricture, pulmonary aspiration and malnutrition.

PROGNOSIS

- Infants and children with reflux oesophagitis will develop stricture.
- Patients who have failed medical therapy will do well with an antireflux procedure.
- Elderly patients are probably better treated by dilatation; however, this is not without risk of perforation or pneumonia.
- One study showed 73% of patients with severe reflux had a good response to surgery compared to 19% treated medically[3].

TREATMENT

Conservative
1. Reduce weight in the obese.
2. Stop smoking.
3. Avoid large meals.
4. Elevate head-end of bed by 18 cm.
5. Avoid physical activity which provokes reflux.
6. Avoid foods which precipitate reflux, e.g. coffee.
7. Avoid all non-steroidal anti-inflammatory drugs.

Medical
1. Give antacids when symptoms arise. High, frequent dosage regimens have not been shown to treat oesophagitis and are of little additional value.
2. Clinical trials have failed to show that metoclopramide is any more effective than a placebo in adults.
3. H$_2$ receptor antagonists are of greater value.
4. Cytoprotective agents such as sucralfate and carbenoxolone show encouraging results.

Surgery
1. Surgery is generally successful, especially if the patient is less than 50 years, fit, and with severe symptoms.
2. Overall success of surgery is dependent on the experience and technique of the surgeon.
3. Most operations act by restoring a zone of high pressure above the cardia. Three common operations are:
   a. 180° wrap and posterior gastropexy of Hill—less than 1% recurrence and less than 0.5% mortality[4].
   b. 270° wrap of the Belsey mark IV—good results in 84% over a 10-year period and a recurrence rate of 11%[5].
   c. 360° wrap of Nissen—87.5% were free of symptoms in the long term[6].
4. Comparisons between Belsey mark IV and Nissen favour the latter[7].
5. Angelchick prosthesis has been used and appears to be as effective as fundoplication for reflux control, but complications are common[8].
6. Polygastrectomy en Roux with vagotomy in presence of stricture and shortened oesophagus.

FOLLOW-UP

Advice should be given on dietary habits and avoidance of gaseous drinks. Elderly patients requiring dilatation should be carefully monitored.

[1] Dodds WJ et al. (1981) Gastroenterology, 81, 376–94.
[2] Sjorgron RW, Johnson LF (1983) Am. J. Med., 74, 313–21.
[3] Behar J et al. (1975) N. Engl. J. Med., 293, 263–8.
[4] Hill LD (1977) World J. Surg, 1, 425–36.
[5] Belsey R (1977) World J. Surg, 1, 475–81.
[6] Rossetti M et al. (1977) World J. Surg, 1, 439–43.
[7] Dilling EW et al. (1977) Am. J. Surg., 134, 730–3.
[8] Morris DL et al. (1985) Br. J. Surg., 72, 1017–20.

Hiatus Hernia

A total of 90% of cases of hiatus hernia are of the 'sliding' variety in which the gastro-oesophageal junction is intrathoracic and predisposes to pathological reflux. In the 'rolling' type the gastro-oesophageal junction is within the abdominal cavity and part of the gastric fundus protrudes through the hiatus into the thoracic cavity.

PROGNOSIS

- Most sliding hernias are asymptomatic.
- The size of the hernia is not related to the severity of symptoms[1].
- Sliding herniae are of little pathological significance apart from the symptoms they cause.
- Rolling herniae carry a significant risk of strangulation.
- Chronic blood loss due to erosive gastritis secondary to venous stasis in the herniated part may occur.
- Less commonly, an ulcer at the neck of the hernia can develop and lead to massive haemorrhage or perforation into the mediastinum.

TREATMENT

1. *Conservative*
   a. Reduce weight in the obese.
   b. Stop smoking.
   c. Avoid large meals.
   d. Elevate head of bed by 18 cm.
   e. Avoid foods which precipitate reflux.
   f. Avoid all non-steroidal anti-inflammatory drugs.
2. *Medical*
   a. Antacids can give symptomatic relief.
   b. H_2-receptor antagonists are of value.
3. *Surgery*
   a. Most patients with sliding hernia require no surgery. Indications for surgery include: failure of medical treatment, dysphagia, ulceration or bleeding[2].
   b. Rolling herniae require surgery because of the risk of strangulation.
   c. Surgery aims to restore a zone of high pressure above the cardia.
   d. 180° wrap and posterior gastropexy of Hill has a recurrence rate of less than 1% and mortality of less than 0.5%[3].
   f. 270° wrap of the Belsey mark IV has good results in 84% of patients over 10 years and a recurrence rate of 11%[4].
   g. 360° wrap of Nissen—87.5% of patients are free of symptoms in the long term[5].
   h. Angelchick prosthesis produces a decrease in postplication ulcers, but further trials are needed[6].

FOLLOW-UP

Follow-up is only necessary for patients with moderate and severe reflux and those who have required surgery. Careful advice should be given on their dietary habits, encouraging patients to chew food properly and avoiding gaseous drinks. The importance of maintaining an ideal weight should be stressed.

[1] Ellis H (1986) *Postgrad. Med. J.*, **727**, 325–7.
[2] Garstin WIH et al. (1986) *J. R. Coll. Surg. Edin.*, **31**, 207–9.
[3] Hill LD (1977) *World J. Surg.*, **1**, 425–36.
[4] Belsey R (1977) *World J. Surg.*, **1**, 475–81.
[5] Rossetti M et al. (1977) *World J. Surg.*, **1**, 439–43.
[6] Green MW (1984) *Br. J. Surg.*, **71**, 681–3.

Dyspepsia

Dyspepsia is a global term used to describe a variety of symptoms such as upper abdominal pain, heartburn, anorexia, nausea and vomiting, flatulence and dysphagia. There are many possible causes including oesophageal disease, gastric ulcer, duodenal ulcer, gallstones, irritable bowel syndrome, alcohol excess, extra-abdominal disease and non-organic dyspepsia. The incidence of non-ulcer dyspepsia is 30–50%[1].

PROGNOSIS

- The prognosis depends on the underlying cause.
- Some 25% of patients with irritable bowel syndrome present with dyspepsia and 5% with dysphagia.
- Patients with pain before diagnosis are significantly more likely to have pain during follow-up.
- Patients taking medication for dyspepsia and the development of gastro-oesophageal reflux are associated with more days of pain.
- Demographic and environmental factors, length of dyspeptic history and past history of ulcer are of no significant prognostic value[2].
- The natural history of non-ulcer dyspepsia is that patients improve.

TREATMENT

1. Accurate history, examination and investigation to elucidate the cause.
2. For dyspepsia caused by gastro-oesophageal reflux:
   a. Elevate the head of bed.
   b. Encourage weight loss.
   c. Decrease smoking and caffeine intake.
   d. Antacids may be of benefit.
   e. Trial of H$_2$ antagonists may be of value.
3. For dyspepsia caused by dysmotility:
   a. Metoclopramide or domperidone can be used.

b. Trials of cisapride show encouraging results[3].
4. For ulcer-like dyspepsia:
   a. H$_2$ antagonists such as cimetidine or ranitidine are used. Treatment with ranitidine for 6 weeks gives complete remission in 80% of patients with non-ulcer dyspepsia[1].
5. For dyspepsia related to aerophagia:
   a. Give advice on sipping fluids.
   b. The condition may be helped by treating underlying depression[4].
6. For idiopathic dyspepsia:
   a. Counselling has a place.
   b. H$_2$ antagonists may be of value. Trials have shown that placebo can decrease pain in 25% and either antacids nor cimetidine improved these results by more than 4%[5].

FOLLOW-UP

Routine follow-up is not required unless the symptoms fail to respond to medical therapy or the patient complains of weight loss. In such cases thorough investigations should be carried out.

[1] Saunders JWB et al. (1986) Br. Med. J., **292**, 665–8.
[2] Talley NJ et al. (1987) Gastroenterology, **4**, 1060–6.
[3] Colin-Jones DG et al. (1988) Lancet, **i**, 576–9.
[4] Editorial (1986) Lancet, **i**, 1306–7.
[5] Nyren O et al. (1986) N. Engl. J. Med., **6**, 339–43.

Oesophageal Cancer

In the UK, the overall incidence of oesophageal cancer ranges from 5 to 10 cases per 100 000 people, or 2.5% of all malignant disease. The incidence varies greatly throughout the world, being highest in China, parts of Africa and the Caspian region of Iran. It is more common in males than females (in a ratio of approximately 4:1) and median age for both is 68 years. The majority of malignant tumours occur in the middle (50%) and lower third (25%) of the oesophagus. They are usually squamous carcinomas but adenocarcinomas occur in the lower third and at the cardia. There is increased incidence of malignancy associated with oesophageal strictures due to corrosive ingestion as well as postirradiation, achalasia, Paterson–Kelly syndrome (hypochromic anaemia and postcricoid web), excessive consumption of alcohol and smoking. Persistent progressive dysphagia with weight loss are the cardinal symptoms. Diagnosis involves radiology and endoscopy. Metastasis is either by direct spread to neighbouring strictures or via lymphatics to local lymph nodes of the liver[1].

PROGNOSIS

- Metastases, mainly to regional lymph nodes, are found in 50% of cases at the time of diagnosis.
- Although preoperative staging for suitability for resection is unreliable, the presence of hoarseness (recurrent laryngeal nerve involvement), aspiration (tracheobronchial fistula) and the involvement of supraclavicular lymph nodes indicate incurable disease.
- Results of surgical treatment depend on the site and histology of the tumour, with mortality varying from 10 to 30%.
- Curative surgery can only be performed in 20% of all cases of oesophageal cancer.
- Selection of suitable cases for surgical treatment remains difficult but has been helped by the advent of computerized tomography scanning.
- Overall 5-year survival for all cases is less than 5%.
- A 20% survival at 5 years following x-ray therapy for squamous carcinoma using megavoltage radiation has been reported. But there is no evidence at present that combining irradiation or chemotherapy with surgery improves prognosis.

TREATMENT

1. *Surgery*
   a. Often only symptomatic palliation is possible.
   b. Dilating the stricture endoscopically and inserting a tube (Atkinson and Celestin) through the tumour is often sufficient for the short life expectancy of the patients.
   c. An alternative approach to maintaining a lumen is by laser photocoagulation. Symptomatic results are satisfactory but this approach may require repeated treatments.
   d. Surgical palliation for squamous carcinoma at any level either by insertion of a tube or by resection and anastomosis of oesophagus and stomach has a high operative mortality (approximately 30%) and long-term results are poor.
   e. Surgical resection is the treatment of choice for adenocarcinoma of the lower oesophageal segment (mortality 10%)[2].
2. *Radiotherapy*
   a. Squamous carcinoma is radiosensitive.
   b. Radiotherapy is mainly favoured for upper-third lesions.
   c. Long-term results of radical treatment are no better than surgery although there is a lower mortality (1–9%)[3].
   d. Long-term problems include fibrous stricture and osteitis of spine.
3. *Chemotherapy:* squamous carcinoma is sensitive to bleomycin, cisplatinum, Mitomycin C and 5FU but chemotherapy has not been shown to improve long-term survival[4].

FOLLOW-UP

This mainly includes advice as to suitable diet of soft and liquidized foods and support and coun-

lling for the patient and relatives. Home care
am or hospice admission may be needed in the
rminal phase.

Vantrappen G et al. (1974) Diseases of Oesophagus.
erlin: Springer Verlag.

[2] Duranceau AC (ed) (1983) Surg. Clin. North Am., **63**, 4.
[3] Pearson JG (1981) World J. Surg., **5**, 489.
[4] Anderson AP et al. (1984) Radiotherapy Oncol., **2**, 179.

Peptic Ulcer

This term describes any break in the mucosa either in the duodenum or the stomach. Some 0% of the population suffer from duodenal ulceration[1] and peptic ulceration accounts for approximately 5000 deaths annually in England and Wales. Peptic ulceration tends to be a chronic illness with relapses and remissions.

Duodenal ulcers tend to present with pain while gastric ulcers may present as a chronic anaemia and tend to be more common between the ages of 55 and 65 years.

PROGNOSIS

Duodenal ulcers
- 65% relapse within 1 year of the ulcer healing.
- 15% give a history of haemorrhage.
- 1% perforate but in the age group 50–60 this figure increases to 10%[2].
- 77% heal after 4 weeks' treatment with H_2 antagonists and 95% after 2 months' treatment.
- Maintenance treatment with H_2 antagonists reduces the relapse rate from 8.5% each month to 2.5%.
- Smoking and non-compliance with therapy have an adverse effect on healing and relapse[4].
- Poor prognostic factors include previous complications and early relapse.
- The risk of a serious complication is 20% with chronic duodenal ulcer.
- Surgery cures duodenal ulcer in 90–95% of patients for 10 years or more.
- Perforation in elderly patients has a mortality rate of up to 30%[5].
- 90% of patients with pyloric stenosis require surgical intervention[6].
- 5% of patients fail to heal with drug treatment.

Gastric ulcers
- If untreated, 45% of ulcers heal by 6 weeks.
- If treated, 60–80% of ulcers are healed by 6 weeks[8–10].
- The recurrence rate is 55–89% in a 12-month period[11].

- The main complications of gastric ulcer are haemorrhage and perforation.
- 15% of gastric ulcers are malignant so all cases must undergo endoscopy and biopsy to exclude this possibility.
- Surgery for benign gastric ulcer gives 95% cure for 10 years or more.

TREATMENT

General
1. Diet: there is little evidence to suggest that dietary manipulation affects ulcer healing. Patients with duodenal ulcer have an exaggerated acid response to eating, so they should eat three normal meals per day and avoid food last thing at night.
2. Smoking delays the healing of gastric ulcers and also of duodenal ulcers treated with cimetidine. Advise patients to stop smoking.
3. Patients should be advised to take alcohol in moderation.
4. Patients should avoid non-steroidal anti-inflammatory drugs, aspirin and steroids.

Medical
1. H_2 antagonists
   a. For duodenal ulcers, cimetidine 800 mg or ranitidine 300 mg nocte are used for 8 weeks[3]. The nocturnal dose has been shown to be as effective as divided daytime

doses[12,13]. Omperazole is a more profound inhibitor of gastric acid secretion and trials have shown complete and rapid healing of duodenal ulcers[14]. Famotidine and nizatidine are also being evaluated. On 400 mg cimetidine nocte, duodenal ulcers recur in 45% of patients in 1 year and 54% at 2 years; half without symptoms[15]. Increasing the dose of cimetidine for chronic ulcers does not increase the drug's antisecretory effect[16,17].

  b. In gastric ulcers cimetidine is given 1 g/day in divided doses or ranitidine 150 mg b.d. for 6–8 weeks. Maintenance therapy of cimetidine 400 mg nocte or ranitidine 150 mg nocte will usually prevent recurrence but is mainly reserved for elderly patients or those unfit for surgery.

  c. It has been suggested that the use of H$_2$ antagonists on demand may provide adequate long-term treatment, without continuous exposure to medication. Long-term studies are awaited.

2. Bismuth: Tripotassium dicitrate bisthmuthate (De-Nol) 1 tablet q.d.s. has been shown to heal gastric ulcers. It may also heal the 20% of duodenal ulcers which fail to respond to H$_2$ antagonists[7,18].

3. Sucralfate 1 g q.d.s. speeds peptic ulcer healing by an unknown mechanism.

4. Antacids are mainly used for the symptomatic relief of dyspepsia.

5. Anticholinergics: Pirenzepine 50 mg b.d. is useful in those who fail to respond to conventional H$_2$ antagonists. When used in combination with ranitidine it increases the antisecretory effect of ranitidine[19].

Surgery

1. Duodenal ulcer
  a. Surgery is indicated if medical treatment fails, or when complications develop. Some 15% of duodenal ulcers require surgery.
  b. The most common operations performed are truncal vagotomy and drainage and highly selective vagotomy. Mortality rates are 1–2% and less than 1% respectively.
  c. Recurrence rate varies from 1–10%.
  d. Epigastric fullness occurs in 33% of patients regardless of operation.
  e. Dumping syndrome is common after truncal vagotomy and drainage and overall can affect 20–40% of patients postoperatively[20]. In many it improves but 5% are incapacitated.

2. *Gastric ulcer*
  a. Partial gastrectomy by Bilroth I or II is the operation of choice.
  b. Mortality following surgery is <1%.
  c. Recurrence rate is 2–4% for partial gastrectomy.
  d. Prepyloric ulcers are treated by vagotomy with atrectomy or partial gastrectomy.
  e. Perforated gastric ulcers have a 10% incidence of malignancy and should not be treated by simple closure.

FOLLOW-UP

1. Gastric ulcer: following medical treatment endoscopy should be carried out at 8 weeks to assess healing, and biopsies should be taken to exclude malignancy. Follow-up should be continued until the ulcer is healed completely.

2. Duodenal ulcer: endoscopy is indicated when the ulcer fails to heal or symptoms are atypical.

3. Surgery: advice is often required for dumping syndrome (early and late). Early symptoms can be avoided by dietary advice, e.g. decreasing carbohydrate in meals and fluid intake. Late symptoms are avoided by sucking sweets. Diarrhoea is helped by dietary advice. Biliary gastritis may respond to metoclopramide or domperidone. Regular blood tests are required to exclude anaemia; vitamin B$_{12}$ therapy may be needed following partial gastrectomy.

[1] Hirschowitz B (1983) *Gastroenterology*, **85**, 967–71.
[2] McKay AJ et al. (1982) *Br. J. Surg.*, **69**, 319–20.
[3] Gough KR et al. (1984) *Lancet*, **ii**, 659–62.
[4] Pounder RE (1981) *Lancet*, **i**, 29–30.
[5] Drury JK et al. (1978) *Lancet*, **ii**, 749–50.
[6] Jaffin BW et al. (1985) *Ann. Surg.*, **201**, 176–9.
[7] Pounder RE (1984) *Gut*, **25**, 697–9.
[8] Littman A (1983) *N. Engl. J. Med.*, **308**, 1356–7.
[9] Isenberg J et al. (1983) *N. Engl. J. Med.*, **308**, 1319–24.
[10] Feely J et al. (1983) *Br. Med. J.*, **286**, 695–7.
[11] Shearman DJC et al. (1982) *Disease of the Gastrointestinal Tract and Liver*. London: Churchill Livingstone.
[12] Burland WL (1980) *Postgrad. Med. J.*, **56**, 173–6.
[13] Ireland A (1984) *Gut*, **25**, A581.
[14] Gustavsson S et al. (1983) *Lancet*, **ii**, 124–5.
[15] Bardhan KD (1981) *Cimetidine in the 80s*. Edinburgh: Churchill Livingstone.

Pounder RE et al. (1975) Lancet, ii, 1069–70.
Peterson WL et al. (1979) Gastroenterology, **77**,
915–20.
Pounder RE (1984) Gut, **25**, 697–9.

[19] Gledhill T et al. (1984) Gut, **25**, 1211–15.
[20] Sleisenger MH et al. (1973) Gastrointestinal Disease.
Philadelphia: WB Saunders.

Gastric Cancer

Gastric carcinoma is the third most fatal cancer in the UK, affecting 20 per 100 000 males per year and is responsible for 10% of all deaths from malignant disease. The highest incidence is found in Japan. Gastric cancer is said to be 'early' when it is limited to the mucosa or submucosa; 50% of patients have symptoms at this point. Early gastric cancer progresses to a more advanced gastric carcinoma with penetration of the muscle coats or beyond[1]. In order to detect gastric cancer at an early stage the Japanese have employed a programme for early diagnosis using barium meal and endoscopy. The diagnostic yield is 1 per 1000 examinees but since more than 50% are early cancers this has led to a reduction in mortality from gastric carcinoma in individuals[2].

Premalignant conditions include dysplasia, atrophic gastritis, adenomatous polyps, pernicious anaemia, intestinal metaplasia and postgastrectomy. There remains an association between gastric ulceration and carcinoma, although it is now thought that the likeliest cause of this association is a secondary ulceration of an enlarging cancer. There is little evidence to suggest that benign gastric ulcers are premalignant, but since ulcerating gastric ulcers are slow-growing and the ulcer appearance is often benign, cancers are commonly misdiagnosed as benign ulcers[3]. Careful endoscopic review of all gastric ulcers with multiple biopsies will minimize this risk. The earliest symptoms may be slight and intermittent. Dyspepsia is a common presenting symptom. In 80% of advanced cancers there may be fullness after meals, loss of appetite and epigastric discomfort relieved by antacids.

PROGNOSIS

- Early gastric cancers have over 90% 5-year survival, even if local lymph nodes are involved.
- Extramural lymphatics allow spread to lymph nodes in more than 50% of operable cases and the presence of involved lymph nodes reduces the 5-year survival rate from 40% to 15%.
- Absolute curative resection has a 77% 5-year survival rate.
- Palliative procedures with proven residual tumour carry a 6% 5-year survival rate.
- Tumour recurrence is the main cause of death after an attempted curative gastrectomy.
- Up to 25% of cases have recurrence in the gastric stump due to multicentric tumours or residual cancer at the anastomotic site.
- Objective evidence of distant spread is the only preoperative indication of incurability.

TREATMENT

1. *Surgery*
   a. This offers the only method of cure but can usually be offered to less than 50% of patients.
   b. Lesions in the distal two-thirds should be removed by subtotal gastrectomy with omentum, spleen and relevant nodes.
   c. Lesions in the proximal third require total gastrectomy with removal of omentum, spleen and relevant nodes en bloc.
   d. The pancreatic body and tail is resected when extension to it or to the retropancreatic nodes is suspected.
   e. A 5 cm microscopic clearance of the tumour is required.
   f. Palliative procedures are all that can be offered in 50% of cases.
   g. Resection (but not total gastrectomy), by-

pass or intubation can be used to relieve obstruction, haemorrhage and pain. Resection provides the best palliation except for proximal tumours. Intubation relieves a proximal obstruction. Endoscopic intubation is best when objective evidence of incurable disease or resectability is present.

2. Radiotherapy is beneficial in a few patients with resected, residual disease or irresectable, localized disease. Studies comparing adjuvant radiotherapy with surgery alone and adjuvant radiotherapy with surgery followed by combination chemotherapy are in progress.

3. *Chemotherapy*
   a. In advanced disease, single-agent therapy is ineffective.
   b. Although 20–30% response rates have been reported with fluorouracil, Mitomycin, carmustine, cisplatin and Adriamycin— there has been no increase in survival.
   c. Response rates are higher with combination therapy but again no improvement in survival has followed their use in advanced disease[4].

FOLLOW-UP

Some 20% of patients experienced postprandial dumping syndrome after gastrectomy and therefore require dietary advice. Supplemental iron and vitamin B_{12} may prevent anaemia developing following gastrectomy. The main requirement for follow-up is support and counselling for the patient and family.

[1] Correa P et al. (1977) Lancet, **ii,** 58–60.
[2] Jass JR (1980) J. Clin. Pathol., **33,** 801–10.
[3] Hisamuchi S et al. (1978) Tokoho J. Exp. Med., **118** (suppl), 69.
[4] Wrigley PFM et al. (1984) Clin. Oncol., **3,** no. 2.

Irritable Bowel Syndrome

The term irritable bowel syndrome describes abdominal pain or discomfort associated with alteration in bowel habit but with no underlying pathology[1]. The prevalence is not known but 20–30% of 'normal' individuals have been found to have symptoms compatible with this syndrome on at least 1 day in 4[2]. The female to male ratio is 2.5:1. The usual presentation occurs in the mid 30s and seldom above the age of 50. Rectal bleeding is not a feature.

PROGNOSIS

- Up to 25% of patients date symptoms to an episode of proven or presumed gastroenteritis although no evidence of persisting infection is found. These patients have a better prognosis and permanent remission is more likely.
- 10% of patients show hypolactasia (the same proportion as in the general population) and do not respond to a lactose-free diet.
- 50% of patients are aware of a link with emotional stress.
- 70% of patients have been found to suffer from depression—especially women—and they are more likely to have considered suicide[3,4].
- Less than 30% of patients will be symptom-free within 1 year of attending a hospital clinic.
- Many patients have symptoms for years.

- The best response to treatment is seen in men, those with predominant constipation and those with a short history[5].

TREATMENT

1. Older patients should have a barium enema and sigmoidoscopy to exclude other pathologies.
2. A response rate of 30–50% has been seen following the use of placebo drugs.
3. A gradual increase in fibre intake is recommended[6].
4. Stool softeners and bulking agents such as ispaghula husk and lactulose may help constipation.
5. Pain and distension may be helped by antispas-

modics, e.g. mebeverine or enteric-coated peppermint oil. Treatment should be for the short term.

- Loperamide 2 mg b.d. or codeine phosphate 30 mg may help diarrhoea[7].
- Relaxation therapy, hypnosis and psychotherapy have all been shown to be useful.
- Antidepressants can cause an impressive improvement.
- Anticholinergics are of limited value and have adverse effects[8].

FOLLOW-UP

Most patients do not require regular follow-up but some may benefit from an occasional supportive review without the need for further investigation or treatment.

[1] Manning KP et al. (1978) Br. Med. J., 2, 653–4.
[2] Thompson WG, Heaton KW (1980) Gastroenterology, 79, 283–8.
[3] Young SJ et al. (1978) Gastroenterology, 70, 162–6.
[4] Barsky AJ (1987) Gastroenterology, 93, 902–4.
[5] Harvey RF et al. (1987) Lancet, i, 963–5.
[6] Conn PA et al. (1984) Gut, 25, 168–73.
[7] Conn PA et al. (1984) Dig. Dis. Sci., 29, 239–47.
[8] Ivey KJ (1975) Gastroenterology, 86, 1300–7.

Crohn's Disease

Crohn's disease is a chronic inflammatory disorder of unknown aetiology which can affect any part of the gastrointestinal tract. It is frequently a recurrent disease and has a tendency to form abscesses and fistulae. It is predominantly found in north-west Europe, North America, Australia, New Zealand and the white population of South Africa. The prevalence is 50 per 100 000 people. It affects young adults—males as commonly as females—and is more common in the higher socioeconomic groups[1]. Genetic factors are thought to be important; 15–40% of patients have relatives with either ulcerative colitis or Crohn's disease. Crohn's disease may present with obstructive symptoms as a result of stricture and 65% of patients have perianal disease with fissures. Most patients complain of diarrhoea (70–90%), abdominal pain (45–66%), and weight loss (65–75%). Colonic disease causes rectal bleeding more commonly than ileal disease and has a higher incidence of extraintestinal manifestations[2].

PROGNOSIS

- Increased disease activity can be diagnosed by finding a reduced serum albumin, a rise in acute-phase reactants (C-reactive protein, orosomucoid), and an elevated erythrocyte sedimentation rate[3].
- A number of indices have been developed in an attempt to standardize assessment. These are the American Crohn's Disease Activity Index and the Dutch Activity Index but they are still at the developmental phase and are too complex for normal clinical use.
- Patients are never cured of Crohn's disease and are subject to relapse and recurrence even following surgical resection.
- Most patients (70–80%) receive surgical treatment at some point during the course of their illness.
- Following resection, the disease recurs in 30% of patients during the subsequent 5 years and in 50% of patients during the subsequent 10 years. Half will require further surgery[4].
- Patients with Crohn's colitis who have proctocolectomy appear to have a lower risk of recurrence than those who have an ileal or ileocolic resection.
- The overall mortality varies from 10 to 15% in different studies. In general, most patients with Crohn's disease have a good prognosis and a mortality which is only about twice that expected, but the disease does carry a considerable morbidity.
- Carcinoma of the colon may complicate

Crohn's colitis with an incidence of about 3–5%, especially in those with extensive long-standing disease.

TREATMENT

1. *Medical*
   a. The role of diet is controversial. Patients should have a well balanced diet: a low residue diet is recommended for those with strictures, and a low fat diet for those with steatorrhoea.
   b. Deficiencies of folic acid, vitamin B_{12} and iron should be treated with appropriate supplements.
   c. Corticosteroids are indicated in symptomatic patients. In the presence of severe disease they may be given intravenously. Patients with less severe disease can be treated with prednisolone 20–40 mg daily by mouth. This should be maintained until a good symptomatic response is achieved. The doses can then be reduced over 4–6 weeks and stopped.
   d. Sulphasalazine (Salazopyrin) has been shown to have some effect on active colonic Crohn's disease but there is no evidence that long-term treatment with either corticosteroids or sulphasalazine is beneficial.
   e. Azathioprine is ineffective in the treatment of active disease and also controversial. It can be used as a maintenance therapy if other treatments have failed or surgical treatment is inappropriate[5].
   f. Other treatments include levamisole, dapsone, transfer factor and cromoglycate but there is little evidence to support their use.
   g. Metronidazole is useful in the treatment of perianal sepsis and abscesses associated with fistulae but it has no direct effect on the disease process.
2. *Surgery*
   a. Indications for surgery include: failure to respond to medical therapy and continuing symptoms; strictures causing mechanical obstruction; fistulae; local complications such as abscess and perforation and toxic megacolon; remote manifestations (iritis, arthritis, erythema nodosum, pyoderma gangrenosum); growth retardation.
   b. Surgery should be limited to removing the most severely affected bowel; end-to-end anastomosis should be performed if at all possible[6].
   c. Bypass procedures, for example ileo transverse colostomy, are associated with a high risk of recurrence.
   d. Proctocolectomy may be required for extensive Crohn's colitis and this operation is preferable to an anastomosis.
   e. The extent of surgical resection depends on the site of the Crohn's disease, but a 10% normal margin on either side of the disease is optimal.
   f. Short bowel strictures may be treated with stricture-plasty at numerous sites along the bowel length.

FOLLOW-UP

There should be regular outpatient attendance under the combined care of both surgeon and physician. These visits are required for correction of deficiencies, psychological support for the patient and family, and stoma care if necessary. Self-help groups are available in various parts of the UK (e.g. CICRA Crohn's in Childhood Research Appeal) offers support for parents of children with inflammatory bowel disease. Contact address: CICRA, 48 Ewell Downs Road, Ewell, Epsom, Surrey, KT17 3BN).

[1] Kirshar JB et al. (1982) N. Engl. J. Med., **306**, 837–48.
[2] Allan RN et al. (1983) Inflammatory Bowel Diseases. Edinburgh: Churchill Livingstone.
[3] Bouchier IAD (1983) Recent Advances in Gastroenterology. Edinburgh: Churchill Livingstone.
[4] Springall R (1986) Br. J. Hosp. Med., **35**, 220–6.
[5] Donald IP, Wilkinson SP (1985) Postgrad. Med. J., **61**, 1047–8.
[6] Kirshar JB et al. (1982) N. Engl. J. Med., **306**, 775–85.

Ulcerative Colitis

Ulcerative colitis is a chronic inflammatory disease of unknown aetiology affecting the rectal mucosa. It can spread proximally from the rectum in a continuous manner to involve part or all of the colon. Incidence is 5–8 per 100 000 of the population; prevalence is 2–3/1000 and the condition develops after puberty. Its course is characterized by periods of remission and relapse. Mucosal changes vary from inflammation to crypt abscesses and pseudopolyps. Cardinal symptoms include the passage of blood per rectum with diarrhoea. Diagnosis is made by sigmoidoscopy and biopsy and the extent of colonic involvement is assessed by barium enema and colonoscopy. Ulcerative colitis can be associated with a seronegative arthritis in 25%. Up to 54% of patients are positive for HLA-B27 typing.

PROGNOSIS

- Approximately 10% of patients suffer from continuous symptoms which vary in severity.
- A few patients will have no further symptoms after the initial attack.
- In all, 70% have chronic, intermittent illness with relapses separated by periods of remission.
- Approximately 10% have a fulminating episode leading to early surgery.
- Prognosis for individual attacks is related to severity, extent of disease and the patient's age. A patient who is over 60 years with severe extensive disease has a poor prognosis.
- Some 20% of all patients with colitis are treated by proctocolectomy within the first 10 years of the illness because of acute or chronic symptoms.
- One-third of patients with extensive disease will have surgical resection at some point.
- There is an association with ulcerative colitis and development of carcinoma, although it is thought that this has been overemphasized[1].

If disease is limited to the left side of the colon there is no increased risk in the development of neoplasm. The risk of developing cancer with extensive disease of 10 years' duration is 1 in 200 each year; when the disease is of 10–20 years' duration, the risk becomes 1 in 60 each year. The main factors associated with this high risk are a severe first attack, involvement of the entire colon, chronic continuous symptoms, and onset of the colitis in childhood or early adult life[2].

TREATMENT

1. *Mild attack*
   a. Oral steroids such as prednisolone 5 mg four times a day should be started, along with Predsol retention enemas nightly[3].
   b. Sulphasalazine is given in a dose of 500 mg four times a day and should be continued as maintenance therapy as the corticosteroids are being decreased.
2. *Moderate attack*
   a. The patient should be admitted to hospital.
   b. Higher doses of oral prednisolone should be given with twice-daily treatment of topical corticosteroid.
   c. This should be continued for a total period of 1 month before being decreased, and sulphasalazine should be continued as maintenance therapy.
3. *Severe attack*
   a. This requires intensive intravenous therapy with electrolytes, blood transfusion and if required, parenteral feeding[4].
   b. Intravenous corticosteroids should be given for 5 days and as the patient responds this should be substituted with oral prednisolone.
   c. The oral steroids should be continued for 1 month and then gradually phased out; again sulphasalazine is used as maintenance therapy.
   d. Failure to respond to this intensive treatment, the occurrence of perforation of the colon, or severe toxic megacolon are indications for emergency colectomy. Subtotal colectomy and ileostomy is the procedure of choice, leaving the rectum in situ. The risk of infection and death is high when more radical surgery is performed.
4. *Maintenance therapy*
   a. Sulphasalazine is the mainstay of treatment in ulcerative colitis and is normally given in

doses of 2 g a day. This results in the recurrence rate being reduced to a quarter of the rate experienced without treatment. The suppressive effect of sulphasalazine appears to persist indefinitely and therefore long-term maintenance therapy is advisable[5].

b. Amino salicylic acid in doses of 400 mg three times a day is also useful in maintenance of clinical remission without the side-effects of sulphasalazine[6].

c. Disodium cromoglycate (Intal or Narcrom) has been shown in large trials to have some limited value.

d. Immunosuppressive drugs, such as azathioprine, have also some limited value in reducing the relapse rate.

5. *Surgery*

Indications for surgery include:

a. Emergency colectomy for reasons indicated above.

b. Elective colectomy for chronic continuous symptoms, frequent troublesome attacks, severe fistula-in-ano, rectal vaginal fistula or other pararectal complications, and cancer of the colon. The surgical procedure most commonly used is proctocolectomy with a permanent ileostomy. When performed electively the operative mortality is about 2%[7].

c. The ileostomy may be a standard ileostomy emptying into a bag or continent ileostomy where the terminal small intestine is converted into an internal pouch opening into the skin as an inconspicuous mucus fistula[8].

d. Colectomy and ileorectal anastomosis runs the risk that the retained rectum may develop carcinoma. But colectomy and ileo-anal anastomosis has shown encouraging results. It is associated with some type of intestinal pouch which acts as a reservoir proximal to the rectum. It has the advantage of preserving defecation through the anus and at the same time avoiding the risk of subsequent cancer inherent in ileorectal anastomosis.

FOLLOW-UP

Patients with mild disease require an annual check-up with sigmoidoscopy. Cancer surveillance should be carried out in patients who have had colitis for more than 10 years. They should have an annual colonoscopy with biopsy at 10 cm intervals. Patients who have proctitis alone require no regular follow-up and those who have a rectal stump following surgery require annual sigmoidoscopy and biopsy. Self-help groups are also available, such as National Association for Colitis, 98A London Road, St Albans, Hertfordshire, AL1 1NX and the Ileostomy Association, Amblehurst House, Black Scotch Lane, Mansfield, Notts NG1 4PF (telephone: 0623 28099).

[1] Allan RN et al. (1983) Inflammatory Bowel Disease. Edinburgh: Churchill Livingstone.
[2] Smart WL, Mayberry JF (1986) Arch. Int. Med., 146, 651–2.
[3] Somerville KW et al. (1985) Br. Med. J., 291, 866.
[4] Jarnerot G et al. (1985) Gastroenterology, 89, 1005–13.
[5] Azad Khan A et al. (1980) Gut, 21, 232–40.
[6] Donald IP, Wilkinson SP (1985) Postgrad. Med. J., 61, 1047–8.
[7] Kirshnar JB et al. (1982) N. Engl. J. Med., 306, 775–82.
[8] Springall R (1986) Br. J. Hosp. Med., 35, 220–6.

Carcinoma of the Colon and Rectum

Carcinoma of the colon and rectum is the commonest gastrointestinal malignancy in the Western world. The lifetime risk of developing large bowel carcinoma is 4%; the risk is low in those aged under 40 and increases steeply each decade thereafter. There are 21 000 new cases in the UK annually with a mortality rate of 30–35 per 100 000 per year[1]. Most colonic carcinomas develop from benign adenomas. The size of the polyps, histological type and degree of epithelial dysplasia determine whether a benign adenoma will undergo malignant change[2]. High-risk groups include those over 40 years of age with first-degree relative affected, those with colonic polyps, those already treated for cancer, those with long-standing inflammatory bowel disease and members of families with polyposis coli and Gardner's syndrome. Sigmoid colon is the most common site for cancer. Presentation includes change in bowel habit, rectal bleeding or obstruction. Right-sided lesions present at a later stage with occult anaemia, vague abdominal pain and a palpable mass. Screening for bowel cancer can be carried out by doing faecal occult bloods and following positive results with colonoscopy.

PROGNOSIS

- Prognosis is influenced by a number of factors present at the time of presentation, such as age of patient, extent of local tumour, histological grade, duration of symptoms, mode of presentation and the amount of tumour removed at the time of operation.
- Specialist centres quote over 90% of cases being suitable for radical or curative surgery with a 5-year survival of 50–60% overall and 90–95% for Dukes' stage A cases.
- Analysis of all surgical centres reduces overall 5-year survival to 20%.
- Dukes' classification is as follows:
  A: Confined to bowel wall, no extension, 5-year survival rate 90–95%.
  B: Full-thickness bowel wall extension to serosa, 5-year survival rate 60%.
  C: i, ii; Spread of tumour which involves lymph nodes, 5-year survival rate 25%.
  D: Distant spread of tumour e.g. liver, 5-year survival rate less than 1%.
- 10% present with Dukes' stage A compared to 40% with stage B and 40% with stage C.
- Well differentiated tumours have a better prognosis than moderately differentiated or anaplastic tumours[3].

TREATMENT

1. Early diagnosis of the tumour is the most important factor for successful treatment[4].

Screening of a population in Nottingham has identified 70% of the tumours as Dukes' A.

2. The mainstay of treatment is surgery.
   a. Right hemicolectomy is performed for lesions on the right side of the colon and proximal transverse colon.
   b. Left hemicolectomy is performed for lesions on the transverse and descending colon.
   c. Anterior resection with end-to-end anastomosis is carried out for lesions in the lower sigmoid, upper and mid rectum.
   d. Abdominoperineal resection with permanent colostomy is carried out for low rectal lesions. The operative mortality of colorectal resections is around 5%.
3. Chemotherapy with 5-fluorouracil alone or in combination with other agents have been assessed but side-effects outweigh the small improvement in survival.
4. Radiotherapy for rectal carcinoma is usually reserved for unfit patients with inoperable tumours, especially for pain relief.
5. Patients who have localized recurrence of disease may undergo a further laparotomy with a view to resection. If recurrence is more widespread then local radiotherapy may be of some benefit.

FOLLOW-UP

After resection of colorectal cancer, follow-up is indicated mainly as a preventive measure since these patients have an increased risk of developing future polyps or carcinoma[5]. Colonoscopy is the preferred technique for patients who require polyp follow-up. A careful proctocolonic examination should usually be made within months of surgery and 2–3-yearly thereafter.

[1] Koch M et al. (1982) J. Chron. Dis., 35, 69–72.
[2] Williams AR (1983) Gut, 23, 835–42.
[3] Chapuis PH et al. (1985) Br. J. Surg., 72, 698–702.
[4] Rehman B et al. (1986) Scott. Med. J., 2, 90–3.
[5] Sherlock P et al. (1980) Am. J. Med., 68, 917–31.

Appendicitis

Appendicectomy is the most common abdominal operation in western countries. Appendicitis can occur at any age with a peak in the teens and early adulthood, and is more common in males. Diagnosis can be difficult at the extremes of age, particularly as only 55% of patients present with classical symptoms of diffuse colicky central abdominal pain which moves to the right iliac fossa[1].

PROGNOSIS

- The usual outcome of acute appendicitis is resolution, with or without fibrosis, followed weeks or months later by another attack.
- If the arterial blood supply is cut off the appendix becomes gangrenous and can perforate. Persistent right iliac fossa pain with tenderness, guarding and vomiting are indications for immediate appendicectomy.
- Incidence of perforation is higher in the very young and very old, presumably because of diagnostic difficulties.
- Some 30% of late cases (perforated and gangrenous) are complicated by wound sepsis, whereas only 7% of early cases become infected[2].

TREATMENT

1. *Surgery*
   a. If diagnosis is certain, appendicectomy through a grid-iron incision should be made.
   b. If the appendix is found to be normal but another pathology is apparent, the appendix should be removed anyway, except in the presence of Crohn's disease.
   c. If diagnosis is uncertain, the patient should be observed as 50% of abdominal pains resolve without a diagnosis being made.
2. *Systemic antibiotics*
   a. Anaerobic infection is abolished with peri-operative metronidazole for 24 hours for a normal or inflamed appendix[3].
   b. Treatment with metronidazole and a broad-spectrum antibiotic over 5 days is indicated for gangrenous or perforated appendices[2].
3. *Appendix mass*
   a. Early mass should be treated by appendicectomy especially in children, pregnant women and elderly patients.
   b. Fixed mass should be treated with bedrest, fluids and antibiotics.
   c. Interval appendicectomy should be done about 6 months after resolution.
   d. Appendix abscess requires drainage[4] followed by interval appendicectomy.

FOLLOW-UP

Follow-up is required for the management of wound infection and also after conservative treatment of an appendix mass until an interval appendicectomy is carried out, usually after three to six months.

[1] Bouchier IAD et al. (1984) Textbook of Gastroenterology. London: Baillière Tindall.
[2] Lau WT et al. (1983) Br. J. Surg., 70, 155–7.
[3] Willis AJ et al. (1976) Br. Med. J., i, 318–20.
[4] Gathney DR (1984) World J. Surg., 8, 287–91.

Diverticular Disease

nly 20% of patients with colonic diverticula develop symptoms so the true incidence of verticular disease is unknown. Incidence increases progressively with age until more than)% of people are affected by the ninth decade; men and women are equally affected[1]. ack of dietary fibre is accepted as the main aetiological factor, as well as other factors ading to constipation. The commonest site of the diverticulum formation is the sigmoid olon (95% of cases). Occasionally the descending colon and, less commonly, the whole olon are involved.

PROGNOSIS

In all, 10–20% of patients admitted to hospital with diverticulitis undergo emergency surgery. Generalized or faecal peritonitis is found in 20–60% of these cases[2].

Other complications include fistula formation, large bowel obstruction and haemorrhage.

In the presence of diverticular disease, coexisting sigmoid carcinoma (5%) or polyps are seen on barium enema.

Acute diverticulitis has a 3% mortality but this rises to 33% when perforation has occurred.

Haemorrhage occurs in 11–17% of cases and diverticulitis is the commonest cause of massive rectal bleeding.

Following hospital treatment 25% of patients will relapse and require re-admission.

TREATMENT

. *Uncomplicated diverticular disease:* a high fibre diet (between 5 and 30 g/day) and/or bulking agents e.g. ispaghula preparations[3,4].

. *Acute diverticulitis:* conservative treatment with bedrest, intravenous fluids and systemic antibiotics, e.g. metronidazole.

. *Localized peritonitis or abscess formation*
   a. Conservative
      i. Systemic antibiotics plus intravenous fluids.
      ii. Surgical drainage may be required.
   b. Surgery if above fails.

4. *Generalized peritonitis*
   a. Treatment of choice is primary resection of colon, peritoneal toilet and systemic antibiotics. The mortality rate is 12%[2].
   b. More conservative surgery, such as defunctioning colostomy and oversew of perforation, has a 25% mortality, and 20% of such procedures result in faecal fistula.
   c. Primary anastomosis should not be performed.

5. *Large bowel obstruction:* if the patient's condition allows, sigmoid resection and primary colorectal anastomosis may be done[5].

6. *Fistula:* the most common fistulae (4%) are colovesical. Treatment is by elective sigmoid resection.

7. *Haemorrhage*
   a. Conservative with blood transfusion.
   b. Sigmoidoscopy excludes other causes and selective mesenteric angiography identifies bleeding in 50% of cases.
   c. If massive haemorrhage occurs, sigmoid resection and colorectal anastamosis may be required.

FOLLOW-UP

Sigmoidoscopy and barium enema must be performed after conservative treatment to exclude any other colonic pathology.

[1] Hughes E (1969) *Gut*, **10**, 336–51.
[2] Krukowski ZH *et al.* (1984) *Br. J. Surg.*, **71**, 921–7.
[3] Bouchier IAD *et al.* (1984) *Textbook of Gastroenterology*. London: Baillière Tindall.
[4] Brodribb AJM (1977) *Lancet*, **i**, 664–6.
[5] Koruth NM *et al.* (1985) *Br. J. Surg.*, **72**, 703–7.

Haemorrhoids

One-half of patients over 50 years have haemorrhoids. In younger age groups haemorrhoids are more commonly seen in males. They can be categorized as first-degree piles which bleed but do not protrude, second-degree piles which protrude on defecation and retract, and third-degree piles which protrude until digitally reduced. Cardinal symptoms include rectal bleeding, prolapse, pain, mucus discharge and pruritus ani. Predisposing factors are heredity, constipation, chronic cough and pregnancy[1].

PROGNOSIS

- Bleeding may cause anaemia. Any rectal bleeding should be fully investigated to exclude other diseases, even in the presence of haemorrhoids.
- In 20% of cases pain is the dominant symptom.

TREATMENT[2]

1. *Medical*
   a. High fibre diet.
   b. Bulking agents may be useful. These measures may control the symptoms in 50% of patients with early disease.
   c. Topical preparations in cream and suppository form are often used and found to be soothing by patients.
2. *Outpatient surgical procedures*
   a. Injection sclerotherapy
      i. The treatment of choice for first-degree haemorrhoids.
      ii. It is the painless injection of 5% phenol in almond oil at the base of the haemorrhoid.
      iii. Repeat treatment may be required 6–8 weeks later.
      iv. Bleeding is controlled in 90% of patients.
      v. Some 10–30% have recurrent symptoms in 1 year.
   b. Photocoagulation
      i. The simplest method for first and second-degree haemorrhoids.
      ii. Some 18% may need further treatment.
   c. Rubber band ligation
      i. The treatment of choice in elderly patients with lax, redundant mucosa, in prolapse and in bleeding second-degree haemorrhoids.
      ii. In younger patients it can cause severe pain; secondary haemorrhage occurs in 1%.
      iii. In all, 90% of first-degree haemorrhoids are improved; 80% are totally symptom-free in 3 years.
   d. Cryosurgery
      i. A total of 50% have persistent haemorrhoids after 1 year.
3. *Surgery*
   a. Anal dilatation—used only in young patients for painful bleeding piles.
   b. Haemorrhoidectomy
      i. A total of 20% of patients will require haemorrhoidectomy.
      ii. The operation may be 'open' where the wound heals by granulation or 'closed' where there is submucosal dissection and the wound is sutured primarily.
      iii. Indications include: large prolapsing piles, recurrent thrombosis, associated external tags or fissures and, failed conservative treatment.
      iv. The recurrence rate is 5% at 5 years.
      v. Postoperative complications include pain, urinary retention, haemorrhage, faecal impaction, formation of skin tags and occasionally incontinence or stenosis.
4. *Prolapsed thrombosed internal piles* are treated by:
   a. Conservative measures with bed elevation, ice packs and analgesia.
   b. Immediate haemorrhoidectomy.
   c. Manual dilatation of the anus.

FOLLOW-UP

This includes review at 6–8 weeks and advice on diet and importance of a regular bowel habit.

[1] Goligher J (1984) *Surgery of the Anus, Rectum and Colon*, 5th edn, pp. 98–245. London: Baillière Tindall.
[2] Thompson JPS (1978) *Br. J. Hosp. Med.*, **20**, 600.

Fissure-in-ano

Fissure-in-ano is a very painful condition which occurs at all ages from infancy upwards but mainly in middle-aged patients who suffer from constipation. An elongated ulcer develops in the midline posteriorly, with its apex at the lower border of the internal sphincter and its base at the anal margin. A 'sentinel' pile may occur at the lower end of the lesion. An anterior fissure is more common in parous women. The cardinal symptom is severe pain on defecation. Stools may be streaked with blood[1].

PROGNOSIS

- In children, relief of constipation leads to spontaneous cure.
- In chronic or recurrent fissure, persistent topical treatment with local anaesthetics may induce skin sensitivity.
- The recurrence rate from both surgical procedures is less than 10%.

TREATMENT[2]

1. *Conservative*
   a. Anaesthetic cream, e.g. Xylocaine 5%, applied before defecation.
   b. Laxatives to soften the stool.
2. *Surgical*
   a. Anal dilatation; however, this is followed by some faecal incontinence in 2–3%.
   b. Sphincter division, usually done as a lateral subcutaneous sphincterotomy. It is a more difficult procedure than above and may be followed by severe bleeding and occasional abscess formation.

FOLLOW-UP

Advice should be given on maintaining regular bowel habits.

---

[1] Passmore R, Robson JS (1975) *A Companion to Medical Studies*, pp. 3, 19, 120. Oxford: Blackwell Scientific Publications.
[2] Goligher J (1984) *Surgery at the Anus, Rectum and Colon*, 5th edn, pp. 98–245. London: Baillière Tindall.

Constipation

Constipation may complicate a large number of medical and surgical conditions and is considered to be present when a patient passes stools less than three times a week and/or passes an average of less than 30 g stool per day. It is caused by failure of colonic propulsion or impairment of normal defecation. Causes include lack of dietary fibre, drugs, dehydration, pregnancy, hypothyroidism, hypercalcaemia, Parkinson's disease, colonic tumours, diverticular disease, haemorrhoids and anal fissure.

PROGNOSIS

- Some 15–25% of intestinal obstruction in the neonate is caused by Hirschsprung's disease.
- Elderly patients with a history of purgative abuse are at increased risk of developing constipation.
- General outlook is good.
- If faecal peritonitis occurs, mortality is 50%.
- Constipation can cause urinary retention.
- Continued straining exacerbates haemorrhoids and anal fissure, and may cause embolism of an iliofemoral venous thrombosis[1].

TREATMENT[2]

1. Dietary advice to increase fibre intake (e.g. to about 30 g/day).
2. Reassurance and explanation of what is 'normal'.
3. Rectal examination and possibly sigmoidoscopy and barium enema should be done to exclude organic pathology:
4. Bulking laxatives, e.g. ispaghula husk, are used in preference to gut stimulants.
5. Simple suppositories may suffice, e.g. glycerine.
6. Faecal impaction may require enemas and/or manual evacuation.
7. Sugar is used to treat intussusception, anterior mucosal prolapse, rectocele and Hirschsprung's disease.
8. Severe idiopathic constipation has been treated by anal myomectomy or even subtotal colectomy.
9. Psychotherapy and biofeedback training to induce normal relaxation of the pelvic floor during defecation are successful in some women with idiopathic constipation.

FOLLOW-UP

No routine follow-up is required but advice should be given on increasing the amount of high fibre foods in the diet and avoiding laxative abuse.

[1] Bouchier IAD et al. (1984) Textbook of Gastroenterology. London: Baillière Tindall.
[2] Sleisenger M et al. (1983) Gastrointestinal Disease, 3rd edn. Philadelphia: WB Saunders.

Gastrointestinal Bleeding

Bleeding is one of the commonest gastrointestinal emergencies in adults, and in the UK accounts for approximately 28 000 hospital admissions per year. Common causes include duodenal ulceration, oesophagitis, duodenitis, varices and Mallory–Weiss tear. Less common causes include carcinomas, bleeding diatheses, leiomyomas, aortic aneurysm and in < 1% hereditary haemorrhagic telangiectasia, pseudooxanthoma elasticum, Ehlers–Danlos syndrome and Meckel's diverticulum.

Most patients present with haematemesis and/or melaena. Endoscopy can identify the bleeding site in 90% of cases. If endoscopy is normal sigmoidoscopy and possibly barium enema and colonoscopy are done. Angiography of the coeliac, superior and inferior mesenteric vessels is useful during an episode of acute bleeding[1].

PROGNOSIS

- Some 5% of patients have massive haemorrhage and may require urgent surgery.
- A total of 90% of patients will stop bleeding spontaneously.
- The mortality rate in developed countries is constant—10%.
- A bleeding ulcer which perforates has the worst prognosis.
- Rebleeding rate and mortality rate are adversely affected by:
  1. Patient's age (> 60 years).
  2. Visible vessel at endoscopy (> 50% rebleed)[2].
  3. Size of initial bleed.
  4. Presence of oesophageal varices.
  5. Presence of gastric rather than duodenal ulceration[3].
  6. Concurrent medical diseases.
  7. Delay in instituting surgery.

TREATMENT

1. Resuscitation if required by transfusion.
2. Bedrest, sedation and fasting.
3. *Upper gastrointestinal bleeding*
   a. Endoscopy: there is no evidence to show that urgent endoscopy has altered the mortality or morbidity of the disease. However, it is indicated to exclude oesophageal varices, patients who continue to bleed and patients who are shocked.
   b. Drugs
      i. H$_2$ antagonists such as cimetidine and ranitidine do not stop bleeding, but some studies suggest they may prevent rebleeding.
      ii. Antifibrinolytic therapy such as tranexamic acid has in a few studies shown a reduction in mortality rate[4].
      iii. Somatostatin is expensive and in its infancy but no trial has yet shown a reduction in rebleeding or mortality rate[5].
   c. Injection sclerotherapy is well established in the treatment of varices.
   d. Diathermy is currently being evaluated. Limitations include inaccessibility of the vessel either by site or active bleeding. Ulcers penetrating the larger splenic and left gastric arteries are not amenable to local therapy and it may, in fact, cause them to rebleed.
   e. Photocoagulation: studies using a Neodynium Yag laser reduced the rebleeding and mortality rate in patients with visible vessels in the ulcer. More controlled trials are needed[6].
   f. Surgery: duodenal ulcer is usually treated with truncal vagotomy and pyloroplasty, or a polygastrectomy. Gastric ulcers require partial gastrectomy.
4. *Other sites of gastrointestinal bleeding*
   a. Angiography may be used to identify the bleeding site and dyes can be injected to localize the lesion.
   b. Colonoscopy will identify, perhaps, diverticulitis and angiodysplasia.
   c. Laparotomy may be required if bleeding continues.

FOLLOW-UP

Patients with no obvious source of their bleeding

require careful follow-up to ensure that a diagnosis is made. Patients with persisting anaemia or rebleeding require full re-investigation.

[1] Protell RL et al. (1981) Clin. Gastroenterol., **10,** 17–64.
[2] Swain CP et al. (1986) Gastroenterology, **90,** 595–608.
[3] Morris DL et al. (1984) Br. Med. J., **188,** 1277–80.
[4] Barer D et al. (1983) N. Engl. J. Med., **308,** 1571–5.
[5] Somerville KW et al. (1985) Lancet, **i,** 130–2.
[6] Tarin D (1978) Br. Med. J., **ii,** 751–4.

Stoma Problems

Stomas can be divided into permanent, e.g. ileostomy and colostomy, or temporary, e.g. gastrostomy, jejunostomy and interim colostomy.

In the UK there are 10 000 people with an ileostomy and 100 000 with a colostomy. In the USA it is estimated that 4000 new ileostomies and 10 times as many colostomies are created each year. Some 30% are done as emergencies, which does not allow full psychosocial preparation of the patient[1].

PROGNOSIS

- Ischaemia can occur if the stoma prolapses repeatedly or if an ill-fitting appliance is used.
- Fistulas can occur due to Crohn's disease, poor surgical technique or local pressure necrosis from a poorly fitting appliance.
- Parastomal hernia is the most common problem: 20% occur with colostomy and 10% with ileostomy.
- Prolapse may require surgical correction.
- Some 30% of patients develop depression.
- Ileostomies may predispose to renal calculi, gallstones, malabsorption and vitamin B_{12} deficiency.

TREATMENT

1. High ileostomy output which can cause salt and water depletion may be helped by codeine phosphate 30 mg t.d.s. or loperamide 2 mg q.d.s. Operations to produce the 'continent ileostomy' such as the Koch operation and Parks' operation are currently being evaluated[2].
2. Bolus obstruction of an ileostomy can result from vegetable residue. Irrigation of the stoma solves the problem.
3. Skin problems

a. Effluent dermatitis.
b. Contact dermatitis from allergy to adhesive or appliance is helped by using a protective layer of carboxymethylcellulose or Karaya gel.
4. Odour and flatus is a common problem, especially in air travellers. Gas filters are helpful and tablets of bismuth subgallate 400 mg help prevent odour. Commercial instillates for stoma pouches include sodium-O-phenylphenate tetrahydrate 0–3%, P-chloro-M-xylenol 0.2% and oxychlorodene.

FOLLOW-UP

Review of the emotional state is as pertinent as review of the underlying medical problem. The district nurse should ensure that specialist stoma nurses assist with follow-up. Further help is available from the Ileostomy Association, 32 Newbury Close, Northolt, Middlesex, UB5 4JF (telephone 0623-28099) and the Colostomy Welfare Group, 38–39 Eccleston Square, London, SW1V 1PB (telephone 01-825-5175).

[1] Devlin HB (1986) Med. Int., **26,** 1071–6.
[2] Hughes E et al. (1983) Colorectal Surgery. Edinburgh: Churchill Livingstone.

Hernia

A hernia is an abnormal protrusion of a viscus or part of a viscus from its containing cavity. It may be reducible or irreducible; if irreducible, it may be obstructed or strangulated. There are various hernias—incisional, inguinal (the commonest), femoral and umbilical. The inguinal to femoral ratio in men is 40:1, and in women 3:1. The incidence of hernia is 0.5–10%. Predisposing factors include obesity, smoking, uraemia, malignancy, age over 60, undernourishment, poor surgical closure, postoperative chest infection or wound infection.

In the UK 112 adults/100 000 present with inguinal hernias. In children the incidence is 1–2% (male to female 9:1). They may be indirect, i.e. come via the deep inguinal ring and obliquely through the inguinal canal, or direct, i.e. through a weakened posterior wall. Direct hernias are rare in women and the overall indirect to direct ratio is 2:1. Some 10% are bilateral, 5% are sliding.

A femoral hernia passes through the femoral canal and medial to the femoral vein in the upper medial aspect of the thigh. The male to female ratio is 1:4.

Umbilical hernia is seen in children at 3 weeks of age due to incomplete closure of the umbilical ring. In adults these hernias occur through the linea alba, and incidence is 6 per 100 000[1].

Inguinal, femoral and para-umbilical hernias are often difficult to feel in the obese or if the patient is small.

PROGNOSIS

- Incisional hernias rarely cause obstruction or strangulation. Recurrence after repair occurs in 10–20% of patients.

Inguinal hernia
- Under 6 months of age, 30% are irreducible on presentation; one-fifth of these are associated with testicular infarction due to spermatic venous occlusion[2].
- The operative mortality for uncomplicated hernias is 1%. This rises to 10% for irreducible or obstructed cases and 30% when bowel resection is done.
- One-half of affected children over 2 years will develop a hernia on the other side.

Femoral hernia
- Most are irreducible and painless; 10% present with obstruction or strangulation[3].

Umbilical hernia
- Complications are rare and in 75% of children there is spontaneous closure.
- Some 20% of adults present as emergency with obstruction.

TREATMENT

1. *Incisional hernia*
   a. Treatment is conservative with corsets or support if the patient is not surgically fit.
   b. Surgery: 60–70% can be repaired by direct opposition of the muscle.

2. *Inguinal hernia*
   a. In children, 75% of irreducible hernias can be reduced under sedation and repaired 48 hours later by herniotomy.
   b. In an unfit adult a surgical truss may be used.
   c. Herniotomy and posterior wall repair is the most common procedure.
   d. Ischaemic orchitis occurs in 0.5% of repairs.
   e. Recurrence rates are 10% for direct, 1% for indirect. Most recurrences are in the first year after repair[4].

3. *Femoral hernia*
   a. Repair should be done. The most popular is the low or crural approach (Lockwood).
   b. Recurrence occurs in 2% of cases.

4. *Umbilical hernia*
   a. Surgical repair should be done if the hernia persists after 3 years of age[2].

FOLLOW-UP

No routine follow-up is required but advice should be given on maintaining an ideal weight and regular bowel habit.

[1] Maingot A (1969) *Abdominal Operations*, 5th edn. Appleton, Century, Crofts.
[2] Gough DCS (1983) *Surgery*, **i**, 13.
[3] Glassow F (1965) *Can. Med. Assoc. J.*, **93**, 1346.
[4] Kidson IG, Britton BJ (1982) *Update*, **24**, 195–209.

Gastroenteritis

Gastroenteritis is characterized by sudden onset of diarrhoea and vomiting. Rotavirus is the most common cause, mainly in infants and children, with a peak incidence in winter months[1]. Norwalk-like viruses are associated with epidemic outbreaks in children and adults. The virus can be found in contaminated food and water but person-to-person transmission is also important. Bacterial causes include *Campylobacter jejuni, Escherichia coli, Shigella* and *Salmonella. Campylobacter* infection is obtained from ingestion of contaminated food or water. Bloody stools are common during *C. jejuni, Shigella* and *Salmonella* infections but not during viral ones.

PROGNOSIS

- Viral gastroenteritis has an incubation period of 24–48 hours.
- The recovery period with rotavirus is 5–7 days.
- Untreated infants may die of dehydration.
- Norwalk–like viral infections last 12–24 hours.
- *C. jejuni* may cause severe systemic symptoms. Most recover in 1 week but 20% have more prolonged illness.
- A few children will develop persistent intolerance to disaccharides such as sucrose, lactose or cow's milk protein after the disease.

TREATMENT

1. Maintain fluid and electrolyte balance with sugar-electrolyte solutions.

2. Young children may need parenteral rehydration.
3. Antidiarrhoeal agents should not be given.
4. Erythromycin is given in *C. jejuni* infection in the presence of systemic illness (i.e. fever and bloody diarrhoea).
5. In postgastroenteritis allergy syndrome exclude milk and sugar products from the diet.

FOLLOW-UP

In secondary milk and lactose intolerance the child should be admitted to hospital for lactose and cow's milk challenge. Growth should be monitored.

[1] Shearman DJC (1982) *Diseases of the Gastrointestinal Tract and Liver*. London: Churchill Livingstone.

Bowel Infections

Gastrointestinal infections are a common cause of diarrhoea which can occur in small outbreaks and simultaneously in several patients. They follow a common epidemiological pattern of faecal–oral transmission. Bowel infections include traveller's diarrhoea, bacillary dysentery, salmonella infection, typhoid and paratyphoid, cholera, amoebiasis, and giardiasis.

PROGNOSIS

Traveller's diarrhoea

- Acute self-limiting illnesses caused by *Escherichia coli*.
- Symptoms start 3–14 days after arrival in the tropics and last for 1–3 days.

Bacillary dysentery

- Seen in developing countries; caused by *Shigella sonnei*, *S. flexneri* or *S. dysenteriae*.
- Outlook is good in *S. sonnei* dysentery.
- Mortality rates of 20% have been reported with *S. dysenteriae*.
- *S. flexneri* also has a poor prognosis.
- Complications include portal pyaemia leading to liver abscesses and portal vein thrombosis, and also peritonitis.
- In children intussusception and rectal prolapse are rare complications.
- Chronic bacillary dysentery can follow an acute attack.

Salmonella

- Symptoms occur 12–72 hours postinfection and vary from mild diarrhoea to septicaemia.
- Achlorhydria predisposes to more severe illness[1].
- Septicaemia occurs in 5% of adults.
- Focal abscesses can occur in soft tissues, bone and viscera.
- Symptoms usually last for a few days.
- Only 0.2% of cases may become chronic and continue to excrete the organism.

Typhoid (see also Infectious diseases)

- Caused by *Salmonella typhi*, the incubation period is 10–14 days.
- Constipation is more common than diarrhoea, which is only present in 20% of cases.
- The relapse rate is <20% and usually occurs 2 weeks after treatment is stopped.
- Perforation occurs in 4% in the second week.
- Occult bleeding occurs in 20% and frank bleeding in 2–8% in the third week.
- Some 1–3% continue to excrete organisms as chronic carriers.
- Intussusception, liver abscesses, appendicitis, osteomyelitis, pulmonary infection and embolism are rare complications.

Cholera (see also Infectious diseases, p. 000)

- Caused by *Vibrio cholerae*, the incubation period is 1–5 days.
- Massive fluid loss can lead to circulatory collapse.
- In untreated cases mortality can be 70%.
- If treated, mortality is <1%.

Amoebiasis

- Caused by *Entamoeba histolytica*, the incubation period is days to years.
- Cases may be mild or asymptomatic.
- Intestinal infection precedes all hepatic infection.
- Amoeboma may occur in the wall of the large intestine in chronic cases and can mimic colonic carcinoma with weight loss, abdominal pain and diarrhoea.
- In severe attacks renal failure can occur.
- Peritonitis carries a high mortality.
- Stricture of colon occurs in 10%.
- Liver abscesses can occur.
- Mortality in the UK is 1–2%.

Giardiasis

- *Giardia lamblia* is a parasite of the duodenum and jejunum.
- In the USA carrier states vary from 1 to 20%.
- Children are most commonly infected in endemic areas.
- Most cases are asymptomatic but giardiasis can cause diarrhoea, failure to thrive and urticaria.
- Spontaneous regression of symptoms may occur after 3 weeks with either complete resolution or milder persisting diarrhoea.
- Giardia may colonize the gallbladder—the frequency of this is unknown.
- Urticaria is cured when giardia is eradicated.

- Folate deficiency can occur with severe diarrhoea.
- A total of 90% of patients respond to treatment and intestinal absorption returns to normal in 4–6 weeks.
- Lactose intolerance may develop but resolves in 1–2 months.

TREATMENT

1. General: In all cases rehydration is important, either by oral sugar-electrolyte solutions or by parenteral means.
2. Specific measures:
   a. *Traveller's diarrhoea*
      i. Avoid contaminated food.
      ii. Doxycycline 100 mg daily started before travelling has given protection to 80% of people visiting tropical countries.
   b. *Bacillary dysentery*
      i. If mild, no treatment is required.
      ii. Depending on sensitivity sulphadiazine 1 g q.d.s. can be given. Alternative antibiotics include nalidixic acid 1 g q.d.s., ampicillin 250 mg q.d.s. or tetracycline 250 mg q.d.s.
   c. *Salmonella*
      i. Antidiarrhoeal agents, e.g. loperamide, may give symptomatic relief.
      ii. In uncomplicated cases antibiotics prolong the period of excretion[3].
      iii. In septicaemia, amoxycillin, chloramphenicol or co-trimoxazole can be given for 10 days.
   d. *Typhoid*
      i. Patient should be barrier-nursed in isolation.
      ii. Chloramphenicol is the drug of choice and is more effective than ampicillin or co-trimoxazole[4,5]. It is given for 2 weeks to reduce the chance of relapse.
      iii. Steroids can be used in conjunction with antibiotics in the absence of intestinal complications for severe toxicity.
      iv. Chronic carriers may require cholecystectomy.
      v. Persistently positive stool cultures require long-term treatment with amoxycillin 1 g q.d.s., along with probenicid.
   e. *Cholera*
      i. Tetracycline 500 mg q.d.s. for 4 days.
   f. *Amoebiasis*
      i. Metronidazole 800 mg t.d.s. for 5–10 days or emetine 1 mg/kg i.m. daily.
      ii. If severe, combine the above with diloxanide 500 mg t.d.s. for 10 days.
      iii. Liver abscesses may be aspirated and metronidazole given.
   g. *Giardiasis*
      i. Metronidazole and tinidazole are the drugs of choice.
      ii. Both can be given as high dose, short course regimens or at a lower dose over a longer period of time.
      iii. For persistent symptoms give two high dose courses of tinidazole two weeks apart.

FOLLOW-UP

Typhoid, cholera, salmonella and bacillary dysentery are notifiable diseases in the UK. Hygiene and health education should be undertaken in all cases.

In bacillary dysentery three negative stool cultures are needed to confirm clearance for food handlers and similar rules apply for cases of salmonellosis and cholera.

For typhoid, three negative faecal and urine samples must be obtained at least 48 hours apart and not earlier than 2–3 weeks after the last possible exposure to infection. If any are positive, culture should be repeated at intervals of 1 month until three negative samples are obtained. For clearance of food handlers, 12 negative faecal samples are needed. Two negative faecal and urine cultures should be obtained from contacts at home.

In cholera, household contacts should be screened for 5 days and possibly given prophylactic tetracycline. Cholera vaccination for travellers only gives minimal immunity for 6 months.

In amoebiasis excretors should be prevented from food handling.

[1] Sharp JCM *et al.* (1982) *Update*, **25**, 213.
[2] Dixon JMS (1965) *Br. Med. J.*, **ii**, 1343–6.
[3] Sharp JCM *et al.* (1981) *Update*, **7**, 737–40.
[4] Snyder MJ *et al.* (1976) *Lancet*, **ii**, 1155–7.
[5] Shearman DJ (1982) *Disease of the Gastrointestinal Tract and Liver*. London: Churchill Livingstone.

Worms

The range of worm infestation found in the gastrointestinal tract are many and varied. These include ascariasis, trichuriasis, enterobiasis, ancylostomiasis and the tapeworms *Taenia solium* and *T. saginata*.

PROGNOSIS

Ascariasis

- Caused by *Ascaris lumbricoides*, it affects mainly young children.
- The adult form can cause volvulus, cholangitis, appendicitis, acute pancreatitis and intussusception.
- Ascariasis causes 20 000 deaths per year worldwide.
- The cure rate with treatment is at least 80%.

Trichuriasis

- *Trichuris trichiura* is known as the whipworm. In warm moist areas 90% of the population is affected[2].
- Infection is usually asymptomatic but occasionally there can be diarrhoea, rectal prolapse and urticaria.

Enterobiasis

- The threadworm *Enterobius vermicularis* infects children.
- Female worms cause perianal itch; if scratched, the ova get beneath the nails; if transmitted to mouth, auto-reinfection takes place.
- Enterobiasis may give symptoms which mimic appendicitis.
- More than 50% of infections are detected by one adhesive tape print from the perianal area.

Ancylostomiasis

- Hookworm disease is caused by *Ancylostoma duodenale* or *Necator americanus*.
- Most patients have no symptoms.
- Ancylostomiasis can cause iron deficiency anaemia and hypoproteinaemia.
- It causes approximately 50 000 deaths per year worldwide from anaemia.

Taeniasis

- The most common form is *Taenia saginata* and *T. solium*.
- Taeniasis is acquired from inadequately cooked meat.
- Most patients are asymptomatic.
- The presence of *T. solium* carries the risk of developing cysticercosis.

TREATMENT

Ascariasis

1. Piperazine (Antepar) is given in a single dose of 500 mg for a child up to 1 year and a maximum of 3 g for an adult.
2. Pyrantel, levamisole, mebendazole and albendazole are also effective.
3. Obstruction should be treated conservatively, if possible.

Trichuriasis/Enterobiasis

1. Cut patients' nails short and educate them on the importance of scrubbing hands after defecation.
2. Bathe a child in the morning rather than at night.
3. Mebenoazole is the drug of choice, given as a single dose to the whole family.
4. Piperazine is also useful.
5. Treatment may need to be repeated weekly.
6. The cure rate from single-dose drugs is 90%.

Ancylostomiasis

1. Anaemia is treated with iron[3].
2. Bephenium in a single dose of 2.5–5 g repeated after 2 days is the drug of choice.
3. Mebendazole 100 mg b.d. for 3 days is effective.
4. Tetrachloroethylene has been superseded by the above treatment.
5. The cure rate with treatment is 70–80%.

Taeniasis

1. Dichlorophen is the drug of choice.
2. Niclosamide and praziquantel are also effective in more than 90% patients.
3. Treatment is regarded as successful if faecal examinations are negative for 4 months for *T. saginata* and 3 months for *T. solium*.

FOLLOW-UP

No regular follow-up is required.

[1] Leading article (1977) *Br. Med. J.*, **i**, 406–7.
[2] Misiewicz JJ *et al.* (1987) Diseases of the Small Intestine, Pancreas and Colon, vol. ii, p. 59. Gower.
[3] Woodruff AW (1964) *Practitioner*, **193**, 138–41.

Jaundice

Jaundice is the term used to describe yellow discoloration of sclerae, mucous membranes and skin caused by accumulation of bilirubin. Jaundice results from either excessive production or defective elimination of bilirubin. It can be defined as prehepatic jaundice, hepatocellular jaundice and cholestatic or posthepatic jaundice[1]. Prehepatic jaundice is commonly due to conditions such as haemolysis from sickle cell anaemia, hereditary spherocytosis and thalassaemia. Familial diseases can cause hyperbilirubinaemia, including Gilbert's disease, Dubin–Johnson's and Rotor's syndromes. Hepatocellular jaundice is usually due to primary biliary cirrhosis, sclerosing cholangitis or parasitic infestations. Drugs (paracetamol, hydralazine and chlorpromazine) and viral hepatitis can also cause hepatocellular jaundice. Posthepatic jaundice includes any condition causing obstruction of the major biliary tree such as gallstones, bile duct stricture, cholangiocarcinoma, or carcinoma of the head of the pancreas.

In the UK, most patients aged 15–20 years who present with jaundice have acute viral hepatitis; the remainder have autoimmune chronic active hepatitis, Gilbert's syndrome, haemolysis or the sequelae of neonatal hepatitis. By the age of 40–50 years over 50% of liver disease is alcohol-related. Over the age of 70 years 50–80% of patients admitted to hospital with jaundice have extrahepatic biliary obstruction[2].

PROGNOSIS

- Prognosis depends on the cause of the jaundice.

Prehapatic prognosis

- Gilbert's disease carries an excellent prognosis.
- Dubin–Johnson's and Rotor's syndromes are benign conditions.
- Crigler–Najjar syndrome is due to a deficiency of glucuronyl transferase and in complete absence of the enzyme carries a poor prognosis leading to kernicterus and early death in most infants.

Hepatocellular prognosis

- These conditions carry a poor prognosis.
- Patients suffering from biliary cirrhosis who have deepening jaundice die within 5 years of the time of diagnosis.
- Acute cholangitis carries a mortality rate of 40%.
- Almost all patients with hepatitis A, 90–95% of those with hepatitis B, and 50–70% of those with non-A or non-B hepatitis have a self-limiting illness from which they recover completely.
- Serum hepatitis occurs in less than 1% of patients and has a high mortality. It occurs most commonly following simultaneous hepatitis B infection and non-A, non-B hepatitis.

Posthepatic prognosis

- Post-mortem studies show that gallstones occur in 15–20% of adults and only a minority cause complications or lead to surgery.
- High bile duct strictures (usually caused following cholecystectomy) carry a poor prognosis but early expert repair improves outcome. Overall mortality is 5–10%.
- Cholangiocarcinoma is uncommon.
  1. Hilar lesions have a poor prognosis with 80% being irresectable at presentation. Overall mortality rates are over 30%.
  2. Bile duct and ampullary lesions have a survival of about 18 months. Some 60–70% are resectable with a 25% 5-year survival.
  3. Adenocarcinoma of the pancreas is increasing in incidence and has a poor prognosis with an overall 5-year survival rate of 1%. In all, 85–90% of patients are dead within 12 months of diagnosis[3].

TREATMENT

1. *General measures*
   a. Pruritus is treated with cholestyramine (up to 4 g t.d.s.). Occasionally ultraviolet lamp treatment is also effective.
   b. In patients with chronic cholestasis a low fat diet with calcium and fat-soluble vitamin supplements may produce weight gain and minimize diarrhoea.

2. *Specific treatment:* this varies according to the individual liver diseases present.

   a. In patients with symptomatic gallstones cholecystectomy is the treatment of choice. Gallstone dissolution with bile acids is possible in 10% of patients who have non-calcified stones within a functioning gallbladder, but this has limited success[4]. Recurrence of dissolved gallstones occurs in 28–64% of patients after 2–12 years[5].

   b. Endoscopic sphincterectomy and stone extraction is valuable in high-risk patients and may be used even if the gallbladder is present. It has a 90% success rate with only 1% mortality.

   c. Benign bile duct strictures can be treated by surgical bypass, that is choledochojejunostomy or choledochoduodenostomy. If surgical resection or repair is not possible dilatation of the strictures (either percutaneous or endoscopic) is possible, but as yet no long-term results are available.

   d. Cholangiocarcinoma is best treated by surgical excision. If irresectable, non-surgical intubation of the area can be performed.

   e. Management of viral hepatitis and primary biliary cirrhosis are discussed in the relevant sections.

   f. Gilbert's syndrome does not require active treatment. Plasma bilirubin levels can be reduced with phenobarbitone, but there is no theoretical benefit to justify its use.

   g. There is no recognized treatment for the Dubin–Johnson or Rotor's syndromes.

FOLLOW-UP

Follow-up is dependent on the cause of the jaundice. Patients with prehepatic jaundice or drug-related liver disease do not require regular follow-up. Follow-up for other causes of jaundice can be seen in the relevant chapters.

[1] Sherlock S (1981) *Diseases of the Liver and Biliary System*, 6th edn. Oxford: Blackwell Scientific Publications.
[2] Elias E, Hawkins CF (1985) *Lecture Notes on Gastroenterology*. Oxford: Blackwell Scientific Publications.
[3] Little JM (1987) *Surgery*, **102**, 473–6.
[4] Leuschner V, Kurth W (1987) *Lancet*, **ii**, 508.
[5] Villanora N *et al.* (1987) *Gastroenterology*, **92**, 1789.

Hepatitis

The term hepatitis is used to describe an acute generalized inflammation of the liver. The most important causes are viral, e.g. hepatitis A, hepatitis B, hepatitis non-A, non-B, hepatitis D and less commonly the Epstein–Barr virus, cytomegalovirus and herpes virus. Drugs, toxins and spirochaetes can also affect the liver.

Virus A has an incubation period of up to 6 weeks and spreads by the oral–faecal route. Virus B has a long incubation period and is spread by blood, blood products and sexual contact. Non-A, non-B has an incubation period of 6–8 weeks and is transmitted by blood transfusion, by the use of coagulation factors and drinking contaminated water. Virus D is an incomplete virus which can only exist in the presence of hepatitis B infection.

PROGNOSIS

- Hepatitis A has a good prognosis with no carrier state. Mortality is about 0.1%.
- Hepatitis B has a poorer prognosis with 5–10% of infected people failing to eliminate the virus. The presence of the virus D causes a more severe hepatitis and worsens the prognosis. Virus B is associated with the development of hepatocellular carcinoma[1].
- Non-A, non-B hepatitis is associated with a carrier state. In the USA 1% of blood donations transmit the virus. Of affected patients, 50% may develop chronic hepatitis and 25% cirrhosis. Mortality is 1%; in the waterborne type it is 12%. Chronicity is higher following transfusion and among drug addicts than in patients without obvious source of infection[2].

TREATMENT

1. Bedrest and isolation for hepatitis B.
2. Avoid alcohol and hepatotoxic drugs, e.g. sedatives.
3. Corticosteroids have been used in cholestatic cases but in hepatitis B there is evidence of virus replication with steroids.
4. Prophylaxis:
   a. Hepatitis B vaccine given in three intra-muscular or subcutaneous injections at 0, 1 and 6 months should be given to those at risk. Immunosuppressed and renal patients may need higher doses[3].
   b. Gammaglobulin is used in patients going to high-incidence areas to prevent hepatitis A.
   c. Antihepatitis B globulin should be given within 48 hours of exposure to those acci-dentally suffering a needlestick injury[4].

FOLLOW-UP

Regular liver function tests should be done. Hepa-titis surface antigen or Australia antigen should disappear after 2–3 months. Hepatitis e antigen should decline but if it remains it is evidence of continuing disease. Advise the patient on graded return to full activity. Alcohol should be avoided for 3–6 months.

[1] Scullard GH et al. (1978) Gastroenterology, 75, 869–74.
[2] Rakela J et al. (1979) Gastroenterology, 77, 1200–2.
[3] Szmuness W et al. (1980) N. Engl. J. Med., 303, 833–41.
[4] Immunisation Practices Advisory Committee (1985) Ann. Int. Med., 103, 391–402.

Cholelithiasis

Gallstones are very common in developed countries and in the over 30 year-olds, 1 in 3 females have gallstones and 1 in 5 males. The incidence increases with age and are commoner in the obese, those on oestrogen or clofibrate therapy, patients with haemolytic disorders, diseases of the ileum, cirrhosis, after ileal resection or vagotomy and those on long-term parenteral nutrition. Most stones consist mainly of cholesterol but 25% are pigment stones associated with haemolysis.

PROGNOSIS

- 50% of gallstones remain silent.
- Only 15% of gallstones lead to cholecystec-tomy[1].
- Only 10% of patients presenting for the first time will develop a complication[2].
- Ductal stones may remain silent but can occur in 10–15% of symptomatic patients with gall-stones and can cause obstructive jaundice, acute cholangitis, and acute pancreatitis.
- 30% of people with gallbladder stones develop biliary carcinoma which is the commonest presentation.
- Acute cholecystitis occurs in 20% of sympto-matic cases.
- Mucocoele of gallbladder is rare.
- Gallstones are strongly associated with carci-noma of the gallbladder although a causal association is not known.
- 5–10% have persistent symptoms after chole-cystectomy.

TREATMENT

1. Gallbladder Stones
   a. If asymptomatic, no treatment required.
   b. If symptomatic, cholecystectomy is the treatment of choice.
   c. Cholecystostomy or subtotal cholecystec-tomy may be sufficient with removal of gallbladder stones and cholecystectomy at a later date.
   d. In high-risk surgical patients analgesics and antiemetics with advice on low fat diet may suffice.
   e. Small, non-calcified (<1.5 cm diameter) stones in a functioning gallbladder may be suitable for dissolution with bile acids but recurrence rate is high.

. Ductal Stones
   a. Exploration of the duct at the time of cholecystectomy is standard.
   b. Choledochoduodenostomy can be useful after exploration of a dilated duct (>15 mm) containing friable stones in older patients.
   c. Endoscopic sphincterotomy and stone extraction is useful in high risk patients even if gallbladder is present. Success rate is up to 90% with 1% mortality and 10% morbidity[3].
   d. Retained stones can be removed under x-ray control if a T-tube is *in situ*.

   e. Dissolution of stones with mono-octanoin has been of limited value.
3. Gallstone Ileus
   a. Enterotomy is required for stone removal.

FOLLOW-UP

Patients on dissolution therapy require regular monitoring for recurrence of stones or side-effects.

[1] Fry J, Sandler G (1986) *Disease Data Book*, Lancaster: MTL.
[2] Ransohoff DF, *et al.* (1983) *Ann Intern Med*, **99**, 199.
[3] Cotton PB (1984) *Gut*, **25**, 587.

Cholecystitis

Cholecystitis may be acute or chronic. Acute cholecystitis may be the initial presentation of cholelithiasis and is associated with gallstones in 95% of cases. Acute acalculus cholecystitis may be precipitated by a bacterial infection or severe systemic infection. Rarely it is embolic in origin or associated with gallbladder carcinoma.

Chronic cholecystitis is characterized by pathological evidence of a chronic inflammatory process and stones are present in a high percentage of patients.

PROGNOSIS

Acute cholecystitis
- A total of 85% of acute episodes resolve on conservative treatment[1].
- Acute cholecystatis can be complicated by perforation with biliary peritonitis (1–2%), empyema (2–3%), gangrene (1–2%) or gallstone ileus.
- The older the patient, the greater the risk of complications and the higher the mortality (10–15%).
- Recurrence of symptoms after an acute calculous cholecystitis is common.
- Mortality for acute acalculous cholecystitis is up to 35%.
- The overall operative mortality for acute cholecystitis is 2%.

Chronic cholecystitis
- The frequency of recurrent attacks varies greatly from patient to patient.

TREATMENT

1. Initial therapy is conservative with intravenous fluids, nasogastric suction, antibiotics and analgesia.
2. An early or delayed cholecystectomy is usually indicated[2]. Some 10% of patients may develop further symptoms while awaiting surgery and 15% default.
3. Failure to respond to conservative measures or development of complications requires urgent surgery.
4. Acute acalculous cholecystitis requires urgent surgery.
5. Cholecystectomy is the operation of choice and in a district general hospital in the UK 200 cholecystectomies will be done each year[3].
6. Perioperative cholangiography at the time of cholecystectomy should be done to detect ductal calculi.
7. Common bile duct exploration is necessary in 10–15% of patients.

8. Cholecystostomy with removal of stones from the gallbladder is indicated following gallbladder perforation or where the patient's condition does not allow more extensive surgery to be done.
9. Gallstone dissolution with bile acids may be possible in 10% of patients with small non-calcified stones (of 1.5 cm diameter) and a functioning gallbladder, but recurrence rates are high.

[1] du Plessis DJ *et al.* (1973) *Surg. Clin. North Am.*, **53**, 1071.
[2] Van der Linden W *et al.* (1981) *Br. J. Surg.*, **68**, 753.
[3] Fry J, Sandler G (1986) *Disease Data Book*. MTP: Lancaster.

FOLLOW-UP

Patients treated conservatively may require later admission for delayed cholecystectomy. Patients on dissolution therapy require regular monitoring for recurrence of stones or side-effects.

Cirrhosis

Cirrhosis is defined as a diffuse irreversible hepatic process characterized by fibrosis and a conversion of the normal liver architecture into nodules as a result of regeneration. There is a loss of the normal relationship of central veins to portal tracts[1]. The incidence of cirrhosis varies greatly in different parts of the world and with changing social conditions. Commonest causes are high alcohol intake, postviral hepatitis and biliary obstruction. The development of portal hypertension is the cause of most complications. In 40–45% of patients presenting with cirrhosis no cause is found—cryptogenic cirrhosis[2].

PROGNOSIS

- Prognosis is dependent on the cause of the cirrhosis and the extent to which the liver is able to compensate[3].
- Liver failure with jaundice, ascites, haemorrhage and encephalopathy has a poor prognosis with death in 2 years.
- Hepatoma develops in 15–20% of patients with chronic cirrhosis. There is a survival rate of 6 months.
- Alcohol cirrhosis: the prognosis depends on abstinence[4]. The 5-year survival is 30% for alcoholics who continue to drink compared with 70% for those who stop.
- Viral hepatitis B or non-A, non-B can cause cirrhosis. The prognosis is good if hepatocellular function is maintained. Hepatoma can be a long-term complication (15–20% of cirrhotics).
- Chronic active hepatitis: survival for 10 years in treated groups is 63% compared to 27% in untreated groups. Mortality is high in the first 2 years after diagnosis and thereafter disease activity lessens. Relapse occurs in 60–70% of patients, especially in those who remain autoantibody(SMA + antinuclear factor)-positive.
- Primary biliary cirrhosis: prognosis is variable. If asymptomatic the average survival has been reported as 12 years. If the bilirubin level rises it may only be 1–2 years.
- Wilson's disease: an acute presentation of liver involvement usually carries a poor prognosis, especially if associated with neurological signs and symptoms.
- α-Antitrypsin deficiency: in homologous patients there is a poor prognosis and a risk of hepatoma. However most adults have minor degrees of portal fibrosis. In children progressive fibrosis is more common in boys than girls and the likelihood of juvenile cirrhosis is greatly increased if there is a history of an affected sibling.
- Haemochromatosis has a 20% risk of hepatoma but with regular therapy usually has a good prognosis.
- Cardiac failure: liver involvement is mild and true cardiac cirrhosis is rare. Prognosis is poor

but death is usually from the consequences of end-stage heart disease.

- Cystic fibrosis: many children now survive into adolescence and may present with the complications of cirrhosis, e.g. variceal bleeding. In these patients a shunt operation is advisable.
- Secondary biliary obstruction: prognosis is dependent on relieving the obstruction.

TREATMENT

Alcoholic cirrhosis
1. The most important part of therapy is abstinence from alcohol.
2. Patients with decompensation may need diuretics for ascites, a low protein diet and lactulose and neomycin for encephalopathy.
3. Studies have shown little value in the use of corticosteroids in the treatment of alcoholic hepatitis.
4. Propylthiouracil is also of limited value.

Postviral cirrhosis
1. There is no specific effective treatment.
2. Antivirals such as interferon, riborivan and adenine arabinoside are still being evaluated.

Primary biliary cirrhosis
1. This requires symptomatic treatment as well as drugs which modify the disease process, such as corticosteroids, azathropine and D-penicillamine.
2. Azathioprine does not increase survival but D-penicillamine has been shown to improve survival after prolonged treatment of 18 months or so.
3. Liver transplantation may prolong survival, but the timing in a disease with such a variable course is extremely difficult.
4. Pruritus is treated by cholestyramine.
5. Intramuscular vitamin K 10 mg may improve bleeding tendencies.
6. Osteomalacia can be prevented by 100 000 i.u. vitamin D intramuscularly or 25-hydroxycholecalciferol 50–100 mg daily by mouth.
7. Painful neuropathy may respond to plasma exchange.

Wilson's disease
1. Penicillamine is the drug of choice given initially as 500 mg t.d.s. and decreased to a maintenance dose of 750 mg per day. Another chelating agent, trientine, is equally effective. The role of zinc is yet to be evaluated.

General
1. There is no specific treatment for α-antitrypsin deficiency.
2. Haemochromatosis is controlled by venesection, initially 1 unit fortnightly increasing to monthly when serum ferritin is normal.
3. There is no specific treatment for cardiac cirrhosis or for hepatic involvement of cystic fibrosis.

Chronic active hepatitis
1. Treatment is corticosteroids 20–30 mg per day for 1 month, decreasing each month until a maintenance dose is established.
2. If side-effects are caused by steroids, azathioprine should be added at a dose of 1–2 mg/kg body weight. Azathioprine on its own has been shown to be ineffective[5].

FOLLOW-UP

Regular liver function tests to monitor hepatocellular damage with clinical examination and alpha-fetoprotein to detect hepatoma are valuable. In haemochromatosis serum ferritin is useful, as is measurement of urinary copper excretion in Wilson's disease.

[1] Rifkind M, Dunn MA (1979) *Gastroenterology*, **76**, 849–63.
[2] Stone WD *et al.* (1968) *O. J. Med.*, **145**, 119–32.
[3] Popper H, Schaffner F (1977) *N. Engl. J. Med.*, **284**, 1154–9.
[4] Sherlock S (1981) *Diseases of the Liver and Biliary System*, 6th edn. Oxford: Blackwell Scientific Publications.
[5] Weatherall *et al.* (1987) *Oxford Textbook of Medicine*. Oxford: Oxford Medical Publications.

6

Psychiatry

B. B. Reiss and J. Draper

Anxiety

Anxiety[1] is a natural reaction to a stressful situation and thus is an experience common to all human beings. Normally it acts as a driving force and produces physiological effects by stimulating sympathetic autonomic activity. Patients not infrequently ask for help with common situations producing anxiety, for example, a driving test.

Inappropriate anxiety may affect or at times virtually destroy people's lives when it pervades all their activities and prevents normal functioning. The sufferer is fearful, irritable, restless, has poor concentration and sleeps badly. Anxiety may also produce unpleasant somatic responses that can in themselves disable. Autonomic overactivity leads to palpitations, dry mouth, bowel and bladder symptoms, and sexual difficulties; hyperventilation effects include dizziness, faintness, paraesthesiae, and chest and muscle pains. Headaches due to tension may occur.

When the symptoms are persistent and disabling, patients are often said to have an anxiety neurosis. The distinction from simple anxiety is one of degree. The term has a pejorative tone and is probably best not used.

Panic attacks are an acute form of anxiety characterized by a sense of impending doom, dizziness, palpitations and other somatic symptoms already listed.

Anxiety is also a feature of other psychiatric disorders occurring invariably in phobic and obsessive compulsive illness and often in depression, schizophrenia and other conditions.

Adolescents and the aged are especially vulnerable to anxiety. Anxiety neuroses and panic attacks usually begin in young adult life. Some people have a lifelong predisposition to be anxious and consult their doctor frequently in search of reassurance.

Anxiety is often a feature of physical illness and many people consult their general practitioner because of anxieties related to physical symptoms. Doctors frequently have to discriminate between anxiety-related somatic symptoms, overanxiety to minor symptoms, and anxiety relating to symptoms caused by serious organic disease.

PROGNOSIS

- Physiological anxiety has a good prognosis. Effective management and education will help future self-care.
- The outlook for anxiety related to other psychiatric conditions depends on their prognosis, outlined in the appropriate section.
- The prognosis of anxiety associated with physical illness varies according to the personality of the individual and to his or her understanding of the condition. In general the greater the understanding the less anxious someone will feel.
- The prognosis in anxiety states or anxiety neuroses is variable. At one extreme are those people with an anxious personality who function effectively but consult frequently. At the other is a smaller group who may have periods of disability on account of their condition. The disablement in a few may be permanent.
- Some anxious people with personality problems may abuse alcohol or drugs, thus adding to their difficulties.
- Many anxious people continue to have symptoms over many years and may be lifelong sufferers.

TREATMENT

1. Listening is a necessary part of all medical care. In the management of anxiety it is particularly important and may be all that is needed. The doctor should listen intently and show concern for the patient and understanding of the problem. This is possible even in quite brief consultations.
2. The significance of symptoms should be explained and followed by appropriate reassurance.
3. Counselling methods are used in all cases of anxiety. They are especially needed for those seeking help before examinations and driving tests etc. and when there are social causes such as marital, housing or work problems. In some cases it is appropriate for the doctor to counsel but others are best referred to a social worker or other trained counsellor.

4. Relaxation training is now being used widely as an aid to control anxiety symptoms, particularly for panic attacks and hyperventilation. People can instruct themselves with self-help booklets or tapes. They can also take part in groups led by a physiotherapist or other suitably trained person. The sharing of problems is often a relief in itself. But sometimes patients find groups too stressful and therefore unacceptable. Yoga or meditation help some.

5. Physical methods are useful. In hyperventilation, breathing into a paper bag will stop or prevent somatic symptoms. Biofeedback machines are used as an aid to relaxation training.

6. Psychotherapy in the wider sense of listening and support is discussed above. In younger patients with personality problems formal psychotherapy can be tried. General practitioners with special training can undertake this or patients can be referred to a therapist.

7. Behaviour and cognitive methods may be useful and are referred to in the sections on phobic conditions (p. 130) and depression (p. 131).

8. Drug treatment
   a. Drugs should usually be avoided. It is a good idea to discuss their use with the patient and explain that at best anxiolytics give only temporary relief of symptoms and are habituating. If they are prescribed, benzodiazepines or other anxiolytics should be used in small doses and for an agreed limited period of time—not more than 2–4 weeks.
   b. Major tranquillizers such as flupenthixol, thioridazine, or chlorpromazine are useful for short-term and occasionally longer-term treatment. They have the advantage of not being addictive.
   c. Antidepressants help anxiety as well as depressive symptoms when both are present together. This is frequently the case. The more sedative ones are useful when insomnia is an additional problem as antidepressants are non-addictive. They need to be tailed off slowly.
   d. Beta-adrenergic blocking drugs may be useful in controlling tremor or palpitations, particularly in the short term, for example, for performing artists.

FOLLOW-UP

Patients with more severe symptoms will be seen regularly. So far as possible self-care should be encouraged; self-help groups are useful for this. Longer-term psychotherapy may be needed for some people.

---

[1] Tyrer P (1987) *Anxiety disorders. Prescribers' Journal*, vol 27. London: HMSO.

Phobias

Phobias are an exaggerated and unreasoning fear of a situation or object which does not normally bother other people. This results in avoidance of the feared situation and leads to varying degrees of handicap. Unfortunately, although phobic patients usually have insight into their disability, this tends to increase rather than decrease their anxiety levels because the insight does not help the sufferer to overcome the difficulty. Agoraphobia, a fear of public places, is by far the commonest phobia presenting to the general practitioner. Other phobias relate to such things as social situations, closed spaces, animals, insects etc. but are relatively less common. Some cases appear to be triggered by a bereavement or other stressful life event.

The lifetime prevalence of agoraphobia is 3–7%. In a general practice population of 2000, about 100 people will suffer from disabling phobias or obsessive compulsive disorders. Not all of these individuals present to the doctor and many people go on for years unable to leave the house or being otherwise disabled by their condition.

Social classes are affected equally but the incidence is higher in women than men. Onset is usually in adults before the age of 40.

PROGNOSIS[2,3]

- People may suffer from phobias that are present for a few months and regress spontaneously without medical intervention. Patients who are seen by a doctor have usually had symptoms for over a year.
- Untreated agoraphobia has the worst prognosis; it is likely to last for many years.
- Specific phobias may also last for years but the outlook is better than for agoraphobia.
- At 5-year follow-up 50% of phobics had improved, 25% were unchanged and 25% were worse[3].
- Phobias, especially agoraphobia, lead to considerable disability. For instance, taking children to school or going to work may be impossible.
- Marital problems and depression are added complications.
- Two-thirds or more of those who accept exposure treatment will obtain appreciable relief[4].

TREATMENT[2]

1. Behavioural treatment by graduated exposure to the feared situation is the treatment of choice and can be supervised by a general practitioner able to give regular time to it. The patient describes the problem. The doctor then clarifies what is being avoided. The information thus obtained forms the basis of a self-exposure programme for the patient to carry out on his or her own. Initially a relatively easy task is agreed between doctor and patient. The longer the exposure—an hour or more—the more effective it is. A diary is kept and progress is discussed with the doctor who encourages and supports the patient. As the level of anxiety decreases so the length of exposure can increase and new tasks can be introduced.

   If this approach is not acceptable or is unsuccessful the patient should be referred to a psychiatrist, clinical psychologist or nurse with special experience of this form of treatment.
2. Often close relatives of a patient cannot understand the problem and may themselves need help.
3. Drugs have a limited place in treatment. Any significant depression may require antidepressants. These drugs may help in the absence of depression but usually have no long-term benefit. No one antidepressant has been shown conclusively to have advantages over any other. Benzodiazepines give only temporary relief of symptoms and because they habituate, are best not prescribed.

FOLLOW-UP

Some patients will need only a few visits and may be able to supervise their own treatment with a self-help booklet. More severe cases will need weekly follow-up with reducing frequency of visits as confidence becomes more secure.

Sireling L (1987) quoted in Marks and Horder[2].

Marks I, Horder J (1987) Phobias and their management. *Br. Med. J.*, **295**, 589.

Reveley MA (1986) Phobic neurosis. In *Treatment and Prognosis; Medicine* (Hawkins R ed). Oxford: Heinemann.

[4] Marks IM (1987) quoted in Marks and Horder[2].

Depression

Depression is a normal experience and only becomes an illness when a constellation of depressive symptoms leads to an impairment of normal activity or is a threat to life. The point prevalence of depressive symptoms is 13–20% of the population. The point prevalence of depressive disorder is 32 per 1000 men and 45–93 per 1000 women. The highest prevalence in women is between the ages of 35 and 45 with a slight increase after 55. In men there is a gradual increase with age[1]. Estimates of the incidence of depression in general practice vary according to doctor and social characteristics of patient population[2]. It is likely however that on average for every 1000 patients on a list a general practitioner will see 10–20 new cases each year. About half of those patients with depressive disorder who attend general practitioners are likely to be undiagnosed[3].

Characteristic features of depression are mood changes, suicidal ideas or plans, anxiety, physical symptoms and hypochondriasis, feelings of guilt or worthlessness, loss of interest, poor concentration and thinking. Biological symptoms include sleep disturbance with intermittent or early waking, diurnal variation of mood, fatigue, poor appetite and weight loss, impaired libido, retardation or agitation. Psychotic symptoms of delusions and hallucinations may occur. In the depressed elderly, biological symptoms are prominent and intellectual capacity is diminished, thus leading to apparent dementia.

PROGNOSIS

- People with depression as a result of life events who visit their doctors are usually helped by one or two visits. Sometimes this type of depression develops into a depressive illness.
- The outlook for those with depressive illness varies greatly.
- Favourable factors are a secure childhood, a supportive spouse or close friend, good social contacts, a stimulating life and activities.
- Unfavourable factors are an obsessional or depressive personality, previous depressive illness, loss of a parent (especially mother) before the age of 12[4], bereavement in later life, no sympathetic close relationship, poor social circumstances, being housebound or tied to the house for family reasons or ill health.
- The mother with young children without a supportive partner, the isolated elderly man or woman whose spouse has died and with physical illness are likely to have a less good prognosis.

TREATMENT

1. It is important to ask about suicidal feelings or fears. If these are substantial (a suicide plan is a danger signal) then admission to hospital, informally or compulsorily, must always be considered.
2. In all cases of depression there should be an empathic exploration of the history of the problem and possible causes. The sharing of the burden with a doctor or other counsellor can reduce anxiety about physical or other symptoms and guilt or self-deprecation. In mild or some moderate cases this supportive psychotherapy is all that is needed.
3. Where depression is the result of isolation or deprivation, possible remedies are by mobilizing statutory or voluntary services; day centres for the elderly housebound; volunteer visitors to old or young; toddler groups; widening the circle of activity or more appropriate employment.
4. Cognitive therapy[5] is a behavioural treatment

aimed at breaking the vicious cycle of depression leading to poor function in daily living, in turn leading to more depression. A detailed diary is kept of a day's activity and mood. The therapist then works on the more negative aspects of the day with the aim of altering the way the patient thinks about them. Positive activities and thoughts are encouraged. The patient is given a limited task to accomplish and report back on each week.

5. Drug treatment: the first tricyclic antidepressants imipramine and amitriptyline have been available since the late 1950s. Many similar preparations have been developed but show few advantages. It is preferable to get to know and use a limited range.

Adequate dosage is essential to ensure effectiveness, e.g. 50–75 mg imipramine or amitriptyline orally, increasing up to 150 mg daily. Immediate side-effects include sedation, tremor, dry mouth, postural hypotension, constipation and blurred vision, but by giving the total dose at night the sedation can be useful therapeutically and the other effects minimized with the exception of dry mouth in the morning. Serious adverse effects are cardiac arrhythmias, especially in the elderly and those with heart disease, anticholinergic effects leading to urinary retention and glaucoma. The side-effects may impair adherence to treatment. In this case it is advisable to reduce dosage and build up slowly.

Antidepressant effects usually take 10–14 days to become apparent. Continue the drug for 6 weeks at an adequate dose before deciding that it is ineffective. Drug treatment for major depression should continue for at least 6 months and may be needed for very much longer. People with lesser degrees of depression may need drugs for only a few months. When stopping treatment, reduce it slowly over a few weeks, especially following longer periods of treatment and higher dosage. Newer antidepressants such as trazodone probably have fewer adverse effects and are useful in the elderly but mianserin may produce bone-marrow suppression and should be used with caution.

Monoamine oxidase inhibitors, e.g. phenelzine, provide an alternative to tricyclics, especially for depression with phobic or atypical features. Drug interactions are numerous and tyramine-containing foods must be excluded. An information leaflet about the food and drugs to be avoided must be given to the patient.

6. Excessive alcohol intake and its withdrawal, prescribed drugs such as beta-blocking agents and organic disease such as carcinoma may be associated with depression. Drugs may have to be stopped but treatment otherwise is similar to other depressive illnesses.

7. Electroconvulsive therapy (ECT) was widely used but is not popular with patients as it affects memory even if only temporarily. Its use is now limited to patients in whom other treatments have failed and to those with marked biological or psychotic features. It may be life-saving in patients refusing to eat or drink.

FOLLOW-UP

Patients with severe depression who are at risk of suicide should be seen every 2 or 3 days; they should also be given an opportunity to seek help when needed between visits. As the intensity of the depression recedes so the frequency of visits can be reduced to weekly and then longer intervals. Patients stabilized on antidepressant medication should usually be seen every 1–3 months. Antidepressants should be continued for several months after remission when depression has been severe but for shorter periods when it is mild.

Depressives Anonymous (36 Chestnut Avenue, Beverley, N. Humberside HU17 9QU) and Depressives Associated offer help and support to those who suffer from depression and their families.

[1] Paykel E (1984) *A Handbook of the Affective Disorders.* Edinburgh: Churchill Livingstone.

[2] Harris CM (1987) In *The Presentation of Depression: Current Approaches* (Freeling P *et al.* eds). Occasional paper 36. London: Royal College of General Practitioners.

[3] Freeling P *et al.* (1985) Unrecognised depression in general practice. *Br. Med. J.,* **290,** 1880.

[4] Brown G, Harris T (1978) *The Social Origins of Depression.* London: Tavistock.

[5] Gelder M (1985) Cognitive therapy. In *Recent Advances in Clinical Psychiatry,* vol 5 (Granville-Grossman K ed). Edinburgh: Churchill Livingstone.

Manic-Depressive Disorder

Manic-depressive disorder is characterized by either periods of mania or depression or both; respectively unipolar or bipolar. The morbid risk (i.e. those vulnerable to the disorder) is about 7.5 per 1000 of the population. The annual incidence is 0.2–0.4 new cases per 1000 per year with a rate slightly higher in women than in men. There is an increased incidence in first-degree relatives, in whom 7–8% suffer from the condition. It is more common in the upper socioeconomic groups[1].

First attacks are less common with increasing age. About 10% of patients with mania have a unipolar illness, 90% are bipolar. 'Mania' is the term used for severe symptoms; hypomania describes less severe symptoms. Patients with this illness are euphoric or irritable in mood and hyperactive. Thoughts and ideas tumble over each other (flight of ideas), are often grandiose and expressed in rapid speech (pressure of speech). There is a decreased need for sleep and patients are easily distracted. They can be disinhibited in sexual behaviour and other ways and spend money recklessly. With more severe degrees of mania, hallucinations and delusions are frequent. Depressive illness is described on page 131. The treatment of a depression with antidepressants sometimes leads to development of manic symptoms.

PROGNOSIS

- Untreated manic episodes may continue over many months.
- Treated manic episodes last less than 3 months[2].
- Nearly all patients recover completely in time, whether treated or untreated.
- Unless preventive measures are taken hypomanic or depressive attacks recur, often with increasing frequency and duration. Manic-depressive disorder can therefore seriously limit a person's life and work and may affect personal relationships and family life.
- Patients often become aware of the impending onset of a manic or depressive episode but lose insight as symptoms become more severe. They then fail to adhere to prophylactic treatment.

TREATMENT

1. Patients with psychotic symptoms who are likely to harm themselves or other people should be admitted either informally or compulsorily under the Mental Health Act.
2. It is important to listen carefully when patients feel another episode is imminent and act accordingly.
3. Hypomania should be treated with phenothiazines. Chlorpromazine in doses of 25–100 mg t.d.s. would be suitable for use at home; haloperidol is an alternative.
4. Lithium carbonate may be used in the acute stage but takes 10 days to be effective.
5. Lithium prevents recurrent attacks in the majority of cases. It is a drug with a small 'therapeutic window'. Serum levels must be measured 12 hours after ingestion and should be 0.5–1.5 mmol/l. Initially blood should be checked for lithium level every 1–2 weeks but when the level is stable every 3 months. Serum urea and electrolytes are checked every 12 months and thyroxine every 3 years.

FOLLOW-UP

During the early stages of an episode of illness patients should be seen every few days. As improvement occurs intervals can be lengthened.

Follow-up is essential in order to monitor treatment as failure to take medication can lead to further acute episodes. Frequency will depend upon the stage of the illness and the reliability of the patient. Maintenance treatment will require regular checks every 3–6 months.

---

[1] Paykel E (1984) *A Handbook of the Affective Disorders.* Edinburgh: Churchill Livingstone.
[2] Reveley MA (1986) Mania. In *Treatment and Prognosis; Medicine* (Hawkins R ed). Oxford: Heinemann.

Suicide and Parasuicide

Suicide is usually associated with mental illness, most commonly depression. Parasuicide or attempted suicide is usually associated with social or relationship breakdown. However there is an overlap in causation and characteristics.

The suicide rate in the UK is estimated to be less than 10 per 100 000 population. Thus in an average general practice list of 2000 a suicide would occur every 5 years or more. The rate is higher in men, the elderly, the unmarried, the unemployed, social classes 1 and 5 and in the months of April, May and June. Many patients who successfully commit suicide have visited a doctor in the preceding week or so.

Parasuicide is most common in adolescent girls and young women in lower socioeconomic groups. It is less common in young males but the rate approaches that of females by the age of 25. The rate declines thereafter in both sexes. In an average general practice of 2000 there are likely to be about 5 cases per year[1]. It most commonly occurs as an impulsive gesture during a relationship problem with a partner. Parasuicide is one of the defining characteristics of personality disorder. It may be related to alcohol problems and drug abuse and is sometimes associated with physical or mental illness. In the young it is usually intended as a gesture or cry for help.

PROGNOSIS

- In most cases of parasuicide there is no further episode but in 15% there is a further attempt during the next year.
- A small number make several attempts and are at considerable risk of suicide. Repetition is more likely in those with previous attempts or a psychiatric history. In repeat attempts the risk of suicide is 1–2%[1,2].
- There is a danger even with a first attempt that an overdose may unintentionally be beyond a safe limit.

TREATMENT

1. Prevention: patients with mental illness showing depression should be carefully assessed (see p. 131. If there are doubts about safety, an urgent consultation with a psychiatrist or admission to hospital should be arranged. Parasuicide by its nature is unpredictable and impulsive and cannot be prevented satisfactorily. Judgement is needed to decide whether someone who has made previous attempts should be admitted when threatening suicide again. When the patient is histrionic and manipulative some risks may have to be taken in the hope of limiting antisocial behaviour.

2. Prevention in the wider sense requires an improvement in the social environment so as to avoid the social circumstances associated with parasuicide.

3. A general practitioner called to see someone who has taken an overdose will have to decide whether to send the person straight to hospital. In an urban area it is usually advisable to do so. In a more remote rural area the doctor may have to take first aid action and then decide. When the overdose was several hours previously, provided the drug is known not to have delayed toxic effects and only a small quantity was taken, it may be safe not to admit the patient. In that case there should be a careful assessment of the circumstances of the attempt. Any mental illness detected will need appropriate action and a social worker can be asked to help find solutions to the difficulties giving rise to the incident. When the patient has been drinking alcohol it is impossible to assess the mental state. This may mean admission to hospital or surveillance by family, friends or police.

4. More often a patient is taken straight to hospital after an overdose and has initial treatment and assessment there. After discharge the general practitioner receives a note with details. If no plan has been made for further treatment the doctor will probably take no action unless called upon to do so by the patient. She or he may however take the opportunity of a visit for some other reason, to

raise the subject and open the door for further exploration of any problems.

5. Drugs should be given with caution after attempted suicide; however, they may be needed for a depressive illness. In such cases they should either be given in small quantities, say, 1 week at a time, or handed to a responsible relative. They should not be given to patients with personality disorders or to those in whom they have been ineffectual in the past.

6. The family of a suicide victim will need continuing counselling and support. There are likely to be similar needs in the families of those who attempt suicide.

FOLLOW-UP

Patients with depressive illness should be followed-up as described on p. 132. Other patients will be followed-up by a social worker until the social circumstances improve. Most patients reject follow-up by a doctor, probably because they feel ashamed of the incident and want to forget it. But if they accept it, continued support and counselling can be helpful.

---

[1] Hawton K (1987) Attempted suicide. *Med. Int.*, **2**, 1786–90.
[2] Reveley MA (1986) Suicide and attempted suicide. In *Treatment and Prognosis: Medicine* (Hawkins R ed). Oxford: Heinemann.

Bereavement[1,2,]

The loss of a close relative or friend is one of the most intense emotional experiences that occurs in human beings. Few will avoid it.

There are characteristic stages in grief after bereavement but they will not be experienced to the same degree by everyone; some stages may not occur at all. Following the death of a much-loved person the first reaction is of numbness and shock. In anything from a few hours to several days this is succeeded by a feeling of intense sadness that is expressed, depending upon differing personalities and cultural backgrounds, as silent weeping or loud lamentation.

Anger may be felt and may be directed at the unfairness that a beloved person has been taken away and the world continues as though nothing has happened. Sometimes the anger is focused on individuals, either family members or medical or nursing attendants who are thought to have been negligent. Feelings of guilt are common. Despite heroic efforts in caring for someone at home, the bereaved person often feels she or he could have done more. Guilt, almost always unfounded, may also be felt by nurses and others with a caring role.

At first intense pangs of grief are felt at frequent intervals and may be triggered by talk about the person who has died. These gradually decrease to a bearable level in the next days and weeks. The imagination of the bereaved person is filled with thoughts of the deceased, and the sense that he or she is still alive and will walk into the room is common. Dreams about the dead person may occur and at times there may be auditory or visual hallucinations. Anxiety or agitation may also occur. Some people develop physical symptoms and insomnia is the general rule.

The funeral is an important landmark as it helps in the process of acceptance. It also coincides with some change from the early intense grief. Gradually a more apathetic phase is entered. Life goes on but seems without purpose or pleasure. This period of apathy and depression may last for many weeks or months. It seems to friends and relatives that it will never end; the bereaved person may not even feel he or she wants it to end. However the burden does eventually lighten and he or she begins to show interest in what is going on and in old or new activities.

Any of the stages following bereavement may be exaggerated or persist. For instance, the feeling of anger can turn to an enduring bitterness that may be lifelong. The depression may turn into a depressive illness.

PROGNOSIS

- Most people do recover from bereavement surprisingly well considering the strains that they suffer. Residual feelings of grief may, however, sometimes linger for life.
- A good prognosis is likely when the bereaved person has a network of family and friends who are able both to share the grief and to give support. A previously wide variety of interests and activities also helps.
- Good anticipatory counselling helps early recovery.
- A poor prognosis is more likely when there is little or no family able or willing to keep in contact and when the bereaved person has a restricted lifestyle. Sometimes when a spouse dies a less than happy relationship may leave the remaining partner feeling persistently angry, guilty or unhappy.
- Anniversary grieving is fairly common and also sadness or depression at Christmas or other times that have special associations.
- The loss of a spouse at a late stage in life means the remaining partner may not fully recover.
- A depressive illness may develop and last for months and perhaps years.
- Sudden unexpected death is more likely to be followed by a longer period of grief than an expected death.

TREATMENT

1. Good standards of care for a dying person, in particular best possible pain relief, high-quality nursing, careful explanation and an opportunity for questioning by the relatives, help the family to accept their inevitable loss. They are thus able to recover more quickly, and the grieving may be less severe.
2. After a death the family, especially the surviving spouse, should be visited by the general practitioner to express and share in the sorrow. At an appropriate moment it can help to go over the last illness so that questions can be asked and guilt or angry feelings expressed. If things have not gone well at any point the doctor should honestly admit to any shortcomings and allow the anger to be dissipated. Letting the bereaved person know that feelings of guilt are understood and to some extent shared can be a great help. Reassurance that the bereaved person had done all that was possible may need to be repeated.
3. Drugs are not often useful. Quite frequently relatives ask the doctor to prescribe for the surviving spouse. This gives an opportunity to explain the nature of bereavement and the grief that has to be worked through before recovery can take place. It is sometimes a good idea to prescribe a sedative to take if desired; this also symbolizes the doctor's willingness to help. If depression is prolonged and severe, antidepressants are fully justified and may need to be continued for many months. A more sedative type of antidepressant taken at night may also be useful for prolonged insomnia.
4. Children who have been bereaved and the parents of a cot-death baby or those who have lost a child in other circumstances need specialized counselling. This is usually best provided through a department of paediatrics and voluntary associations. The general practitioner should continue to be involved and ensure that the specialized help is being made available.

FOLLOW-UP

Follow-up will depend a great deal on the family and social support system. Where it is good, little more need be done after initial visiting than offer and encourage further contact if needed. If the support system is not so good or a person has been badly shaken by the loss of someone close there should be positive follow-up by home visits or surgery appointments. This task can be shared with a health visitor or trained volunteer. Sometimes health visitors establish contact during the terminal illness.

Cruse (National Organization for the Widowed and their Children, Cruse House, 126 Sheen Road, Richmond, Surrey TW9 1UR) is a national organization that exists to help the bereaved. There are branches throughout the UK. They offer a valuable voluntary service to individuals by counselling and sharing the experience of bereavement. Other support organizations (see *Health Directory, 1990,* published for Thames Television's Help! programme by Bedford Square Press, London) exist for people with particular needs.

Parkes CM (1986) *Bereavement*, 2nd edn. London: Tavistock.

[2] Parkes CM, Weiss RS (1983) *Recovery from Bereavement*. New York: Basic Books.

Schizophrenia

Schizophrenia is a condition characterized by delusions and hallucinations—usually auditory—and abnormal, illogical thought processes. These occur in the absence of organic brain disease or intoxication with drugs or alcohol which might otherwise account for the symptoms.

The diagnosis of schizophrenia can be difficult as a wide variety of symptoms may occur and many are shared with other mental states. In order to overcome the diagnostic difficulties certain symptoms are called 'first-rank'[1]. These are: thought insertion or withdrawal (a thought put into or withdrawn from the mind); thought broadcasting (being known to others); feelings of passivity (emotions, sensations, bodily movement and impulses being under external influence); the patient hearing voices discussing his or her thoughts or behaviour as they occur, sometimes carrying on a running commentary; voices discussing or arguing about the patient, referring to him or her in the third person as 'he' or 'she'; voices repeating the patient's thoughts out loud; delusional perceptions, that is delusions arising from perceptions which themselves are normal. The presence of one or more of these symptoms makes the diagnosis likely. In addition there may be flattened or inappropriate affect or paranoid delusions of persecution. At times the patient may be apathetic, at others overactive or irritable. Behaviour may be grossly disorganized with deterioration of the personality. In schizoaffective psychosis affective symptoms are prominent and whilst recovery is usually complete, relapse is common. 'Schizophreniform psychosis' is a term used to describe an acute illness somewhat atypical in form and from which recovery is rapid[2].

Schizophrenia has a point prevalence of 2–4 per 1000 population and a first episode of illness incidence of about 0.2 per 1000. The mean age of onset is in the early 20s, and it rarely occurs for the first time after age 45. Although relatively uncommon, the early age of onset and tendency to become chronic or recur make it a significant cause of disability for both the individual and the family.

PROGNOSIS

- There is a tendency for schizophrenia to relapse or become chronic.
- Some 20% of patients have one or two acute episodes and then remain well; 35% are well for long periods but have relapses from time to time; 35% have mild and persistent symptoms; 10% show rapid deterioration[3].
- Good prognostic features are: a good premorbid personality in a person with stable home and work environment; being married; no family history of schizophrenia; acute onset; older age at first episode; a known precipitation cause; short duration of episode; prominent affective symptoms such as depression, and the presence of perplexity and confusion.
- Bad prognostic features are: a shy, isolated and aloof premorbid personality; 'blunted affect', that is a lack of emotional responsiveness and normal variation in mood, and a high level of stormy, hostile 'expressed emotion' in the home environment.

TREATMENT

1. An acute episode of schizophrenia is a disturbing and upsetting experience for the family of the patient as much as for the patient, and often results in an emergency call to the family doctor. One of the first tasks in management is to make a calm appraisal of the situation and in doing so, to reduce anxiety and tension in both

patient and family. With first episodes, and often with later acute relapses, the patient will need to be admitted to hospital. This may be on an informal basis but may have to be compulsory under a section of the Mental Health Act. In this case a social worker and a psychiatrist will have to be called in to support the enforced admission.

2. Drug treatment with phenothiazines has changed the previously poor outlook in both the acute and long-term management of the condition. Chlorpromazine is most widely used for the acute episode; 100–200 mg t.d.s. might be given to the patient managed at home but sometimes larger doses are needed in severe cases in hospital. Other phenothiazines such as thioridazine, fluphenazine, trifluperazine or haloperidol (a butyrophenone) are alternatives for the acute episode. The most frequent and troublesome side-effects are extrapyramidal symptoms which occur more with some preparations, e.g. haloperidol, than others. Some drugs, e.g. chlorpromazine or thioridazine, have a more sedative effect which can be useful for patients needing sedation.

3. Long-term treatment by drugs is essential for most patients for a year or longer following an acute episode. Relapse can occur even after several years of freedom from symptoms, so the decision to stop drugs must be taken with care. Medication can either be given orally or as a depot injection of fluphenazine decanoate (or enanthate) or flupenthixol decanoate by the practice or community psychiatric nurse. A serious adverse-effect of long-term use of phenothiazines is tardive dyskinesia, a condition characterized by involuntary movements of face, trunk and limbs. The risk of this can be minimized by using the smallest possible dose for the shortest possible time.

4. Anticholinergic drugs such as procyclidine are sometimes used to prevent extrapyramidal side-effects. However there is evidence that they can contribute to the development of tardive dyskinesia and they should be given for a limited period, if at all.

5. The social treatment of schizophrenia is an important part of its management. The patient is liable to be rejected by family, at work and by his or her normal social circle, so every effort should be made to maintain and foster these relationships. The risk of relapse is lower when the patient returns to a peaceful home environment and when a high level of expressed emotion in the family has been reduced. Family tensions may also be reduced by the patient attending a day centre. Rehabilitation services help patients to return to their normal community or if recovery is incomplete provide workshops and continuing occupational therapy. Sheltered housing is needed for patients with a chronic illness who lack a supportive home.

6. Electroconvulsive therapy may be indicated for severe depressive symptoms or catatonic stupor.

FOLLOW-UP

Patients on treatment need careful follow-up to ensure that medication is continued. This applies in particular to young patients who are liable to feel that they are being 'damaged' by receiving drug treatment and plead to stop their medication. It is a matter for agreement as to whether care is supervised by the general practitioner or psychiatrist.

Community psychiatric nurses are invaluable in maintaining contacts with patient and family and links between hospital and community-based services. Social workers also have an important role in continuing care. Voluntary organizations such as the National Schizophrenia Fellowship (78/79 Victoria Road, Surbiton, Surrey KT6 4NS; telephone 01-390 3651) can provide support for families of schizophrenics.

---

[1] Schneider K quoted by Cooper JE[2].
[2] Cooper JE (1987) Schizophrenia and allied conditions. *Med. Int.*, **2,** 1773–8.
[3] Goldberg D *et al.* (1987) Psychiatry in medical practice. London: Tavistock Publications.

Personality Disorders

Personality disorder' is a term used to describe persistent abnormal behaviour in an individual in the absence of mental or physical illness, drugs or alcohol. As it depends on subjective judgement it is an inexact term. What to one observer is a personality disorder, to another is merely an unusual trait. An essential element in the definition is the effect the person has on other people—usually a damaging or unpleasant one.

At one extreme is the person with an antisocial personality who from an early age gets into difficulties with truancy from school and breaking the law. She or he is unable to form stable close relationships and has an amoral behaviour pattern. There may be outbursts of uncontrolled aggression and an inability to learn from experience. At the other end of the scale, people with personality problems may be excessively dependent, withdrawn or passively aggressive. There may be associated dependence on drugs or alcohol, or mental illness. This can make diagnosis difficult because it may not be clear which is the primary disorder.

The abnormality manifests itself in adolescence in the case of antisocial personality but sometimes in the 20s or 30s with other varieties of the disorder.

PROGNOSIS

- By definition personality disorder is persistent and in general, is resistant to attempts at modification. However improvements often occur after the age of 45 and in some people the abnormality may disappear almost entirely[1].
- In others abnormalities persist. The effects of alcohol abuse or associated mental illness can add to the problem of the patient, family and community.

TREATMENT

1. Prevention: the cause of personality disorder is not known. Some varieties may be genetically determined. In others it is probable that the lack of a secure and loving childhood background predisposes to personality problems and disorders in adolescent and adult life. Both these aspects may offer hope for prevention.
2. Antipsychotic drugs, e.g. flupenthixol or haloperidol, may have a limited place in treatment but should be used with care because of the risk of abuse[2].
3. Psychotherapy and behavioural treatments are unlikely to help. There is some evidence that group therapy in a therapeutic community may modify behaviour in some people with personality disorders.
4. To help someone with a personality disorder the doctor has to develop tolerance to difficult behaviour. However it is essential to set boundaries as to what is acceptable. There should be a consistent, supportive yet firm approach. This may make it possible to develop a relationship which is of benefit to the patient and acceptable to the doctor.

FOLLOW-UP

Patients with personality problems frequently do not keep follow-up appointments. However if the person is prepared to attend regularly this implies some possibility of making progress.

---

[1] Reveley MA (1986) Antisocial personality. In *Treatment and Prognosis Medicine* (Hawkins R ed). Oxford: Heinemann.
[2] Tyrer P (1987) Personality difficulties and disorders. *Med. Int.*, **2**, 1839–45.

Drug Abuse

The abuse of drugs means the repeated misuse of a drug which may have damaging consequences to the user, often his or her family and sometimes the society in which he or she lives. Dependence on a drug may be physical. This means that sudden withdrawal leads to unpleasant or even dangerous physical effects. Psychological dependence means the compulsive use of a drug with few physical consequences on withdrawal but with a tendency to relapse. Some people become dependent on a drug but maintain a stable relationship with it and continue a normal working and social life. Others live in a world dominated by drug-taking and its tragic consequences of personal destruction, mental and physical illness, crime and suicide. In this group multiple drugs may be used, including the abuse of alcohol.

Illicit drug-taking usually begins in adolescence or early adult life. Cannabis is the most widely used and many who take it do not succumb to further drugs. For some, however, it is the starting point of abuse of other drugs such as opiates. Solvent abuse is particularly common in children with a deprived background. Cocaine and hallucinogens tend to be the choice of the more privileged groups in society.

Injected drugs can lead to the transmission of hepatitis, human immunodeficiency virus, or development of local infections or endocarditis. Evidence of needle marks and thrombosed veins may be found in those who inject drugs. The use of drugs should be suspected when there is a change in behaviour of a young person or an otherwise unaccountable decline in performance at school or at work.

PROGNOSIS[1]

- Prognosis depends upon the type of drug, age and social personality characteristics of the patient.
- Follow-up studies of opiate users show that after 7 years about 25–33% are abstinent, while 10–20% have died due to drug-related causes.
- However, 95% of soldiers who became addicted during the Vietnam War were abstinent on follow-up, indicating the importance of personality and social factors on outcome.
- Barbiturate dependence is similar to alcoholism in its tendency to relapse and become chronic. There is a high risk of death by accidental overdose. Withdrawal can lead to the occurrence of seizures.
- Stopping cannabis produces no definite withdrawal syndrome, nor is there evidence of tolerance to this drug. Its deleterious effects are principally due to intoxication. High doses may lead to psychotic symptoms.
- Amphetamine dependence can lead to a paranoid psychosis indistinguishable from paranoid schizophrenia.
- Cocaine, hallucinogens and phencyclidine tend to be recreational drugs whose principal risk is from life-threatening behaviour during the acute intoxication, particularly psychotic episodes leading to suicide.
- Solvent abuse may lead to death through toxic effects and trauma, asphyxia or inhalation of stomach contents. A total of 169 deaths were reported from 1971 to 1981 in the UK[2].

TREATMENT

1. A common presentation of a drug user is to register as a temporary resident and to request a prescription for a drug which she or he has run out of when away from home. The alternatives for the general practitioner are either to refuse a prescription or to telephone the patient's own doctor to confirm the authenticity of the story. A small quantity only should be supplied.

2. A history should be taken before treating a regular drug user and any relevant psychological or physical assessment should be made.

3. Diamorphine, dipipanone and cocaine may only be prescribed for users by doctors holding a special licence at treatment centres. Patients needing these drugs must therefore be referred to a centre. It is often also advisable to refer users of other illicit drugs because

facilities and expertise are needed to treat them.

4. The treatment of established drug users is based on a plan agreed by both taker and prescriber to reduce the dose at regular intervals at a rate that avoids withdrawal symptoms. It is in the nature of a contract, binding on both user and prescriber. Any change in the contract must be renegotiated.

5. For those withdrawing from opiates, methadone is prescribed in liquid form in a dose of 20–70 mg/day depending on the level of opiate taken. The dose is adjusted to avoid both intoxication and symptoms of withdrawal. There is then a regular small reduction of dose over the next few weeks until it can be stopped altogether. Methadone is given in liquid form to avoid tablets being crushed and taken intravenously.

6. Toxicological screening may help management[3].

7. Other drugs are dealt with in a similar way by gradual reduction. Sometimes medication is given for withdrawal symptoms.

8. Inpatient treatment enables a more rapid reduction in drugs to be made, combined with psychotherapy, and a start on rehabilitation that can be continued as an outpatient.

9. There are various organizations and other approaches available to drug users and their families. Some are residential therapeutic communities whilst others are based in the general community.

10. Some drug users are unwilling to stop altogether. They should be maintained on the lowest dose that they can manage.

11. There is a legal obligation to register a person who uses or is suspected of using controlled drugs. Details may be found in the British National Formulary[5].

FOLLOW-UP

Whilst they require prescriptions patients will continue to attend. After treatment is complete it is vital that help from social worker, groups and voluntary bodies is maintained.

The doctor can assist by offering personal support and ensuring that the patient makes use of rehabilitation services.

[1] Reveley MA (1986) Drug dependence. In *Treatment and Prognosis; Medicine* (Hawkins R ed). Oxford: Heinemann.
[2] Anderson HR et al. (1982) *Hum. Toxicol.*, **1**, 207.
[3] Skidmore CA et al. (1987) Toxicological screening in heroin users: implications for management of drug misuse. *J. R. Coll. Gen. Pract.*, **37**, 397–9.
[4] *Guidelines of Good Clinical Practice in the Treatment of Drug Misuse. Report of the Medical Working Group on Drug Dependence* (1984) London: DHSS.
[5] British National Formulary. Br. Med. Assn. and R. Pharm. Soc. Great Britain.

Alcohol and its Problems

Recent reports on alcohol suggest it should be treated as a risk factor in the development of health problems[1]. At one end of the scale light social drinking has few risks; at the other end heavy uncontrolled drinking leads to disastrous physical, psychological and social consequences. In England and Wales in 1980 27% of men drank 21 or more units* of alcohol in a single week; in the same week 3% of women drank 21 or more units and 10% drank 11–20 units[2].

On average a general practitioner is likely to have on the list about 55 people whose drinking is at a level of high risk and over 200 who are at intermediate risk. Heavy drinkers consult general practitioners twice as often as light drinkers[3]. Drinking rates are higher in the young and in men[1,2,4]. Heavy and even moderate alcohol consumption can have widespread physical effects[1,5]. In primary care these may present in a variety of ways, including gastrointestinal upsets and otherwise unexplained vomiting or diarrhoea, blackouts and trauma, sometimes as a result of traffic accidents or fights. At 80 mg per 100 ml blood alcohol, the UK legal limit, the road traffic accident risk is twice the sober level.

Depression, anxiety and insomnia are common and alcohol reduces sexual function. Adverse effects are felt by the family and there is liable to be marital disharmony: work suffers.

Heavy drinking in pregnancy results in the fetal alcohol syndrome. The relative risk of second-trimester loss is 1.03 (not significant), 1.98 and 3.53 in women taking less than 1, 1–2 and more than 3 units of alcohol daily compared with non-drinkers[6].

Withdrawal from alcohol may result in shakiness, nausea, sweating and anxiety; more severe symptoms are illusions, a sense of dread and auditory hallucinations. Generalized epileptiform fits may occur, as well as delirium tremens.

PROGNOSIS

- Recent recommendations[1] suggest that there is minimal risk to health at a weekly intake up to 15 units for women and 20 units for men. There is a moderate risk from 16 to 35 units for women and 21–50 units for men. Regular weekly intakes above these levels, if continued, carry considerable risks.

- Those dependent on alcohol have a compulsive urge to drink and have increased tolerance and symptoms on withdrawal. They therefore find it more difficult to stop or reduce drinking and thus are at greater risk.

- The longer the history of drinking and the heavier the weekly consumption, the more likely there are to be adverse effects.

- Women are more vulnerable than men at a given level of alcohol intake. The reason for this has not been finally established.

- Some patients with mental illness such as phobic anxiety or patients with personality disorder are more prone to continue drinking.

- Some occupations carry a high risk of heavy drinking and alcohol-related damage—in particular for those who work in the drink industry.

- Good prognostic features include a previously good personality, a stable and supportive family and friends, a steady job, insight and motivation.

- The 10-year death rate for those in middle age who drink 36 units of alcohol or more per week has been estimated to be twice the rate of those who drink 10 units or less[1].

TREATMENT

1. One of the first tasks is to determine as accurately as possible how much the patient is drinking. This may need to be established over several consultations. It can be facilitated by the patient keeping a daily diary of intake over 1 week; this diary might include other information about diet, exercise etc.

---

* 8 g absolute alcohol = 1 unit = ½ pint beer = 1 glass wine = single measure of spirits = 1 glass sherry or port.

2. In the moderate or heavy drinker assessment should include relevant physical examination and laboratory tests and enquiry about psychiatric symptoms and social background.

3. The patient's attitude to his or her own drinking is fundamental to successful treatment and may take time and several visits to establish. The attitude of the spouse is of scarcely less importance and she or he should be included so far as possible.

4. A planned reduction is then worked out with the patient. This may be on a stepped basis over several weeks at a rate the patient feels he or she can manage. For the moderate drinker the goal can be a lower safer level. Heavy drinkers, especially with evidence of alcohol-induced damage or past failures, should aim at complete abstinence.

5. When consumption has been very high and particularly when the patient is hallucinating, it is often best to admit the patient to hospital for the initial drying out.

6. Sedatives such as diazepam are sometimes used over the initial phase of reduction but should be given for a few days only. Chlormethiazole is used for the treatment of acute withdrawal symptoms in hospital but for no more than 9 days, as otherwise dependence will result.

7. Vitamin B preparations should be given during detoxification by injection and later by mouth.

8. Disulfiram (Antabuse) can be given to heavy drinkers wanting to abstain. It causes flushing, palpitations, nausea and vomiting in the presence of alcohol. It carries some risk and should not be given to anyone with heart disease.

9. An essential part of treatment is to provide support to patient and family. Rehabilitation should aim to create a wider social life so that other activities fill the time that was spent drinking. Group therapy with others who have been heavy drinkers is very helpful to some.

FOLLOW-UP

Careful follow-up is essential as patients need continuing support and encouragement. When patients are being treated at a drinking-problem unit the general practitioner can fulfil a useful function by providing additional support and continuity of care when the patient is discharged from the clinic.

Alcoholics Anonymous (General Service Office, PO Box 1, Stonebow House, Stonebow, York YO1 2NJ; telephone 0904 644026; Greater London, telephone 01-834 8202) is a self-help organization for those wishing to maintain long-term abstinence. Al-Anon and Alateen (Al-Anon and Alateen, 61 Great Dover Street, London SE1 4YF; telephone 01-403 0888) provide support for the spouses and teenage children of problem drinkers.

[1] Alcohol—A Balanced View. Report from General Practice 24. (1986) London: Royal College of General Practitioners.

[2] Wilson P (1980) Drinking in England and Wales. London: HMSO.

[3] Office of Population Censuses and Surveys (1984) General Household Survey 1982. London: HMSO.

[4] Wallace PG et al. (1987) Drinking patterns in general practice patients. J. R. Coll. Gen. Pract., 37, 354–7.

[5] Reveley MA (1986) Alcoholism. In Treatment and Prognosis: Medicine (Hawkins R ed). Oxford: Heinemann.

[6] Harlap S, Shiono PH (1980) Alcohol and smoking and the incidence of spontaneous abortion in the first and second trimester. Lancet, ii, 173.

Eating Disorders

Anorexia nervosa is characterized by loss of 25% of original body weight in the absence of identifiable physical cause. The patient (usually female) is fearful of being fat and has a distorted body image so that despite being excessively thin she sees herself as too fat and feels that she must reduce her food intake still further. The anorexic is obsessed with food and will often prepare large meals for the family whilst not eating herself. She may weigh herself several times in the day.

Amenorrhoea is almost invariable and may be a presenting symptom; without it the diagnosis must remain in doubt. The skin is rough and dry, and a soft down-like lanugo hair develops, whilst there is loss of hair from axillae, pubis and sometimes head. The patient feels the cold and stays wrapped up in thick clothes despite warm weather. The extremities are cold and blue. There is hypotension and bradycardia, and leg oedema when weight loss is severe. Patients are often overactive and restless and may exercise excessively in order to lose weight. Episodes of bulimia (bingeing) may occur with self-induced vomiting or taking of purgatives.

Patients often show obsessional traits, are hardworking, perfectionist and may be described as 'good' children by their parents. They are usually inexperienced sexually and may become socially isolated.

Anorexia nervosa is a condition associated with affluence; it is commoner in higher socioeconomic groups and does not usually occur in third-world countries. It is a condition affecting young people, with an onset between the ages of 12 and 30, peaking at 15–16. Typically it affects adolescent girls amongst whom the prevalence is 0.3–1% depending on social class, with a male-to-female ratio of approximately 1:15. Milder symptoms of anorexia are common, only in some instances progressing to a more severe illness.

Bulimia is a closely related condition in which a pattern of gorge-eating occurs. This may be associated with self-induced vomiting and features of anorexia or with a sometimes gross increase in weight. In some instances bulimia is a symptom of or associated with a depressive disorder. The episodes of overeating are kept secret and there are feelings of guilt. Severe bulimia can lead to metabolic disturbances, dental caries, swollen parotid glands and other physical effects. The mean age of onset is somewhat later than for anorexia but there is an even more marked preponderance of females. The prevalence is similar to anorexia. Minor episodes of bingeing and vomiting are quite common in adolescent girls but few if any of these reach the doctor.

PROGNOSIS

- Unfavourable prognostic features are late age of onset, long illness, severe weight loss resistant to treatment, bulimia, vomiting and purging, depression, marked anxiety, obsessional features and difficulties with relationships.
- Follow-up studies of anorexia show that with active treatment 70% of patients have reached 90% or more of standard weight after 10 years. Of the other 30% a small number die of starvation or suicide and the remainder continue to have eating or other problems.
- In 86% of cases the illness lasts 2 years or more[1].
- Bulimia without anorexic episodes carries a better prognosis.

TREATMENT

1. There should be a full clinical examination with biochemical and other tests as necessary.
2. Inpatient care is needed when weight loss is more than 25% so as to restore weight to normal as soon as possible. It is usually preferable to admit the patient to a psychiatric unit that specializes in treating anorexia. Separation from the family seems to be an important element in the treatment. A strict regimen of regular meals is instituted with privileges granted as progress is made.
3. Psychotherapy is begun once the refeeding programme is established. Family therapy is usually the preferred method for the sufferer

who is not yet living independently, but on an individual basis for the person who has left home. Following discharge psychotherapy is continued.

4. In milder cases treatment can be on an out-patient basis. One of the aims is to change behaviour in the patient by altering set patterns in the family.
5. Drugs have little place in the treatment of anorexia.
6. Bulimia is usually treated on an outpatient basis by psychotherapy or group therapy. Anti-depressant drugs have also been shown to be effective.

7. The patient and family may feel shame and guilt. They must be firmly told that no one is to blame. The parents or spouse need support as the illness may last many years.

FOLLOW-UP

Treatment may have to continue for several years.

Once independent self-management has been achieved no further follow-up is needed. However relapses may occur and require treatment.

[1] Dally P, Gomez J (1979) *Anorexia Nervosa*. London: Heinemann.

Psychosexual Problems[1,2,3]

In the female the commonest sexual problems are dyspareunia, failure to achieve orgasm and vaginismus. In the male erectile impotence and premature ejaculation are the commonest; failure of ejaculation occurs occasionally. In either sex libido can be lacking as a primary complaint or it may develop in the course of a relationship. Non-consummation of a marriage may result from male or female difficulties or a combination of the two. It should raise questions about the sexual orientation of one or other partner or both. Sexual difficulties may be solely due to physical disorder, drugs or alcohol but are usually the result of a complex situation that includes psychological factors.

PROGNOSIS

- Early experiences are of the utmost importance for later sexual health. An upbringing in which there are warm loving relationships, free expression of emotions and uninhibited discussion of matters related to sex are positive indicators.
- An early background of marital discord, inconstant relationships, distaste for sex by either parent, of inhibited rigid attitudes or of sexual assault or abuse almost inevitably leads to sexual difficulties.
- In the early stage of a marriage between a previously inexperienced couple there may be a sexual failure. This usually responds to simple advice and encouragement.
- Erectile impotence due to physical causes has less chance of recovery than that of psychological origin. Loss of nocturnal and morning erections and a progressive organic illness indicate a poor outlook. Impotence due to drugs should improve following withdrawal but may persist in the heavy drinker after stopping alcohol consumption.
- Premature ejaculation is amenable to treatment but success depends to a considerable extent on co-operation by the female partner.
- Following acute illnesses such as myocardial infarction or strokes sexual function often ceases. Although initially it may do so for physical reasons anxiety perpetuates the situation. Function can usually be restored in part if not completely.
- Few women attain orgasm at each act of sexual intercourse. Counselling can help many women who do not or only infrequently have an orgasm. But about 10% of women are likely never to experience one.

TREATMENT

1. Many patients are embarrassed by their sexual problems which in any case may result from inhibitions. They therefore need a sympathetic response to cues that indicate the nature of the problem. A detailed description and history, to include alcohol and drugs, should be obtained and a physical examination made. This will require adequate time and much of the detail is best left to a second or third interview. In erectile impotence organic causes such as diabetes mellitus should be sought. Talking about the difficulty is often therapeutic in itself.

2. It is almost always a good idea to interview both partners together to gain insight into how they relate to each other. It can also help them to talk freely about problems in a way that has not until then been possible. Improvement in communication is one of the most important aspects of treatment.

3. The physical aspects of the problem are dealt with appropriately. In the case of dyspareunia a painful episiotomy is treated by gentle self-stretching with a finger or sometimes injection of a local anaesthetic. Other causes of dyspareunia are investigated and treated. Anxiety often surrounds physical problems. It is usually possible to dispel this by explanation and reassurance and by advice for specific diseases such as heart disease, multiple sclerosis, or arthritis of the hips.

4. Mental illness should be treated but with due regard to the possible effects of drugs.

5. Psychological treatment is based on the concept that sexual arousal leads to anxiety about intercourse and in turn to failure. This in turn raises the level of anxiety. The couple are instructed not to attempt intercourse for a few weeks. At first they enjoy the pleasures of physical stimulation but avoid the genital areas. In controlled stages, as agreed with the therapist, increasing stimulation of sexual areas is allowed. Only when both partners are completely relaxed with this stage and after several weeks is full intercourse allowed.

6. Premature ejaculation may be treated by the squeeze technique of Masters and Johnson[1,2]. The couple begin with a period of non-sexual stimulation as described above. Sexual stimulation is then allowed but without penetration. When ejaculation is approaching it is inhibited by the woman squeezing the penis below the glans. When control at this stage has been achieved then penetration is allowed with the woman astride the man. Ejaculation is again inhibited by withdrawing and squeezing the penis.

FOLLOW-UP

A series of usually joint interviews are needed for treatment. Once success has been achieved it can be left that either member of the couple can return if necessary.

[1] Bancroft J (1983) *Human Sexuality and its Problems*. Edinburgh: Churchill Livingstone.
[2] Kaplan HS (1974) *The New Sex Therapy*. London: Baillière Tindall.
[3] Hawton K, Oppenheimer C (1981) Sexual problems In *Women's Problems in General Practice* Oxford General Practice Series : 12 (McPherson A ed.) Oxford: Oxford University Press.

Obesity

Obesity is defined as an excess weight of 20% or more above the normal range for height and build and overweight as 10% above the range[1]. Obesity is not a disease but can be regarded as a risk factor for many medical conditions such as hypertension, cardiovascular disease including varicose veins, diabetes mellitus, gallstones and arthritis of weight-bearing joints, especially the spine and knees in pregnancy.

Surgery is more hazardous in the obese. Genetic, dietary, economic, cultural and psychological factors may be implicated in its development.

Obesity may also be a feature of endocrine disease, for instance Cushing's disease or myxoedema. It may result from treatment with corticosteroids, psychotropic or other drugs or from excessive intake of alcohol.

The prevalence of obesity varies with age and culture. By the mid 20s in the UK 31% of men and 27% of women are substantially overweight[2].

PROGNOSIS

- Many overweight individuals do not see a doctor and are able to lose weight without professional help.
- Poor prognostic features are a family history of obesity, whether it be genetic in origin or as a result of eating habits or beliefs; living in a culture in which wealth and status are associated with food and obesity; physical disability so that locomotion is diminished; psychological dependence on food in depression and emotional deprivation; a need for continued psychotropic medication as in schizophrenia; a past history of failed treatment; a business lifestyle that involves eating and drinking.
- Good prognostic features are high motivation, a previous lack of information about obesity and a supportive spouse.

TREATMENT

1. National food policies and the interests of the food industry play a part in the diet of a country. Obesity could in part be prevented by changing policies to improve nutrition.
2. Health education starting in early childhood and continuing throughout school age into adult life should be vigorously pursued.
3. In the treatment of established obesity it is important to assess the reasons for the obesity and confirm the patient's own motivation and goals. Depression may need treatment but preferably without drugs. Psychotherapy or behavioural methods may be appropriate in some instances.

4. Diet: the treatment of established obesity is essentially to reduce intake below requirement. In uncomplicated cases simple dietary advice is given to exclude refined carbohydrate, to reduce fat intake and include a high fibre content. In resistant cases a more detailed diet of 800–1000 calories is needed. It is helpful to ask the patient to write down every item of food and drink taken over, say 1 week. This should focus his or her thoughts on keeping to a diet and actual intake can then be calculated.

Very low calorie diets of about 400 kcal or below are now commercially available. They are liquid preparations with the necessary mineral content to prevent the dangers associated with hypokalaemia. They lead to impressive reductions in weight not always maintained in the long term. They should be used with caution in people with cardiovascular disease.

Diet and weight reduction can be supervised by a doctor, nurse, dietician or trained counsellor or within a group. Regular visits every 2–4 weeks may be helpful.

For obese children or adolescents dietary advice should in the first place be confined to sensible eating, in particular limiting sweets and sugars. More detailed diets may be worked out with the help of a dietician. In extreme cases referral to a paediatrician may be necessary.

5. Groups: one of the best forms of treatment for the obese is by joining a group. This is a form of self-help but with the advantage of support from other members of the group who help

each other and maintain motivation. Some groups are run on a commercial basis; others by health visitors, nurses or dieticians. Successful groups are also run by patients themselves and are thus genuinely self-help.

6. Drugs, once widely used, are now rarely considered advisable as long-term results have been poor. It is sometimes appropriate to give an appetite-suppressant such as diethylpropion for a limited period to initiate loss of weight. Drugs should be avoided in people with personality problems or depression. Bulk-forming agents such as methyl cellulose have a small place in treatment.

7. Exercise helps people to lose weight. It is likely that if exercise is taken before or within 2 hours after a meal some of the food is turned into heat rather than fat. Walking 5 km a day can reduce excessive appetite.

8. Heroic surgical measures are sometimes used as a last resort, e.g. intestinal bypass operations or adipectomy.

FOLLOW-UP

When obesity is a contributory factor in, for instance, cardiovascular disease, follow-up will relate to the other condition. It is for negotiation as to how often and for how long a period people with simple obesity should be seen. Some patients are oppressed and some are helped by regular visits.

[1] James WPT (1987) Obesity. In *Oxford Textbook of Medicine*, pp. 8.35–8.51 (Weatherall DJ *et al.* ed). Oxford: Oxford University Press.
[2] Royal College of Physicians Report on Obesity (1983) *J. R. Coll. Phys. Lond.*, **17**, 3–58.

Dementia[1,2,]

Dementia (chronic brain syndrome) occurs in 6–7% of people over 65. Of those over 75, 12–15% are affected, and 20% of those over 85. Alzheimer's disease is the commonest variety of degenerative dementia, representing about 55% of cases. It is commoner in women and there is a higher incidence in families. Multi-infarct dementia, as its name suggests, results from cerebrovascular accidents and accounts for about 20% of cases of dementia. It is characterized by a stepwise progression of the dementia and by neurological deficits, often transient, such as hemiplegia. The ratio of men to women is about 3:2. There may be physical signs of past damage, for example altered reflexes or upgoing plantar responses. A further 20% are of mixed degenerative and cerebrovascular type. The remaining 5% are made up of Pick's disease, in which personality changes and dysphasia occur early; Huntington's chorea, in which psychotic and neurological features and personality changes appear before dementia; and least commonly, Creutzfeldt–Jacob disease, in which different parts of the brain are affected with consequent differing clinical features but characteristic myoclonic jerks and abnormal electroencephalogram.

Dementia is characterized by memory impairment without clouding of consciousness, decreased ability to think and concentrate and deterioration of personality in some but not all sufferers. Affective symptoms may occur as a consequence of the intellectual decline, especially whilst there is still some insight. In the later stages when insight is lost the patient may be totally unaware of and unconcerned by failure of performance in thought or daily living.

Dementia presents in a variety of ways depending on the area of brain most affected. Some or all of the following may occur: a decline in behaviour and social skills; poor judgement; loss of abstract thought; emotional lability; impaired personal hygiene; incontinence; perplexity; agitation or apathy; aphasia; apraxia; agnosia, or loss of constructional skills.

If the age of onset is under 65 dementia is called presenile or early-onset. Alzheimer's disease after 65 is known as senile dementia Alzheimer's type. The effect on the spouse, other family members and sometimes neighbours is profound and may be disastrous in the later stages of the disease.

PROGNOSIS

- There are a number of non-degenerative causes of dementia. Many of these are reversible and include vitamin B_{12} and other vitamin deficiencies; endocrine disease such as myxoedema; metabolic disease; some cases of cerebral anoxia; some chemical toxins including drugs; the earlier stages of alcohol damage; normal-pressure hydrocephalus and other reversible types of cerebral pressure, and some infections.
- Non-degenerative causes that are not reversible, or only temporarily reversible, include brain metastases; alcohol damage leading to atrophy; other chemical toxins; some types of encephalitis; trauma, for instance boxing injuries; brain damage due to severe traffic accident, or after a major intracranial haemorrhage.
- There is no hope of significant recovery in any case of dementia of degenerative origin. In those with an early onset more severe symptoms develop relatively early, usually with dysphasia and dyspraxia and often with aggressiveness, rages, and other disinhibited behaviour.
- The average lifespan from diagnosis of Alzheimer's disease is 3–10 years but there is little or no shortening of life expectancy in the late-onset type. The lifespan in multi-infarct dementia is variable; the average is about 5 years.

TREATMENT

1. A complete physical assessment should be made. Appropriate treatment should be given for any disorder that is found and offending drugs withdrawn.
2. In some cases of dementia physical causes, hearing or visual difficulties, constipation, infections or lack of stimulation may make matters worse. These conditions should be treated or ameliorated if possible.
3. The patient's mental state should be assessed formally.
4. Sometimes depression mimics dementia (pseudodementia) and should be treated.
5. Disturbed or disturbing behaviour may require sedatives such as thioridazine or haloperidol.
6. It is usually a good idea to refer a patient for psychogeriatric assessment at a fairly early stage to enable services to be made available.
7. Relatives require support and relief. They can help each other by meeting in organized groups.
8. Day centres, intermittent admissions and regular visiting by social worker or community psychiatric nurse can all help maintain home care. Eventual long-stay admission to residential home or hospital is often needed.

FOLLOW-UP

Patients with dementia require regular monitoring to assess progress and to give relatives the necessary support.

[1] Levy R, Post F (eds) (1982) *The Psychiatry of Late Life*. Oxford: Blackwell.
[2] Wattis J, Church M (1986) *The Practical Psychiatry of Old Age*. London: Croom Helm.

Mental Conditions Following Childbirth

The increased incidence in mental illness following childbirth is a well recognized phenomenon and may be classified separately into 'the maternity blues', puerperal psychosis and postnatal depression, although there are several features common to all three conditions. Mental illness in the puerperium is not confined to western society; postnatal depression with similar features to that found in Europe has been studied in Uganda[1].

Maternity blues is a transitory condition occurring during the first 2 weeks following delivery. It affects 50–80% of women. Symptoms include weeping, mild perplexity and disorientation, restlessness, irritability and exhaustion. The cause is thought to be due to the profound biological changes occurring after parturition but most studies have failed to show any association with hormonal status.

Postnatal depression is an important cause of misery and debility in mothers with very young children. The incidence may be as high as 30% in the first 3 months after childbirth[2]. A general practitioner should therefore look for about five new cases every year. The symptoms usually develop between 2 and 6 weeks after delivery but may be as late as 6 months. Depressed mood, sleep disturbance, anxiety, irritability, low self-esteem and worry about competence are common symptoms. The mother may experience frightening thoughts about self-harm, abnormal identification feelings with her baby, and feelings that she may harm or reject the baby. She may continue to be exhausted, lack libido, and be unable to carry out simple household tasks.

The Edinburgh 13-point postnatal depression scale is a useful aid in diagnosis. It is a self-completed questionnaire which can be administered either at home by the health visitor or filled in before a mother sees her general practitioner for the 6-week visit[3].

There is no evidence that biological factors play a major part in aetiology. The incidence is increased in first-time mothers over the age of 30, and adverse life events during pregnancy or the puerperium may precipitate depression in a vulnerable personality. Some mothers may have particular problems adjusting to the psychological and physical demands of a new baby.

Puerperal psychosis is an uncommon condition and occurs in 1–2 women in 1000 livebirths. The risk is increased in primiparous women. Symptoms begin between 3 and 10 days after delivery and develop rapidly. Insomnia and perplexity are important first symptoms. Depression and mania may occur and are often mixed with first-rank symptoms of schizophrenia. The mother may be fearful for the health of her baby and express suicidal or infanticidal ideas.

PROGNOSIS

- Maternity blues usually resolves in a few days. If severe, it may herald puerperal psychosis.
- There is evidence that many women with postnatal depression remain undiagnosed.
- The majority of women with postnatal depression recover within 6–12 months but some women take longer[4] and may be vulnerable to depression after subsequent deliveries.
- Severe untreated depression may seriously disrupt a marriage and impair a mother–infant relationship.
- Suicide and infanticide are definite risks in puerperal psychosis but rare in postnatal depression.
- The subsequent risk of future puerperal psychosis is 30%.

TREATMENT

Maternity blues does not require formal treatment. Women and their partners need to be prepared for it. Midwives are in a good position to give support and reassurance to a mother who is worried about herself and the baby.

Postnatal depression

1. Early diagnosis is important. Midwives, health visitors and general practitioners need to be aware of the problem.

2. Treatment should focus on counselling and support for the mother and her partner. The general practitioner is ideally placed to organize this together with the primary health care team. Initially the doctor needs to review the situation frequently and may need to give ongoing support for many months. Three organizations, the National Childbirth Trust, 9 Queensborough Terrace, London, W1 3TB. Tel. 071-221-3883 the Association for Postnatal Illness, 7 Gowan Ave, London, SW6 6RH. Tel. 071-731-4867 and Meet-a-Mum, c/o Kate Goodyer, 3 Woodside Ave, South Norwood, London SE25 5DW, Tel. 081-654-3137 offer support locally and nationally.

3. Antidepressants should be used for the usual indications in adequate doses for an adequate length of time. Women who are breastfeeding can be reassured that tricyclic antidepressants are not excreted in breast milk to any great extent. There is no evidence at present that progesterone is effective either in the treatment of postnatal depression or for prophylaxis against developing it.

4. Primary prevention includes basic information, the opportunity for discussion of postnatal depression prenatally and the identification of women with a previous history of mental illness who are at increased risk.

Puerperal psychosis is a major psychiatric emergency. Most mothers are now admitted with their babies to a mother-and-baby unit in the local psychiatric hospital. Standard treatment with major tranquillizers is effective. Expert nursing and supervision of the mother's access to the baby are important.

FOLLOW-UP

It is important to continue giving support until recovery is secure. This task can be shared between the general practitioner and health visitor.

---

[1] Cox JL (1986) *Postnatal Depression*, pp. 10–11. Edinburgh Churchill Livingstone.

[2] Cox JL, Connor YM, Kendall RE (1982) Prospective study of the psychiatric disorders of childbirth. *Br. J. Psychiatry*, **140,** 111–17.

[3] Cox JL (1986) *Postnatal Depression*, pp. 26–30. Edinburgh Churchill Livingstone.

[4] Nott PN (1987) Extent, timing and persistence of emotional disorders following childbirth. *Br. J. Psychiatry*, **151,** 523–7.

Mental Handicap

'Mental handicap' is the term used to describe a lifelong intellectual impairment with a consequent impairment of social skills and abilities in daily living. Severe mental handicap refers to that group with an intelligent quotient (IQ) of less than 50. In mild mental handicap the IQ is in the range 50–70. The overall prevalence of severe mental handicap is slightly in excess of 3 per 1000[1]. Mild mental handicap is 10 times as common[2]. This categorization by IQ has limitations as it is social functioning that determines needs, especially with lesser degrees of handicap.

There are many causes of mental handicap: genetic, for example phenylketonuria; chromosomal, for example Down's syndrome; prenatal infections, for example rubella; developmental abnormalities of the nervous system, for example neural tube defects and damage due to drugs, chemical toxins, and anorexia. Postnatal causes include postmeningitis, trauma and cerebral damage due to tumours or other space-occupying lesions. In most mild and some severe cases there is no identifiable cause.

Down's syndrome is the commonest chromosomal disorder with an overall incidence of 1 in 600 births. But the range varies between 1 in 2000 births in younger women to 1 in 50 in those at the upper end of the childbearing years. The characteristic physical appearances enable the condition to be diagnosed early.

The majority of cases of mental handicap cannot be diagnosed at birth. Many individuals who later prove to be handicapped show no abnormalities at first; it is only when the milestones of development are not reached at the correct age that handicap is suspected and later confirmed. Sometimes mental retardation is not suspected until the child has reached school age.

With improvements in general care many more of the severely handicapped are living to maturity. This poses increasing problems in their care and in their relationships with each other and with society as a whole.

Physical abnormalities, epilepsy and problems of sphincter control often accompany the more severe degress of handicap.

PROGNOSIS

- Prognosis depends on the type and severity of the disorder. It is particularly difficult to make a diagnosis in the first months of life and thus the prospect for future development must be approached with caution.
- Mild degrees of mental retardation are compatible with living a normal life in the community, including employment in an appropriate occupation.
- More severe mental retardation inevitably means a future restricted to a degree of dependence.
- Active treatment and help with disabilities together with imaginative education makes it possible for handicapped people to reach their full potential. Those from deprived backgrounds have particular needs in this respect. If not too severely handicapped, they can be enabled to look after themselves, enjoy life and to be appropriately employed.

TREATMENT

1. The first crucial requirement is for medical staff to establish good communication with the parents. Parents remember for ever how the news was first broken to them and it colours their future relationship with doctors.
2. In the case of a condition such as Down's syndrome which is evident at birth the parents must be warned of the possibility in the gentlest way. They can then be told for certain when the diagnosis is confirmed.
3. When the diagnosis is suspected at a later stage the parents must again be warned of the suspicion of a developmental defect or of future learning problems. Whilst it is important not to raise alarm unnecessarily it is equally important to prepare parents for possible difficulties.
4. The general practitioner is not likely to see the baby until some time after birth. If a defect has been found it is vitally important to

see the parents and ascertain their understanding of what has been said to them. Working from their level of understanding the general practitioner should help them to extend their knowledge and come to terms with the implications. Many parents of mentally handicapped children have a sense of shame and guilt about their child. It is important to explore these feelings. These tasks are usually shared with the health visitor. It is vital that paediatricians, other professionals and general practitioners communicate with one another about what the parents have been told.

5. Much of the care of the mentally handicapped is provided by the community health services and the local education authority (LEA). In most localities there is a mental handicap team with a multidisciplinary membership.

6. Under the Education Act (1981) LEAs have a duty to provide for children with special educational needs in ordinary schools whenever appropriate facilities can be made available. It is also the duty of the district health authority (DHA) to inform the parents of children under 5 and the LEA if there is reason to believe a child may have special educational needs. Those over the age of 2 must then be formally assessed under the provision of the Act. Those under the age of 2 may also be assessed with the consent of the parents.[1] The general practitioner should ensure that these steps are being taken.

7. Almost all those with mild handicap and many with more severe handicap live in their own homes with their families. For those not able to live at home the present policy is to place them in small houses with a home-like atmosphere managed by the Local Authority in conjunction with the DHA. Medical care is provided by general practitioners with visits at intervals by specialist paediatricians.

8. Many severely handicapped people need continuing care for epilepsy and care for skeletal disabilities. They also suffer from a wide range of common and uncommon medical problems. There is evidence that needs are not always met satisfactorily by general practitioners.[3] There is a case therefore for a regular screening examination especially of sight and hearing and checks of anticonvulsants and other medication.

9. As well as special educational needs and general care needs, the mentally handicapped frequently have defects of motor function including speech. These problems require skilled physiotherapy and speech therapy. Occupational therapy also has an important place in management.

10. Psychiatric illness occurs in the mentally handicapped but the mode of presentation is modified by their level of intellectual and verbal ability. Especially sympathetic management is required and drug treatment may be needed.

11. Those caring for the mentally handicapped at home need support. They may also require relief from the tasks, at times burdensome, of caring. This can be achieved by holiday breaks with admissions to hospitals or LA homes, or to the family homes of those who have offered to help.

FOLLOW-UP

All those with severe mental handicap should have regular contact with the primary health services. The general practitioner should feel responsible for ensuring that regular checks are made of physical disabilities, medication, organic or psychiatric illness and difficulties in care. There are a number of voluntary bodies that assist the handicapped and their families and promote research and political activity on their behalf. These include Mencap and Down's Syndrome Association. There are many self-help organizations other than those listed. These may be found in Health Directory 1990 (p. 136).

[1] *Mental Handicap: Partnership in the Community* (1986) Office of Health Economics/Mencap.
[2] Craft M, Bicknell J, Hollins S (1985) eds *Mental Handicap: A Multi-Disciplinary Approach*. London: Baillière Tindall.
[3] Howells G (1986) Are the needs of mentally handicapped adults being met? *J Royal College of General Practitioners*, **36**, 449–453.

7

Neurology

F. D. R. Hobbs

Epilepsy

Epilepsy is a seizure due to a paroxysm of abnormal electrical activity in neurones. One classification divides it into primary generalized seizures (tonic/clonic, petit mal, absences or myoclonic) and partial seizures (simple or complex). The incidence of epilepsy is around 4–6 per 1000 population[1]. However, since around 4–5% of the population will suffer a non-febrile convulsion during their lifetime, most people who suffer a seizure do not develop chronic epilepsy. Prevalence rates are highest among children (2% of all children under 2, and 7% of under 5-year-olds in the UK).

Some 60% of cases are idiopathic. The commonest identifiable causes are head injury (15% of cases), brain tumours (10–15% of late-onset epilepsies), vascular lesions, meningitis/encephalitis, neonatal trauma, drug therapy (lignocaine or tricyclics), metabolic upset (hypoglycaemia) or drug/alcohol withdrawal.

PROGNOSIS

- The risk of further seizures after a single fit is between 60%[2] and 82%[3]. The prognosis is poor if there is a positive family history, abnormal EEG, neurological lesion, focal seizures, psychiatric or social problems.

- Some 80–90% of second seizures occur within 12–24 hours.

- There is a 65% chance of remission within 10 years of diagnosis[2]; this reduces to a 33% chance at remission if epilepsy continues for 5 years after diagnosis[2].

- Relapse risk at 20 years is 6% for petit mal, 21% for grand mal, 32% for focal fits; it is 13% for patients under 9; 22% for 10–19 year-olds and 32% for the over 20s[2].

- Standardized mortality is 2.5 times greater than in the non-epileptic population (12% due to status epilepticus, 55% to fatal accident during seizure and 12% to suicide[4]). The risk of death is unchanged in petit mal and complex partial, but 4 times greater in myoclonic and 2.5 times greater in generalized seizures.

- The suicide risk is 5–7 times that of matched subjects[5].

- The prognosis for seizure control is worse with focal than tonic/clonic seizures.

- Multiple seizures in the first year of disease carry a worse prognosis for chronic attacks, therefore good early control may improve the prognosis[6].

- EEG is limited in establishing diagnosis (about 20–40% of new patients have normal EEG and 15% of normal persons have abnormal EEG) but it is invaluable for classification and assessment.

- Computerized tomography (CT) scan is normal in 80% but shows a high yield in partial seizures, neonatal and adult-onset seizures and patients with focal EEG changes or neurological signs.

TREATMENT

1. The patient's family, school or employer all need help to act reasonably. Life should be lived as normally as possible, although swimming alone or climbing heights should not be attempted.

2. Having decided to take medication, patients must realize the importance of regular compliance with therapy. Serum phenytoin levels are worth monitoring (a defined therapeutic range exists and the drug has a narrow therapeutic:toxic ratio). Monitoring all other drugs is only of value in checking compliance.

3. Patients should be assessed 2 weeks following any therapy change and then 6-monthly.

4. The patient must inform the DVLC if they drive. The licence requires them to be free of fits for 2 years. Nocturnal fits do not prevent driving, if the patient has demonstrated a 3-year period of being free from daytime convulsions. Any change in medication requires a ban from driving for 6 months. If a fit occurs, then the ban operates until the driver has been free of fits for another 2 years. A heavy goods vehicle licence is not possible after even one non-febrile convulsion over the age of 5 years.

5. If the patient is fit-free for 3 years then consider tailing off therapy (although the patient may prefer to continue if a driver). The recurrence

rate after stopping is 30%. Recurrence is more likely if seizure onset is before a child is 6 months or in adults with a long history of epilepsy, frequent attacks, partial seizures, or associated cerebral lesion.

6. Epileptic women who are pregnant should continue their treatment, although they have a higher risk of congenital malformation (6–11% compared to 2–3% in non-epileptic mothers). All the drugs listed are compatible with breastfeeding since drug concentrations are extremely low.
7. The British Epilepsy Association is based at Crowthorne House, New Wokingham Road, Wokingham, Berks, RG11 3AY; telephone 0344-773122.

Status epilepticus (fitting for longer than 15 minutes)

TREATMENT

1. Ensure an adequate airway.
2. Call for an ambulance on 999 emergency.
3. Administer rectal diazepam 1 mg per year of age up to 5 mg in children; 10 mg in adults. This dose is repeatable after 15 minutes.
4. Alternatively, give intravenous diazepam 5–10 mg as a bolus, repeatable hourly.
5. Alternatively or additionally administer Paraldehyde 1 ml per year of life up to 5 ml in children, 5–10 ml in adults i.m. into the buttock.
6. The patient should be admitted urgently to hospital and the airway maintained if he or she is still unconscious.

Grand mal epilepsy (tonic/clonic)

This is the commonest type of epilepsy, although no reliable figures are available. The main feature is loss of consciousness, which may be preceded by a prodromal period of vague sensation (aura). Tonic (rigidity) and then clonic (jerking) contractions usually follow the collapse. Incontinence occurs in around 50% of cases. The duration of the unconscious period is variable and the patient is often drowsy or confused afterwards. Grand

mal epilepsy usually occurs between birth and 15 years of age or over the age of 50, when there is an increased risk of cerebrovascular or neoplastic disease.

PROGNOSIS

- In the young, metabolic (heavy alcohol consumption or drug ingestion) and hormonal factors (menstrual cycle) are more common and therefore may be avoidable.
- Neoplastic, cerebrovascular or toxic causes are commoner in the elderly.

TREATMENT

1. Avoid obvious precipitants.
2. A decision to accept therapy should be taken by the patient after consideration of the benefits and potential side-effects.
3. In all, 70–80% of patients will be controlled on monotherapy. Only 10–15% will require two or more drugs. Choice is largely personal preference. Therapy should be titrated in slow increments according to seizure control.
4. In children or young adults, carbamazepine 100–400 mg t.d.s. can be prescribed. The drug may cause marrow suppression, usually in the elderly. Side-effects include skin rashes (3%), dizziness or drowsiness. Carbamazepine appears to be non-teratogenic.
5. In elderly patients, phenytoin 300 g daily to 500 g b.d. may be given. Phenytoin is safe, but numerous side-effects include skin rashes, confusion, ataxia, gum hypertrophy, tremor and macrocytosis. Rarely phenytoin can be teratogenic.
6. Sodium valproate 250 mg t.d.s. to 500 mg q.d.s. may cause skin rashes, gastrointestinal effects, alopecia, oedema and weight gain. It may be teratogenic, and can rarely cause hepatic failure or pancreatitis.
7. Any of the above can be substituted if there is no relief at therapeutic maximum doses.
8. All will cause drowsiness, ataxia, diplopia and nausea in toxic dosages.

Petit mal epilepsy (absences)

This is a rare form of epilepsy occurring in 1–20% of epileptics. It has a probable genetic factor with a family history of epilepsy in 34%. Usually there is no warning before onset. There is a short-lived (5–60 second) impairment of awareness, associated with 2–3 cps spike wave on EEG. Immediate full recovery follows, but the patient will be unaware of the attack. A brief clonic jerk of eyelids and arms occurs in 75% and short automatisms (chewing, swallowing, finger-fumbling) in 88%[7].

PROGNOSIS

- Fewer than 2% of attacks continue into adulthood[7].
- Remission usually occurs by the age of 17.

TREATMENT

1. Since it is extremely rare in adults, therapy can be withdrawn at the age of 12–14 or after 3 years of full control.
2. Ethosuximide 250 mg b.d.–500 mg q.d.s. is the treatment of choice. Drowsiness, dizziness, ataxia, headache and gastrointestinal effects can occur. Rarely psychosis and agranulocytosis occur.
3. Sodium valproate 250 g t.d.s.–500 g q.d.s. can be given.

Temporal lobe epilepsy (complex partial)

This accounts for 33% of new epilepsies, but as prognosis for remission is poor it has a higher prevalence. It is the commonest type of seizure from adolescence to middle age and the commonest cause of focal epilepsy. There is an alteration of consciousness during attacks with sudden changes in mood, behaviour or personality. Repetitive movements can follow, like fiddling with objects, lip-smacking, chewing or unilateral jerking from hand to arm to leg and face (jacksonian seizure). Sensory (paraesthesiae or numbness) and psychic (dizziness, hallucinations, *déjà vu*) symptoms often precede the attack and can eventually be recognized by the patient.

PROGNOSIS

- Temporal lobe epilepsy has a poor prognosis since seizures are difficult to control.

- There is a strong association with psychiatric and physical morbidity.
- It has been postulated that a major aetiology is anoxic damage to the temporal lobe during a prolonged febrile convulsion in childhood[8].
- Some 10% of patients have a cerebral neoplasm[8].

TREATMENT

1. Temporal lobe epilepsy is difficult to treat successfully.
2. Carbamazepine 100 mg b.d.–400 mg t.d.s. is the drug of choice.
3. Phenytoin 300–500 mg daily can be used, particularly in the elderly.
4. Support will be needed for the family if there are associated psychiatric disorders.

Myoclonic seizures

Myoclonic seizures consist of brief jerks of a muscle or several muscle groups, in single jerks or rapidly repetitive. Patients may fall but recovery is immediate and consciousness is not lost. Seizures occur on wakening, in the early morning or when dropping off to sleep.

TREATMENT

1. Sodium valproate 200–600 mg at night can be given.
2. Clonazepam 0.5–2 g at night is an alternative.

Neonatal seizures

Neonatal seizures occur in 0.5–1% of neonates and are always symptomatic. In all, 90% are due to birth complications, hypoglycaemia, hypocalcaemia or meningitis.

PROGNOSIS[9]

- 22% of babies having seizures die during the first month of life.
- 24% become mentally retarded.
- 16% continue to suffer from seizures.

Infantile spasms

This is a serious syndrome occurring in infants aged between 1 and 12 months (peak at 5 months). It is characterized by spasm, intellectual decline and specific EEG changes. The incidence is 1 in 6000 livebirths.

PROGNOSIS

- 20% die in infancy.
- Of the 80% that survive[10]
    - 20% develop normally.
    - 70% develop mental retardation.
    - 30% develop physical handicap.
    - 50% continue to have seizures.

Febrile convulsions

Febrile convulsions are seizures associated with fever between the ages of 6 months and 5 (usually 2–4) years. Around 30% of children will have at least one febrile fit.

PROGNOSIS

- Recurrence of febrile fits will occur in 33% of children[11].
- Recurrence is more likely if the initial fit occurs before the age of 15 months, in females and with a positive family history[11].
- Only 3% of children with febrile fits will develop epilepsy (1.5% if the fit is uncomplicated, 3% if the fit lasts more than 15 minutes, 7% if the fit occurs with focal signs, 15% if there is neurological deficit).

TREATMENT

1. Immediate treatment is unnecessary if the convulsion stops within 15 minutes.
2. Prolonged fits should be treated by rectal diazepam 0.5 mg per kg body weight.
3. The child should be admitted to hospital immediately if he or she remains floppy or drowsy after the fit or is less than 18 months old. Older children should be admitted if fits are prolonged (over 15 minutes), multiple or focal, or if they have persisting neurological deficit.

FOLLOW-UP

1. Parents will need much reassurance over the prognosis.
2. Parents should understand the importance of reducing the risk of further fits by treating fevers promptly with paracetamol syrup 120–240 mg q.d.s. and tepid sponging.
3. The immunization schedule should proceed normally with the exception of pertussis (but note that pertussis is not then contraindicated in siblings). Any vaccine should be covered by paracetamol 120–240 mg q.d.s.

[1] Crombie DL et al. (1960) Br. Med. J., ii, 416.
[2] Hauser WA, Kurland LT (1975) Epilepsia, 16, 1.
[3] Goodridge DMG, Shorvan SD (1983) Br. Med. J., 287, 641.
[4] Laidlow J, Richen AL (eds) (1982) A Textbook of Epilepsy. London: Churchill Livingstone.
[5] Editorial (1980) Br. Med. J., 281, 530.
[6] Shorvan SD (1983) In Research Progress in Epilepsy (Rose FC ed). London: Pitman Books.
[7] Patten JP (1986) In Treatment and Prognosis; Medicine (Hawkins R ed) pp. 102–4. Oxford: Heinemann.
[8] Currie S et al. (1971) Clinical course and prognosis of temporal lobe epilepsy. Brain, 94, 173.
[9] Holden KR et al. (1980) Advances in Epileptology, p. 155. New York: Raven Press.
[10] Bellman M (1983) Recent Advances in Epilepsy. London: Churchill Livingstone.
[11] Hobbs R, Williams A (1988) Management of episodes of altered consciousness. Update, 2, 1499–1504.

Headache

In a random sample of British adults 28% reported a headache during the 2 weeks prior to the survey[1]. This was the commonest symptom volunteered. A total of 16% of the same sample took analgesics for migraine.

Headaches account for 2–4% of all surgery consultations[2]. Causes of headache include simple tension, migraine, fever, trauma and excess alcohol. Less common and more serious causes include vascular (hypertension, cerebral bleeds), metabolic (hypothyroidism, anaemias), infective (meningitis, encephalitis), tumour, glaucoma, and temporal arteritis. Facial pain and neuralgia can also present with headache.

Commonest causes in general practice[3] are tension (36%), migraine (30%), fever (10%) and in hospital practice[4] tension (35%), migraine (61%) and sinuses (1%).

PROGNOSIS

- Depression is often associated with headache (probably due to serotonin deficiency)[5].
- In the absence of physical signs, investigations such as CT scans and routine skull x-rays are not cost-effective[6].
- Exclude temporal arteritis and glaucoma in the elderly. These will both lead to blindness if undiagnosed.
- The probability of an isolated headache being due to a cerebral tumour is less than 1%.
- A total of 85% of children with headaches due to cerebral tumours developed abnormal neurological signs within 2 months of headache onset[7].
- Some 25% of patients will get a headache after lumbar puncture or epidural anaesthesia.

TREATMENT

1. The reassurance of a thorough examination can be therapeutic.
2. Generally patients with headache and no physical signs can be initially reassured that no organic disease is present. Exceptions include severe headache in the elderly (consider erythrocyte sedimentation rate to check for polymyalgia rheumatica or temporal arteritis) or those over 50 (consider chest X-ray).
2. Simple analgesics can be advised, such as paracetamol 0.5–1 g q.d.s., soluble aspirin 300–600 g or ibuprofen 200–400 g q.d.s. (aspirin in children under 12 is contraindicated).
3. Patients' fears should be sought and explored.

This is inevitably time-consuming, but may be the only opportunity the doctor has to improve the patient's headache.

4. Relaxation classes or tapes can help tension headaches. Discussion on aspects of lifestyle which are causing stress may well be useful. This can help patients to avoid or cope more effectively with areas of conflict in their personal or working environments.

FOLLOW-UP

Patients with no prior presented headache should be followed up at 3–4 weeks to check for resolution or developing signs. Referral should be made if signs are present, or considered if severe headaches have persisted despite therapy. Consider depressive illness in patients with recurrent simple headaches with no physical signs.

A delay in diagnosing the rare headache due to cerebral tumour will rarely affect the prognosis. Recurrent prescriptions should be regularly reviewed.

[1] Dunnell K, Cartwright A (1972) *Medicine Takers, Prescribers and Hoarders*. London: Routledge & Kegan Paul.
[2] Hodgkin K (1978) *Towards Earlier Diagnosis in General Practice*. London: Churchill Livingstone.
[3] Lance JW et al. (1965) *Med. J. Aust.*, 2, 909–14.
[4] Jerrett WA (1979) *Practitioner*, 222, 549–55.
[5] Editorial (1984) *Lancet*, i, 495.
[6] Larson EB et al. (1980) *J.A.M.A.*, 243, 359–62.
[7] Honig PJ et al. (1982) *Am. J. Dis. Child.*, 136, 121–4.

Migraine

Migraine' is the term used for recurrent episodic headache usually accompanied by visual disturbance, nausea and vomiting. Headaches last between 2 and 72 hours[1]. Attacks can be preceded by an aura with visual or sensory symptoms. The cause is unknown, but popularly presumed to be vasoconstriction of cerebral blood arteries (leading to focal signs) followed by vasodilatation (leading to the headache).

In all reported series, migraine is the commonest cause of headache. The suggested annual incidence in the USA is 250 per 100 000[2] with a frequency of 5–20% in the population (probably 10% is the closest UK figure). Migraine is a common cause of headache in children, and women are affected more frequently than men (in a ratio of 60:40). Maximum incidence is in the 20–30-year age group. Some 25% will have their first attack by the age of 10; migraine rarely presents after the age of 55. There is a strong familial tendency (46%) and a link with motion sickness.

Migraine can be subdivided into several types. *Classical* migraines start with an aura of major visual disruption (including scotomas), and paraesthesiae leading to a severe, throbbing, unilateral headache accompanied by nausea, vomiting, photophobia and prostration. Attacks last 8–24 hours. *Common* migraine is usually a generalized and severe throbbing headache with nausea and photophobia. Pain usually lasts hours to days.

PROGNOSIS

- Hemiplegic migraine (hemiparesis or plegia followed by severe headache) can produce focal signs that last days or weeks, suggesting a stroke has occurred. Most patients will recover fully. Rarely, deficits will persist and CT scans then suggest multi-infarct damage[3].
- All other migraines are not associated with permanent or progressive neurological damage.
- The avoidance of trigger factors can reduce the recurrence rate (although up to 60% of patients may be placebo-responders[4]).
- In classical migraine, nausea occurs in 89%, vomiting in 60%, photophobia in 82% and giddiness in 72%[5].
- In common migraine, 90% feel nauseated and 10% vomit.
- Visual disturbance occurs in 30% of patients.
- In all, 75% of attacks last less than 24 hours[6].

TREATMENT

1. Advice should be given on avoidance of trigger factors. The commonest are eating substances containing tyramine, amines or additives, like monosodium glutamate. These include chocolate, cheese, citrus fruits, onions, nitrites and spiced food. Other triggers include bright sunlight, stress and exertion.

2. Exclude a drug precipitant. Oral contraceptives can worsen attacks (although occasionally they will improve them) and should be stopped immediately if the attacks become more severe or occur with neurological signs. Nitrites can cause migraine.

3. Excessive ergot preparations will cause headaches, as can ergotamine withdrawal in habitual users.

4. Simple analgesics, particularly paracetamol (1 g 4-hourly), can be helpful if given early enough.

5. If these are ineffective then co-codamal (codeine phosphate 8 mg and paracetamol 500 g) 2 tablets q.d.s. or a non-steroidal anti-inflammatory like ibuprofen 400 mg t.d.s. or mefenamic acid 500 g t.d.s. should be tried.

6. Studies have demonstrated that drug absorption is reduced during migraine attacks and several preparations combine an analgesic with an antiemetic (Migravess, Paramax, Migraleve). There is however no evidence that they are any more effective than simple analgesics.

7. Ergot preparations if taken early enough can reduce the severity of the headache in 50% of patients with some prodrome. The dose of 2 mg repeated after 1 hour and then after 4–6 hours (to a maximum of 6 mg in 24 hours, 10 g in a week) should not be exceeded. Ergot can cause vomiting and diarrhoea, with a risk of

habituation leading to withdrawal headache. Excessive use can result in vascular insufficiency and gangrene.

8. Prophylaxis for frequent or severe attacks is through 5–hydroxytryptamine antagonism.
   a. Pizotifen 1.5 mg nocte (maximum 1.5 g b.d.) can cause drowsiness, weight gain and aggravate urinary retention or glaucoma. It takes 2–3 weeks to work.
   b. Propranolol 20 g b.d. to 40 mg t.d.s. or 80–160 mg SR daily can also reduce underlying anxiety. Side-effects include nausea, cold extremities and tiredness. Propranolol is to be avoided in heart failure or bronchospasm.
   c. Clonidine 50–75 mg b.d. has a variable effect and can cause dry mouth, dizziness, insomnia and depression.
   d. Methysergide maleate 1–2 mg t.d.s. is the most potent prophylactic with 25% resolution and 50% improvement in patients. Side-effects include nausea, giddiness, blurred vision and peripheral vasoconstriction. The rare serious complication of retroperitoneal fibrosis can be reduced by not giving the drug continuously for more than 12 weeks at a time.

9. Antidepressant therapy should be considered in some patients.

FOLLOW-UP

Prophylaxis should be continued for 1-2 months after symptoms have resolved. Repeat courses may be required. Patients on repeat prescriptions for acute therapy should be reviewed regularly and drug use monitored, particularly when ergots are being given.

[1] Blau JN (1982) *Lancet*, **i**, 444–5.
[2] Kurtzee JF (1982) *Neurology*, **32**, 1207–14.
[3] Fowler T (1987) *Headache*. Lancaster: MTP Press.
[4] Grant ECG (1979) *Lancet*, **i**, 966–8.
[5] Selby G *et al.* (1960) *J. Neurol. Neurosurg. Psychiatry*, **23**, 23–32.
[6] Patten JP (1987) *Diseases of the nervous system in Treatment and Prognosis, Medicine* (Hawkins R ed). Oxford: Heinemann.

Migrainous Neuralgia

Cluster headaches are recurring attacks of intense pain behind or around one eye. Pain can radiate to the forehead, gum or face. Pain is severe and lasts 20–120 minutes. These headaches are mainly nocturnal and wake the patient. Associated vasomotor symptoms include ipsilateral ptosis, miosis, conjunctival suffusion, epiphora and blocked nose. Cluster headaches mainly affect males between the ages of 35 and 45; onset is from 10 to 55 years[1].

PROGNOSIS

- Attacks can occur 2–3 times per night.
- Cluster headaches rarely occur during the day.
- Clusters of pain occur over a few weeks (occasionally up to 3 months) and then patients are free from pain for months or even years.
- Attacks are likely to recur annually during middle age.
- Alcohol during the evening can precipitate attacks.

TREATMENT

1. Reassurance can be made that attacks are short-lived and never proceed to neurological deficit.
2. Ergotamine suppository can be given once at night for 5 successive nights. No treatment should be given on the next 2 nights, but if the cluster has persisted a further 5-night course can be given.
3. Methysergide maleate 1–3 mg nocte can be added to the ergotamine suppositories in non-

responders. This should not be given for longer than 12 weeks continuously.
. Pizotifen 0.5–3 mg nocte can be tried.
. Lithium carbonate 250 mg b.d./t.d.s. can be used[2] as last-line therapy (with methysergide maleate nocte if necessary). Drug levels should be monitored.

FOLLOW-UP

Follow-up is as for migraine headaches. Persistent facial neuralgias should be seen at intervals for support, medication review and to exclude the development of depression.

[1] Sacks O (1981) *Migraine*. London: Pan Books.
[2] Peatfield RC (1981) *J. R. Soc. Med.*, **74**, 432–6.

Cerebral Tumours

The brain is a rare site for tumours, which can be primary (65%) or secondary (35%)[1]. The commonest sites for primary tumours are the supporting tissues producing gliomas or astrocytomas (35%), oligodendrogliomas and ependymomas (both benign). Other primary sites are the meninges, producing meningiomas (15%), and blood vessels, producing angiomas and angioblastomas. Secondary tumours arise from the bronchus, breast, kidney, colon, ovary, prostate or thyroid, in order of frequency. Symptoms depend on age and speed of tumour growth. Young patients will normally present with signs of raised intracranial pressure (ICP), particularly with rapid growing malignant tumours. Signs classically include frontal dull, aching morning headaches associated with nausea, vomiting and later papilloedema. Other pressure effects are changes in levels of consciousness, sixth nerve palsy (diplopia) and third nerve palsy (dilated pupil). Older patients are less likely to have raised ICP, even with large tumours, since they will have some cerebral atrophy. They usually present with epilepsy or focal neurological signs like dementia (prefrontal tumours), contralateral hemiplegia (precentral) or spatial disorientation and dysphasia (parietal).

PROGNOSIS

● Although malignant tumours will rarely metastasize outside the central nervous system, they carry a significantly worse prognosis due to their rapid growth and infiltration of brain tissue (making treatment difficult).
● *Malignant gliomas* have an untreated prognosis of a few weeks or months. Treatment is likely to extend this to 12–18 months. Prognosis depends on age, focal signs and site.
● Young patients do better than middle-aged and older patients.
● Absence of focal neurological signs carries a better prognosis.
● Frontal tumours fare better than parietal tumours. Parieto–occipital tumours carry the worse prognosis.
● *Cerebral metastases* have a short history, unless they are solitary, which is rare. Removal of the primary tumour will extend survival, particularly if it is in the breast[2].

● *Meningiomas* are benign, but will commonly recur.
● Raised ICP will only produce papilloedema in 50% of cases[1].
● Epilepsy occurs in 30% of tumours, particularly frontal or temporal lobe ones[3].
● Large tumours may develop with few or no signs in the frontal lobes, non-determinant temporal lobe, or posterior fossa.

TREATMENT

Glioma

1. The aim of treatment is removal of the tumour with minimal or no deficit. Recurrence is almost always inevitable.
2. Life expectancy is unlikely beyond 12 months with surgery alone. Adjuvant radiotherapy should extend life beyond 12 months.
3. Although there is no statistical evidence that

163

additional chemotherapy will increase the relapse-free interval, the few patients who survive longer tend to be those in whom chemotherapy has been used[4].

4. Dexamethasone helps to reduce cerebral oedema and cranial irradiation symptoms. Symptomatic improvement can be dramatic in a short time with 10–20 g dexamethasone i.m. stat then 4 mg q.d.s. orally. Maintenance dosages vary from 2 to 4 mg daily (alternate-day therapy reduces Cushing's complications).

5. Treatment of status epilepticus: rectal diazepam 10 mg stat, repeated after 10 minutes if necessary, should be used to control fitting lasting more than a few minutes. Relatives can be instructed in this use.

6. Fit frequency can be reduced by anticonvulsants. The type of epilepsy will dictate the most appropriate medication (see section on epilepsy, p. 156).

7. Analgesia should be provided for headaches. Narcotic drugs may be needed for intractable pain, although the use of dexamethasone will normally avoid this.

Metastases

1. Surgical removal is successful if the tumour is truly solitary on CT scans or magnetic resonance imaging, and the primary tumour is eradicated[5].

2. The use of radiotherapy in patients without other secondary tumours produces a longer survival[2].

Meningioma

1. This tumour is benign but almost impossible to remove surgically entirely.

2. Recurrence is reduced by postoperative radiotherapy.

FOLLOW-UP

Follow-up frequency will be dictated by the type of tumour. Shared care is likely in most cases: emotional support and information on the disease should be given by neurosurgeon, radiotherapist and general practitioner.

[1] Sharr MM, Fowler T (1987) Subacute headache. In *Headache* (Fowler T ed). Lancaster: MTP Press.
[2] Sharr MM (1983) *J. Neurol. Oncol.*, **1**, 307–12.
[3] Rubenstein D, Wayne D (1976) *Lecture Notes on Clinical Medicine*. Oxford: Blackwell Scientific Publications.
[4] Thomas DGT et al. (1985) *Br. J. Cancer*, **51**, 525–32.
[5] Galicich JA et al. (1980) J. Neurol. Surg., **53**, 63–70.

Pituitary Tumours

Pituitary tumours constitute 10% of cerebral tumours[1]. The commonest lesion is the chromophobe adenoma which presents with hypopituitarism (lethargy, cold intolerance, amenorrhoea and polydypsia) and associated visual signs. The common visual field defects from the enlarging tumour pressing on the optic chiasm are bitemporal hemianopia (60%), scotomas (15%), uniocular blindness (15%) and homonymous hemianopia (10%)[1]. Headache will occur in 50% of patients[2]. Less common pituitary tumours are microadenomas which can produce excess prolactin (amenorrhoea, gynaecomastia) or excess growth hormone (acromegaly). These can occasionally grow to produce visual or hypopituitary symptoms.

PROGNOSIS

● Tumours producing visual changes require rapid treatment to avoid permanent visual loss.
● Headaches associated with acromegaly will frequently not settle despite adequate treatment of the pituitary tumour.
● Prognosis largely depends on the resultant endocrine deficits.
● Life expectancy is unaltered in successfully treated tumours.

TREATMENT

1. Bromocriptine is often effective in medically controlling pituitary microprolactinomas (See page 303). It may need to be followed by a course of radiotherapy.
2. If vision is endangered, surgery is mandatory. Transethmoidal or trans-spheroidal approaches are safer and have better results than frontal craniotomy. Postoperative radiotherapy to the pituitary fossa will reduce recurrence.
3. Surgery is preferably preceded by bromocriptine to reduce the tumour mass. Bromocriptine can also be used as a postoperative adjuvant.

FOLLOW-UP

Patients should be carefully followed up by the specialist to assess their endocrine status with a view to replacement therapy for any deficiencies.

---

[1] Sharr MM, Fowler T (1987) Subacute headache. In *Headache* (Fowler T ed). Lancaster: MTP Press.
[2] Moore KP *et al.* (1986) *Br. Med. J.*, **293**, 609–10.

Motor Neurone Disease

Motor neurone disease is a neuromuscular condition with progressive destruction of motor neurones in the brain and spinal cord. This leads to weakness and wasting in the corresponding muscles. It has an incidence of 1 in 50 000–100 000 people[1] and a prevalence of 5 per 100 000. Sporadic outbreaks occur; endemic clusters are well recognized in Japan and Guam[2]. Only 5% of patients show a familial tendency[3]. The death rate is 50 per 100 000[4]. The aetiology is unknown. There is little evidence for previous theories which have included slow viruses or autoimmune disease.

Motor neurone disease is a condition of the middle-aged; peak incidence is between 40 and 60 years (range 20–70). Men are affected more than women in a ratio of 1.7 to 1[4].

Diagnosis is established by the mixture of upper and lower motor neurone signs in one limb. Muscle fasciculation is common—it is rarely seen in other diseases.

There are three types of motor neurone disease. *Amyotrophic lateral sclerosis* (ALS) is the commonest form with a mixture of upper and lower motor neurone signs. Signs include both spasticity and flaccidity, muscle weakness, and fasciculation. Symptoms develop first in the hands and feet; the patient has a tendency to drop objects or trip up. *Progressive bulbar palsy* (PBP) affects 25% of patients, particularly the elderly, and presents with speech, chewing or swallowing difficulties (early symptoms are slurred speech or choking on certain foods). Signs include flaccid or spastic tongue with fasciculation. *Progressive muscular atrophy* (PMA) is a rarer but relatively benign form. It starts with lower motor neurone symptoms (weakness, wasting and fasciculation), but upper motor signs can develop late in the course of the disease.

Motor neurone disease does not affect intellectual or sensory function. Bladder, bowel and eye functions are unimpaired.

PROGNOSIS

- PBP and ALS are malignant forms. Of these patients, 50% will be dead within 3 years; maximum likely prognosis is 5 years. Progression can take as little as 6–9 months[4].
- PMA is benign with a history of up to 20 years[4] (normally 8–10 years).
- Deterioration in PBP and ALS is frequently constant at around 3–8% of function per month.
- Elderly patients presenting with bulbar signs have a particularly poor prognosis.
- Death is usually due to secondary complications, particularly pneumonia. Aspiration pneumonia is common, as bulbar involvement necessitates the consumption of liquidized food; there is difficult respiratory clearance due to intercostal muscle involvement.

TREATMENT

1. This is a disease which requires a particularly close primary care team approach.
2. The patient should have physiotherapy to avoid cramps and reduce spasticity and flexures. Carers should be advised on lifting techniques.
3. Occupational therapists should be involved so that they can advise on beds, chairs and walking aids.
4. Speech therapy exercises can delay dysarthria. Various speech aids, including computers, can extend employment. There is a facility available from the Manpower Services Commission, Moorfoot, Sheffield who loan out the more expensive speech aids. Speech therapists can also advise on swallowing techniques to reduce the risk of aspiration.
5. General nursing care will be required by most patients. Carers may need help from bathing nurses. Macmillan nurses provide practical support in the terminal phase. Contact address is Cancer Relief MacMillan Fund, Anchor House, 15/19 Britten St, London SW3 3TY.
6. The general practitioner will need to co-ordinate adequate services and should provide a valuable counselling role to patients and carers. Relief admissions on a regular basis can assist patients remaining in the community. These

admissions may be in Cheshire Homes (Leonard Cheshire Foundation, 7 Market Mews, London W1Y 8HP, Tel. 071-499-2665), young disabled units or hospices. Substitute carers are also available through organizations like Crossroads Care Attendants Scheme Trust, 11 Whitehall Road, Rugby, Warwickshire, CV21 3AQ, Tel. 0788 61536.

. There are no drugs that will modify the disease. Spasticity may be improved by baclofen 5 mg t.d.s., increasing until maximum benefit is achieved or side-effects become unacceptable.

. In a few patients life can be extended by a cricophanyngeal myotomy for swallowing purposes or a feeding gastrostomy for major difficulties. The need for these procedures will require careful counselling between family, patient and general practitioner.

FOLLOW-UP

Patients and families will need close and structured support from the full primary care team. Further support is available from the Motor Neurone Disease Association, 38 Hazelwood Road, Northampton, NN1 1LN.

[1] Caroscio JT (1986) *Amyotrophic Lateral Sclerosis—A Guide to Patient Care*. New York: Thieme Medical Publishers.
[2] Malamud *et al.* (1961) *Arch. Neurol.*, **5,** 401–15.
[3] Horton *et al.* (1976) *Neurology*, **26,** 460–5.
[4] Munsat T (1984) Adult motor neurone diseases. In *Merritt's Textbook of Neurology* (Rowland L ed). Philadelphia: Lea & Fabinger.

Multiple Sclerosis

Multiple sclerosis (MS) is a syndrome of diffuse neurological disturbances, occurring in exacerbations and remissions. Progressive disability will generally occur. The cause is unknown and degenerative, toxic or inflammatory agents have all been implicated. Much research into viruses with long latent infections (slow viruses) has been inconclusive, but these are believed to be the most likely causative agents.

The widespread disabilities are caused by scattered plaques of demyelination that can occur throughout the brain or spinal cord. The onset is rare before puberty (5% of cases) and over 50 years of age (10% of cases)[1]. The incidence varies around the world with 1 per 1000 in the UK and Europe and 4 per 1000 in Japan[2]; peak age of onset is 20–35 years. Women are affected more frequently than men in a ratio of 1.5–2:1.

PROGNOSIS

- In all, 90% of patients will have disease remissions lasting from months to years; the remainder will progress without remission.
- Early remissions tend to complete functional recovery (particularly single symptoms). Later remissions tend to be partial.
- Possible presenting signs may be: acute transverse myelitis (20% will develop MS) or acute retrobulbar neuritis (35% will develop MS)[2].
- Common problems encountered are sensory paraesthesiae (35% of patients), painful dysaesthesiae (20%), cerebellar symptoms (50%) or nystagmus (42%)[2].

- Bladder problems will eventually affect 90% of patients.
- Depression is common, but euphoria can occur as well.
- Average survival time after onset of symptoms is 27 years. Reduced life expectancy is 9.5 years in men and 14.4 years in women[3].
- The prognosis for developing a major disability is 40% within 5 years, 50% within 10 years and 66% within 15 years.
- Only 5% of pregnant MS patients will relapse in the puerperium.
- High temperatures increase the relapse rate so patients should avoid living in tropical countries or taking very hot baths.

TREATMENT

1. The diagnosis should not be given to the patient until there is absolute certainty. There will usually have been several episodes of demyelination.
2. There is no rationale for performing investigations, such as CT scans, in an attempt to establish the diagnosis, since this may only increase the uncertainty and anxiety felt by the patient.
3. Initial optimism is recommended in view of the variable and often extended remissions.
4. There is no evidence that treatment to influence immune mechanisms improves the prognosis.
5. Studies purporting to show disease stabilization or remission are all contradictory and mostly uncontrolled, even for the most popular treatments such as adrenocorticotrophic hormone and steroids, immunosuppression (azathioprine or cyclophosphamide), plasmapheresis or desensitization[5].
6. The long-term use of steroids can worsen the prognosis. Immunosuppression carries major side-effects.
7. There is no evidence of benefit from any dietary changes. Linoleic acid should be avoided since it can be carcinogenic[6].
8. Hyperbaric oxygen has no demonstrated benefit, and no obvious theoretical basis. It can be hazardous.
9. Retention of urine may require the use of self-catheterization or a long-term catheter. Treatment can be attempted with propantheline (Pro-Banthine) 15–30 mg t.d.s. or phenoxybenzamine hydrochloride (Dibenyline) 10 mg b.d.
10. Urinary incontinence may require catheterization but urological referral is advisable. Flavoxate hydrochloride (Urispas) 200 mg t.d.s. can be effective.
11. Spasticity can be helped by baclofen 5–20 mg t.d.s. or diazepam 2–10 g t.d.s.
12. Constipation is common and requires faecal softeners (lactulose 10–15 ml b.d.) or stimulants (senna 2–3 tablets b.d.).
13. Walking aids or a wheelchair may be needed.
14. Impotence can sometimes be helped by the use of erectile implants.

FOLLOW-UP

The role of the general practitioner is very important in the management of this disease. Patients should be seen by their general practitioner at each attack for assessment and in between, as required, for support counselling. As the disease progresses support for the principal carer should include the possibility of relief hospital admission to enable breaks or holidays.

The general practitioner may need to involve neurologist, urologist and rehabilitation specialist. Admission to special facilities such as a Cheshire Home (address see p. 167) or a hospice may be required at the end-stage of the disease.

[1] Patten J (1986) Disease of nervous system and voluntary muscle. In *Treatment and Prognosis, Medicine*, (Hawkins R. ed.) p. 107. Oxford: Heinemann.
[2] Reder T (1983) *Med. Clin. North Am.*, **1**, 573.
[3] Poser CM (1979) Multiple sclerosis: a critical update. *Med. Clin. North Am.*, **63**, 729.
[4] Hart RG, Sherman DG (1982) The diagnosis of multiple sclerosis J.A.M.A. **247**, 498.
[5] Anon (1986) The management of multiple sclerosis. *Drugs Ther. Bull.*, 41–4.
[6] Editorial (1986) Managing multiple sclerosis. *Neurology*, **25**, 703–4.

Myasthenia Gravis

Myasthenia gravis is characterized by weakness or exaggerated fatigue of the bulbar innervated muscles on sustained effort due to impairment of neuromuscular transmission by antibodies to the neural end-plate. Anticholinergic receptor antibodies are present in the sera of 90% of patients[1]. The main muscle groups affected are extraocular (lid ptosis or diplopia), facial and pharyngeal muscles (slurring of speech, choking or dysphagia). Proximal limb weakness or easy fatigue can occur. The most serious effect is when respiratory muscles are involved. The condition is intermittent with a wide variation in severity of attacks.

Incidence is 1 per 10 000 population. The commonest affected groups are women between the ages of 20 and 30 and men between 50 and 70[1].

The diagnosis is confirmed by a positive edrophonium (Tensilon) test carried out in hospital during an attack of weakness: 0.6 mg atropine i.v. is given to prevent bradycardia and nausea, followed by 1 mg i.v. test dose, proceeding to 5 mg edrophonium i.v. The weakness should respond completely in a positive test. Resuscitation equipment must be available for the test. Some 5–10% of patients produce a false negative result[3].

PROGNOSIS

- Without treatment, 30% will die in 3 years. At 10 years after diagnosis, 57% have persistent disease and 13% have incomplete remission[4].
- The prognosis with modern management is uncertain.
- Difficulty achieving successful management of the condition in the first few years is associated with a poor prognosis for frequency and severity of attacks.
- Death is usually secondary to respiratory failure.
- There is a strong association with the auto-immune diseases: 10% of patients are also thyrotoxic[3]; there is also an increased incidence of myxoedema, pernicious anaemia, polymyositis, rheumatoid arthritis and diabetes mellitus.

TREATMENT

1. Patient and family will need sympathetic support until the disease pattern is established, when an estimate of the prognosis can be made.
2. Any intercurrent infection should be treated promptly and vigorously to avoid additional fatiguing. Patients will need easy and rapid access to their general practitioner at all times. The patient's notes should indicate this ease of access.
3. Treatment should be decided only after neurological opinion has been obtained.
4. Pyridostigmine (anticholinesterase) can be prescribed for symptomatic treatment at 30–120 mg daily in divided doses. This has cholinergic side-effects (excessive salivation, colic and diarrhoea) which may require the addition of an anticholinergic agent.
5. Direct treatment involves autoimmune suppression:
   a. *Thymectomy*: this is effective in 50% of under 50-year-olds[5]. The response is slow, but there are no side-effects after surgery recovery.
   b. *Corticosteroids*: this is effective treatment for 80% of patients[6]. A high dose is given until there is an improvement (usually at 3 weeks); then this is tailed off to low-dose maintenance. The patient often suffers transitory worsening (for 7–14 days) and will require close neurological monitoring.
   c. *Plasma exchange*: this is second-line therapy for crises, steroid worsening or as an adjunct to other treatments[7]. Plasma exchange produces striking but temporary remissions.
   d. *Cytotoxic immunosuppressants*: usually azathioprine or cyclophosphamide is prescribed, but response is slow. This should be second-line therapy because of major side-effects.
   e. *Splenectomy*: this is rarely used and should be third-line treatment.
6. The patient may require intensive care for several crises, such as respiratory failure or severe bulbar dysfunction.

169

Patients will need some sort of regular review by the general practitioner. The interval between visits will be dictated by the level of concern and frequency of attacks. Further support may be obtained from the British Association of Myasthenics, 38 Selwood Road, Brentwood, Essex (telephone 0277-218082).

[1] Cohen MS (1987) *Monogr. Allergy*, **21,** 246–51.
[2] Engel AG (1986) *Ann. Neurol.*, **16,** 529–34.
[3] Lindstrom LH (1976) *Neurology*, **26,** 1054–9.
[4] Editorial (1985) *J. Neurol.*, **232,** 202–3.
[5] Buckingham MJ (1986) *Ann. Surgery*, **184,** 453–7.
[6] Pascuzzi RM (1985) *Ann. Neurol.*, **15,** 291–8.
[7] Newson-Davis J (1979) *Lancet*, 464–8.

Parkinson's Disease

Parkinson's disease is a progressive incurable disease of the extrapyramidal motor system. It is the most common disabling neurological condition after stroke. It is caused by a degeneration of dopamine-containing neurones in the midbrain, as a result of which there is an imbalance between the increased activity of the cholinergic transmitter system and the decreased activity of the dopaminergic system, leading to progressive disability.

The incidence is 130 per 100 000 and the annual death rate in England and Wales is 1600[1]. Parkinsonism may be idiopathic (paralysis agitans) with no familial tendency or sympotomatic and secondary to encephalitis, drugs (e.g. phenothiazines, prochlorperazine or metoclopramide), atherosclerosis, or trauma.

Idiopathic parkinsonism rarely presents before the age of 40. It affects both sexes equally. About 1% of people will be affected by the age of 50. Parkinson's disease presents initially with stiffness, muscle aches and slowed movement and progresses to resting tremor (usually mild), muscle rigidity (cogwheel) and bradykinesia.

Parkinsonism is usually an asymmetrical disease and can be unilateral. The most problematic symptoms tend to be bradykinesia (slow movements) or akathisia (restlessness).

PROGNOSIS

Idiopathic parkinsonism

- Slow deterioration over 3–30 years (usually 5–10).
- Some 20–30% of patients over the age of 70 (60% of all Parkinson's sufferers) also exhibit progressive dementing states.
- The worst prognosis occurs when Parkinson's is combined with other brain diseases, like Alzheimer's or Steele–Richardson syndrome.
- Poor prognostic indicators include rapid progression to bilateral disease and poor response to initial medication.
- Depression is a very common sequela.
- Ultimately the effect of medication decreases, the patient becomes bed-ridden and dies of some intercurrent infection.

Secondary parkinsonism

- Postencephalitic parkinsonism and arteriosclerotic parkinsonism have a bad prognosis.
- Drug-induced parkinsonism—normally related to phenothiazines—usually disappears when the offending drug is withdrawn.
- Some 3% of patients treated for over 3 years with phenothiazines may develop irreversible tardive dyskinesia[2].

TREATMENT

1. Any possible drug precipitant should be stopped. If a psychiatric patient requires continued phenothiazines then a reduced dose or an alternative drug may be tried, or an anticholinergic should be added (benzhexol 4–15 mg

daily in young or orphenadrine 100–300 mg daily in elderly patients).

2. Counselling of the patient and relatives should include the fact that there is no perfect drug.

3. Exercise is beneficial, particularly walking and deep breathing exercises. Bedrest during illness should be kept to a minimum.

4. Drugs should be withheld until reasonable activity is disabled. Treatment should be the minimal acceptable to keep the patient independent, not symptom-free.

5. *Drug treatment in mild Parkinson's disease*
   a. Early tremor may respond to a beta-blocker, such as propranolol 40 mg b.d.
   b. Early rigidity in the young should be treated with an anticholinergic like benzhexol (Artane) 4–15 mg per day or orphenadrine (Disipal) 100–300 mg per day in divided doses, or benztropine (Cogentin) 0.5–6 mg per day, as a single night-time dose. Common side-effects are dry mouth, constipation, urinary retention or blurred vision. Confusion is common in the elderly.
   c. Amantadine hydrochloride (Symmetrel) has a mixed action and is safe. It is particularly effective in hypokinesia but has no effect on tremor. Initial response should be seen in 2 weeks, but there is a gradual decline to loss of effect in 3–6 months. Maximum dose is 100 mg three times daily, with the last dose no later than 6 p.m. Common side-effects include hallucination, oedema and mottled skin rash on legs (livido reticularis).

6. *Drug treatment in moderate Parkinson's disease*
   a. Once disability has occurred (or earlier in the elderly), levodopa is indicated. This is combined with carbidopa (Sinemet) or benserazide (Madopar) to prevent metabolism of levodopa outside the central nervous system. Thus gastrointestinal and systemic side-effects are lessened.
   b. Levodopa is particularly helpful for bradykinesia. Tremor and rigidity should show an improvement.
   c. Low doses of levodopa should be used since tolerance occurs with time. The maintenance dose is usually 400 mg to 1.5 g daily in

divided doses. It is usual to start with a small dose of Madopar 62.5 capsules or Sinemet-Plus once or twice daily and then increase every 1–2 days until maximal improvement without side-effect is achieved.
   d. Side-effects include dyskinesia (abnormal involuntary movements), painful cramps, 'on–off' attacks (under- to overactivity) or nausea. Confusion can occur in the elderly.

7. *Drug treatment in severe Parkinson's disease*
   a. The maximum tolerated levodopa combination is recommended.
   b. Bromocriptine is longer-acting but similar to levodopa. Patients should receive a test dose of 2.5 g after a meal, thereafter 2.5 g b.d. after food, increased by weekly increments of 2.5 g up to 15 g daily and then by 5 mg increments up to 30–40 mg daily (10–20 g in the elderly). Levodopa should be tailed off. Side-effects include nausea and vomiting, hypotension, painful erythema of the extremities and serious confusional states.

FOLLOW-UP

Depression is very common and may require treatment with tricyclic antidepressants. Constipation should be expected. Dietary advice should be given and faecal softeners prescribed as necessary. Speech therapy can help—two-thirds of patients have some speech defect[3]. Aids are required by 75% of patients in time[3]. A zimmer frame is not recommended as a walking aid, but a wheeled Delta-aid or Rollator is helpful. Parkinson's is a relevant disability for driving and patients should inform the DVLC and their insurance company. The Parkinson's Disease Society is based at 36 Portland Place, London W1N 3DG (telephone 071-323-1174/5).

[1] Quinn N, Husain F (1986) *Parkinson's Disease*. Br. Med. J., **293,** 379–80.
[2] American College of Neuropsychopharmacology (1973) Neurologic syndromes associated with antipsychotic drug use. N. Engl. J. Med., **289,** 20.
[3] Godwin-Austen RB *et al.* (1982) *Parkinson's Disease*. London: Scientific Projects.

Peripheral Nerve Disorders

Damage to single nerves (mononeuritis) is usually due to trauma or compression and the signs are limited to that particular nerve's distribution. Multiple isolated nerves (mononeuritis multiplex) are affected by patchy inflammation (sarcoid, amyloid) or vascular disorders (diabetes, polyarteritis nodosa). This rare condition will produce paraesthesiae and pain over the sensory distribution with associated muscle-wasting and weakness. It is often asymmetrical and the symptoms are distal. Diffuse generalized nerve involvement produces the true peripheral neuropathy which may be acute or chronic.

The commonest causes are diabetes mellitus, infection, vitamin B deficiency, carcinomatosis, or toxic due to drugs or chemicals. In 50% of peripheral neuropathies the cause will be unknown. Only the commonest single nerve entrapments or peripheral neuropathies are considered further.

Isolated nerve palsies[1]

Carpal tunnel syndrome (see p. 274)

Ulnar nerve compression

Damage will usually occur at the elbow (due to mechanical stretching or pressure or joint deformity) but occasionally is seen at the wrist (from trauma or compression, as in carpal tunnel syndrome). Symptoms include pain and paraesthesiae over the little and ring fingers. Motor fibres to the small muscles of the hand are disrupted, causing problems with fine movements like sewing, writing and buttoning up. A claw hand can develop.

PROGNOSIS

- Acute compression will normally resolve completely.
- Chronic compression with weak or wasted muscles is unlikely to recover function.

TREATMENT

1. Treatment is conservative initially with avoidance of full elbow flexion and leaning on the elbow.
2. For chronic symptoms, decompression or anterior transposition of the nerve should be considered.

Radial nerve compression

Pressure on the nerve occurs in the spiral groove of the humerus, usually by hanging one arm over the back of a chair, frequently during alcohol or drug excess. Symptoms are mainly confined to the motor innervation of brachioradialis and finger extensors, producing wrist and finger drop.

PROGNOSIS

- Recovery will usually occur within 6–12 weeks, unless the nerve has been accidentally ligated.

TREATMENT

1. Splintage of the hand is necessary to avoid contractures developing whilst resolution is awaited.
2. Surgery is only indicated where the cause is a complicated fracture.

Lateral popliteal nerve palsy

This is usually caused by compression of the nerve over the lateral aspect of the knee during prolonged sitting cross-legged, squatting or occasionally from an overtight plaster cast. The resultant weakness of foot dorsiflexion and eversion leads to foot drop and a tendency to trip.

PROGNOSIS

- If external pressure is the cause then complete recovery is likely within 3 months.

TREATMENT

1. Splintage of the foot prevents tripping and contractures.

. Surgery is only indicated for resistant cases.

Lateral cutaneous nerve of thigh compression

This produces a purely sensory deficit due to pressure under the lateral end of the inguinal ligament. Symptoms include pain, paraesthesiae and numbness over the lateral thigh (meralgia paraesthetica). Precipitants include obesity and pregnancy.

PROGNOSIS

● No complications or permanent deficits occur.

TREATMENT

1. Injection of local steroid under the inguinal ligament is usually effective.
2. Surgery to free the nerve is reserved for resistant cases.

Peripheral neuropathies

Diabetic neuropathy

Nerve disorders complicate diabetes mildly in around 50% of cases and severely in 10% of patients. They include isolated palsies and mononeuritis multiplex but are predominantly peripheral neuropathies. The symptoms tend to be symmetrical and sensory, especially impaired vibration sense and burning or tingling of the feet. The pain that can develop may be severe. Late autonomic neuropathy frequently occurs with postural hypotension, nocturnal diarrhoea, neurogenic bladder and sexual dysfunction.

PROGNOSIS

● Once presented, generalized neuropathy will progress despite therapy.
● Recovery of isolated palsies and mononeuritis occurs, but more slowly than in non-diabetic individuals.
● Autonomic neuropathy can severely compromise lifestyle and lead to depressive illness.

TREATMENT

1. Good diabetic control should be attempted,

although there is no evidence that this is protective.
2. Pain control may require regular analgesia. Severe cases may respond to amitriptyline 50–100 g daily and carbamazepine 100–200 mg t.d.s.
3. There is no specific therapy to improve nerve function and no treatment that will prevent further loss.

FOLLOW-UP

Assessment of the diabetic patient must include at least an annual check for the presence of a neuropathy. Patients will need to understand the dangers of developing neuropathy to avoid secondary damage to denervated structures. Scrupulous foot care is essential, including avoidance of walking with bare feet. Great care should be taken to avoid scalds, overhot baths and pressure injuries. Patients who develop autonomic neuropathy will need careful counselling and may require a variety of aids.

Guillain–Barré syndrome

This is the commonest acquired neuropathy (around 30% of acute cases) with an annual incidence of 1–2 per 100 000 population[2]. It usually presents as an acute motor demyelinating polyneuropathy 1–2 weeks after a febrile illness (in 60% of cases) or an event such as surgery. Pain in the back and legs progresses to weakness over a few hours or weeks. Proximal, bulbar and facial muscles are mainly affected. Respiratory muscles are involved in 50% of cases. Paralysis may become complete.

PROGNOSIS

● 20% of patients will suffer sufficient respiratory compromise to require ventilation.
● 50% will progress over 2 weeks, with 90% at their worst by 4 weeks[3].
● Spontaneous resolution is likely within 3–6 months, although it can take up to 2 years.
● 35% of patients will remain with some permanent deficit (usually weakness of distal muscles or a facial paresis)[2].
● Recurrence occurs in 2% of patients[4].

TREATMENT

1. Patients should be admitted to hospital for observation of respiratory function.
2. Patients in respiratory difficulty should be ventilated early.
3. Patients with bulbar dysfunction may require tube-feeding.
4. No specific therapy exists. Claims are made for plasmapheresis and steroids but no controlled trials exist.
5. Strict rest during the progression of disease symptoms should be followed by physiotherapy once the condition starts to remit.

FOLLOW-UP

Patients should be reassured that the possibility of relapse is extremely remote. Recovery of full function may take some months.

Alcoholic neuropathy

The neuropathic consequences of alcohol abuse are related to deprivation of essential nutrients as much as to the effects of the alcohol. The main vitamin depleted is B (thiamine). Principal symptoms include pains and paraesthesiae in the feet and calves. This can lead to motor weakness of the distal leg muscles. A sensory loss occurs below the wrists and knees with loss of ankle jerk and an increase in other reflexes.

PROGNOSIS

● Prognosis is poor as long as drinking continues.
● If drinking has ceased full recovery of neurological deficit can take years.

TREATMENT

1. Support for giving up alcohol is essential. Patients may benefit from referral to agencies like Alcoholics Anonymous, P.O. Box 1, Stonebow House, Stonebow, York YO1 2NJ (telephone 0904-644026) or local support groups.
2. Vitamin supplements should be routinely prescribed to all heavy drinkers. Maintenance vitamin B_1 therapy requires a dose of vitamin B compound strong, 6 tablets per day.
3. Assessment of other vitamin deficit, including B_{12}, should be made.
4. There is no specific therapy for the neuropathy.

[1] Dyck PJ et al. (1975) Peripheral Neuropathy. Philadelphia: WB Saunders.
[2] Neury D (1980) Br. J. Hosp. Med., 24, 206.
[3] Loffel NB et al. (1977) J. Neurol. Sci., 33, 71.
[4] Rowland LP (ed) (1984) Merritt's Textbook of Neurology. Philadelphia: Lea & Febiger.

Bell's Palsy

Bell's palsy is a unilateral lower motor neurone facial paralysis of sudden onset, unrelated to disease elsewhere. Frequently patients will have associated pain around the ear or neck (50%), disturbance of taste (35%), hyperacusis (30%), tears and gustatory sweating (10%). The whole of one side of the face is affected; the degree is equivalent to the extent of nerve damage—there is complete paralysis in 75%. Signs include the inability to wrinkle the forehead or close an eye, and drooping of the mouth. Incidence is 22.8 per 100000[1]. Bell's palsy is more prevalent in the third, fourth and fifth decades. A total of 30% of affected patients have a family history[2].

PROGNOSIS

- Deficit is maximal within 48 hours.
- A total of 80% will attain a good or full recovery within 3–6 weeks.
- In all, 80% will achieve reasonable facial symmetry.
- Recovery takes 9–12 months in 15% of cases.
- There is residual muscle weakness in 30%, with a contracture in 5%[2].

TREATMENT

1. Steroids are of no proven value.
2. Surgical decompression of the nerve is sometimes tried but has no proven benefit.
3. The cornea must be protected if the eyelid cannot be closed.

FOLLOW-UP

Patients can be reassured that significant improvement is likely to occur without any need for treatment.

---

[1] Hauser WA *et al.* (1971) *Mayo Clin. Proc.*, **46,** 258.
[2] Pryse-Phillips W, Murray TJ (1982) *Essential Neurology*. New York: Medical Examination.

Transient Ischaemic Attacks

A transient ischaemic attack (TIA) is an acute loss of focal brain or ocular function, with symptoms lasting less than 24 hours, produced by microemboli from atheromatous plaques in the internal carotid or vertebrobasilar arteries (ratio of 2:1) in 80% of cases or emboli from heart lesions in 10–15%. Incidence is at least 31 per 100000[1]. There are 25000 patients in the UK presenting for the first time with a TIA every year.

Symptoms include mono-ocular visual loss (whole or part-field), unilateral weakness or paraesthesiae(arm, leg or face), language disturbance, dysarthria, dysphagia, falls, confusion or vertigo.

PROGNOSIS

- In all, 90% of first strokes have had a previous TIA[2].
- Risk of subsequent stroke; the most frequently quoted figures for the risk of stroke following TIA (from the Framingham Study) put the risk at 21% within 1 month, 51% within 1 year and 85% within 5 years[1]. However this was a moderately small patient cohort. Extrapolating figures from the five main studies with more than 100 patients of all ages, the risk does not appear as great. The expected rate of stroke following a TIA is probably around 7% per year (30–40% within 5 years)[3].
- Risk of stroke is five times that of the non-TIA population[4].
- There is only a marginal decrease in survival in patients following TIA compared to the age/sex-matched random population[1]. Mortality is usually due to cardiovascular disease.
- TIA patients have a five times greater risk of cardiovascular disease, 50% will die from a myocardial infarction.
- Angiography carries a 0.4–0.8% risk of death and a 1–2% risk of stroke.
- The mortality rate from surgery is 3.5%.
- The overall morbidity/mortality risk of angiography, endarterectomy and anaesthetic is 11%.

TREATMENT

1. Prevention of TIA must involve the same strategy as for stroke (pp. 178–179).
2. Patients with artificial heart valves should be anticoagulated for life on warfarin (prothrombin time 3–3.5 times normal control).
3. Patients with clearcut mitral valve disease and atrial fibrillation should also be anticoagulated.
4. Other cardiac emboli should probably not be treated by anticoagulation since:
   a. in 40–60-year-olds there is no significant reduction of embolic episodes following anticoagulation[5].
   b. over the age of 60, there is a substantial reduction in cerebral infarction, but also a major increase in haemorrhagic risk[6]. The risk of haemorrhagic complications is 8.2% with 0.4% risk of death from cerebral haemorrhage[7].
5. Surgery by carotid endarterectomy has yet to demonstrate conclusive benefit. The prognosis of patients who survive surgery would not appear to alter.
6. Medical treatment with aspirin (300 mg daily) significantly reduces the subsequent risk of stroke[8]. It is highly probable that low-dose aspirin (75 or 150 mg daily) will be shown to confer similar benefits with a lower incidence of side-effects.

FOLLOW-UP

The patient and carers will need continuing support over their uncertain prognosis. Hypertensive patients should be monitored carefully. The prothrombin time should be checked regularly in patients on warfarin.

[1] Whisnant JP et al. (1973) Mayo Clin. Proc., 48, 194–8.
[2] Matsumoto N et al. (1973) Stroke, 4, 20–9.
[3] Millikan CH, McDowell FH (1978) Stroke, 9, 299–308.
[4] Greenhaulgh R, Clifford Rose F (1979) Progress in Stroke Research. London: Pitman Medical.
[5] Hildan T et al. (1961) Lancet, ii, 327–31.
[6] De Vries WA et al. (1979) Med. T. Geneesk, 123, 1211–12.
[7] Forfar JC (1979) Br. Heart J., 42, 128–32.
[8] UK TIA Study Group (1988) Br. Med. J., 296, 316–20.

Subarachnoid Haemorrhage

Subarachnoid haemorrhage (SAH) is due to the rupture of an intracranial saccular aneurysm. Transient loss of consciousness in 45% of patients (in 10% for several days) and there is abrupt onset of severe headaches in 40%, often with vomiting. Up to 5% of the population have cerebral aneurysms over 3 mm in size[1]. The incidence of SAH in the UK is 10.3 per 100 000[2], (6000 people suffer SAH per year). Peak age range is 55–60 years (range 35–65). Unlike stroke, SAH is not declining in incidence. There is a familial tendency. SAH is more likely to occur in patients with polycystic kidneys, coarctation of the aorta and in hypertensive subjects. Warning leaks produce an acute severe headache with vomiting and neck or shoulder pain. Expanding aneurysms produce cranial nerve palsies, particularly of the third (lid or eye muscle palsy, dilated pupils) or sixth nerve (diplopia).

PROGNOSIS

- 6% of all strokes are due to SAH[3].
- 10% of all those who have SAH will die without warning.
- 20–30% of those with SAH will rebleed, with a mortality rate of 20% within 2 weeks.
- 45–50% of all patients with SAH will die within 3 months[4].
- 35–40% of patients with catastrophic haemorrhage will die without regaining consciousness.
- Only 30% of patients survive a rupture without major disability[5].
- 75% of patients have evidence of bleeding on CT scan within 48 hours[6].
- 10–20% will develop epilepsy post-SAH.
- The mortality risk of surgery to a ruptured aneurysm is as low as 2% in major centres.
- 54% of patients never achieve their previous quality of life following obliteration of the aneurysm[7].
- The risk of rupture in asymptomatic aneurysm is 15% in 10–50-year-olds[8]. The risk is reduced in patients over the age of 50, and substantially reduced if the aneurysm is smaller than 1 cm in size.

TREATMENT

1. Early recognition of patients with warning leaks or expanding lesions is the major priority for general practitioners.
2. Patients with sudden-onset severe headaches and vomiting, without a history of migraine, or acute cranial nerve palsies should be referred for diagnosis by CT scan, cerebral angiography or magnetic resonance imaging and early surgical clipping of the aneurysm.
3. Following SAH, surviving patients are treated with absolute bedrest, with head elevated, for 3 weeks.
4. Patients may be sedated with chlormethiazole.
5. Patients should be formally considered for neurosurgery. If blood loss is high, surgery should take place within 48 hours. Smaller bleeds are usually left 14 days before surgery, although the risk of a rebleed is high.
6. Long-term medical treatment with antifibrinolytics has no place.
7. Short-term tranexamic acid or epsilon can be considered in patients for delayed surgery. Epsilon will reduce the risk of rebleeding from 24 to 9%, but increases the risk of cerebral infarction[9].

FOLLOW-UP

Follow-up is as for stroke patients. (See p. 179)

[1] Chason JL et al. (1958) Neurology, **8**, 41.
[2] Garaway WH et al. (1979) N. Engl. J. Med., **300**, 449–52.
[3] Mohr JP, Kase CS (1983) Rev. Neurol., **139**, 99.
[4] Pritz MB et al. (1978) Neurosurgery, **3**, 364.
[5] Kassall NF, Drake CG (1983) Neurol. Clin., **1**, 73–86.
[6] Ojemann RG et al. (1983) Surgical Management of Cerebrovascular Disease. Baltimore: Williams & Wilkins.
[7] Ropper AH, Zerras NT (1984) J. Neurosurg., **60**, 909.
[8] Dell S (1982) Neurosurgery, **10**, 162–6.
[9] Sengupta RP et al. (1976) J. Neurosurg., **44**, 479–84.

Strokes

A stroke is an acute disturbance of cerebral function of vascular origin causing death within or disability over 24 hours. The incidence of first stroke in the UK is 2 per 1000 per year[1]. Recurrent strokes occur in 2.6 patients per 1000 per year. The majority of strokes occur in those over 65; the incidence for over 75-year-olds is 47.41 per 1000 per year[2]. More men are affected than women (in a ratio of 1.3:1). The incidence of stroke is declining in most developed countries, probably as a consequence of the recognition and treatment of hypertension[3].

The prevalence of stroke is 5–10/1000 population. A general practitioner will see 5 new cases of stroke per year and have 15–20 chronic stroke patients in the community. Altogether 1 in 3 people will develop cardiovascular disease.

Most strokes are due to cerebral infarction secondary to thrombosis or embolism (65–80%). Other causes are cerebral haemorrhage (10–15%) or subarachnoid haemorrhage (5–10%), which causes 50% of strokes in those aged under 35.

Main risk factors for strokes are age, hypertension (systolic blood pressure over 180 mmHg has an 8 times greater risk than systolic blood pressure below 120 mmHg), transient ischaemic attack (10-times greater risk), smoking (3-times risk), diabetes (3-times risk), and elevated cholesterol in the under-50 age group.

PROGNOSIS

- Stroke is the third commonest cause of death in England and Wales. The probability of ultimate death from stroke is 1 in 8[4].

- Following a stroke, approximately 20% of patients will die within a month—this figure increases to 25–30% if recurrent strokes are included.

- Of those who survive 1 month, approximately 10% will be unimpaired, 40% will be mildly disabled, 40% will require special care and 10% will need residential care[5].

- Some 50% of survivors have minor problems, 35% have speech disorders and 25% have sensory deficits[3].

- Stroke is the leading cause of disability in the world.

- In 60% of stroke patients the neurological deficit is maximal at 1 hour of onset. Deficit will progress in less than 10% after 24 hours.

Prevention

- Good control of moderate or severe hypertension will lower the incidence of stroke from 2.6/1000 patient years to 1.4/1000[6].

- This control of blood pressure has no effect on overall mortality or cerebrovascular mortality, but non-fatal cardiovascular events are reduced by 50%[7].

- Older, higher-risk hypertensive subjects gain benefits from prevention, with a reduction in stroke incidence of 26 per 1000 between the treated and placebo groups[8].

Recovery

- The fastest recovery takes place in the first few weeks; 50% of the recovery over 3 months is made in the first 2 weeks[1].

- After 6 months little further recovery is likely, although 5–10% will improve slowly.

- A patient who is continent of urine at 2 days post-stroke is likely to regain independent mobility.

- A patient with a good hand grip at 3 weeks should regain useful arm function.

- A patient who is not walking at 5 weeks is likely to continue with poor gait.

TREATMENT

Prevention

1. Preventing strokes is the absolute priority. This involves the population adopting healthier lifestyles, which must include cessation of smoking, lower cholesterol intake and weight moderation through diet and exercise.

2. The general practitioner can assist this process through health education on an opportunistic basis or via well-person clinics, involving the practice nurse and reception staff. Poster displays and handouts may be effective in promoting good health.

3. Identification of the hypertensive subjects in the general practitioner's practice must be organized formally to have impact, either through opportunistic blood pressure checks in all patients over the age of 35 or through call/recall checks using an age/sex register.

4. Diabetic patients should have vigorous follow-up to ensure good blood sugar control and avoidance of other risk factors.

Following a stroke

1. No treatment has been conclusively shown to be beneficial in limiting the neuronal damage associated with stroke[9]. There is insufficient evidence to validate the use of any drugs in the immediate post stroke period.

2. Neurosurgery may be indicated in a few patients with haemorrhage due to an aneurysm or arteriovenous malformation (see p. 177).

3. A few strokes will be due to an underlying disease which may respond to treatment (e.g. cranial arteritis, myelomatosis or polycythaemia).

4. Care should be taken to avoid the early complications of stroke including chest infections, deep vein thrombosis, urinary infections, pressure sores, dehydration, constipation and falls.

5. Patients may require hospitalization, physiotherapy, occupational therapy or speech therapy. Many patients can be managed at home if there is sufficient support from a carer.

6. Recurrent ischaemic strokes can be reduced by treatment with an antiplatelet drug like aspirin 75–150 mg/day. However, intracerebral haemorrhage should be excluded first.

7 Recurrent stroke can also be reduced by adequately treating hypertension, reducing a high cholesterol level, stopping smoking and reducing alcohol intake.

FOLLOW-UP

Rehabilitation should aim to maximize independence through multidisciplinary support. This will require close co-operation and effective communication between the primary care team and therapists. The general practitioner will need to respond to patient and carer alike in providing an explanation (of the cause, treatment, prevention and realistic goals), practical advice (helps, housing needs, aids, financial allowances) and social support (providing a listening ear, coping with family role changes). Depression amongst patients (or carers) is common and must be continually assessed for. Treatment with antidepressants should be early if mood or sleep disturbance occurs. Support for carers may require organizing a day centre or day hospital place for the patient, or arranging relief admissions to Part III or hospital. Voluntary help may be obtained through the Chest, Heart and Stroke Association, Tavistock House, Tavistock Square, London WC1H 9SE (telephone 01-387-3012) or Association of Carers, Medway Homes, Balfour Road, Rochester, Kent ME4 6QU.

[1] Warlow C et al. (1987) Strokes. London: MTP Press.
[2] Kannal A (1987) A Colour Atlas of Stroke. London: Wolfe Medical Publications.
[3] Gordan T et al. (1971) The Framingham Study: A 16-Year Follow Up. Washington DC: US Govt Printing Office.
[4] Wylie CM (1970) Stroke, 1, 184.
[5] Kuller L et al. (1970) Stroke, 1, 86–9.
[6] MRC Working Party (1985) Br. Med. J., 291, 97–104.
[7] Amery A et al. (1978) Lancet, i, 681–3.
[8] Amery A et al. (1985) European Working Party on Hypertension (EWPHE) in the elderly. Lancet, 1, 1349–54.
[9] King's Fund Forum (1988) Treatment of stroke. Br. Med. J., 297, 126–8.

Trigeminal Neuralgia

'Trigeminal neuralgia' is the term used to describe sudden clusters of intense unilateral pain lasting seconds or minutes over the second (maxillary) or third (mandibular) divisions of the trigeminal nerve. Rarely the first division is affected or the pain is bilateral. Attacks are often triggered by touch or contact (60% around the mouth to ear, 30% are nose to orbit). Spasms may become continuous with time. Trigeminal neuralgia is commoner is the elderly (mean age of onset is 50) and in females (in a ratio of 3:2 female to male)[1]. Most cases are idiopathic and there should be no physical signs. If sensory loss is apparent in the trigeminal territory, then investigation for an irritative cause (tumour or aneurysm) is indicated.

Rarely trigeminal neuralgia may be a presentation of multiple sclerosis in the young, especially if accompanied by a tic.

PROGNOSIS

- Even if the pain remits it is almost certain to return.
- Trigeminal neuralgia can be one of the most severe of all possible pains.
- Depression is a common sequela.
- A total of 75% of patients will show some response to carbamazepine.

TREATMENT

1. Management should include explanation and reassurance.
2. The drug of choice is carbamazepine. The initial dose should be 100 g daily, increasing every 2 days until relief is obtained, to a maximum of 200 mg q.d.s. Side-effects include unsteadiness, diplopia or gastrointestinal effects. Complications include skin rashes, liver disturbance and marrow suppression.
3. Phenytoin 200–300 g daily can be added to carbamazepine, or used separately.
4. Clonazepam 2–6 mg daily has also been used effectively.
5. Baclofen is occasionally helpful, particularly when there is an associated tic (two-thirds improve). The dose is 5 mg b.d. up to 20 g t.d.s.
6. Antidepressants should be considered.
7. Non-responders may well require surgical destruction of the trigeminal nerve, although this involves a craniotomy and results in sensory deficit.

FOLLOW-UP

Regular follow-up may well be necessary even if it is only to provide counselling and support. Referral to a pain clinic may be needed. The patient's (and carer's) mood should be regularly assessed.

[1] Hobbs FDR (1988) Treatment of facial pain. In *Treatment* (Drury M *et al.* eds). London: Kluwer Publishing.

Postherpetic Neuralgia

Persistent burning or gnawing pains will occur in about 15% of patients who have suffered an attack of herpes zoster. Trigeminal involvement is usually over the first division (the forehead and around the eye). Most patients are elderly and become depressed.

PROGNOSIS

- If the neuralgia persists over 18 months, improvement becomes unlikely.
- Treatment is difficult.

TREATMENT

1. Acute therapy in zoster infections with acyclovir may reduce the incidence of postherpetic neuralgia, although this is not proven.
2. Moderate analgesics and an antidepressant (like dothiepin 75–150 mg nocte) should be tried first, but the painkillers are unlikely to provide much relief.
3. Carbamazepine can be added, 100 g daily, increasing gradually to control pain to a maximum of 1.6 g daily (usually in doses of 600–800 mg).
4. Rarely transcutaneous nerve stimulation is effective and has no side-effects.
5. Surgical destruction of the nerve has not demonstrated benefit.

FOLLOW-UP

Follow-up is as for trigeminal neuralgia.

8

Paediatrics

D. R. Morgan

Heart Defects

Atrial Septal Defect

Atrial septal defect occurs in 0.6/1000 livebirths. Most cases (53%) are the ostium secundum type, where the defect lies in the fossa ovalis; two-thirds of these cases involve a central defect. The remainder consist of an ostium primum defect where the opening is either in the lower part of the septum, usually involving a cleft in the mitral valve, or in a common arteriovenous canal where there can be a variety of atrial and septal defects as well as defects in the mitral and tricuspid valves.

The majority of patients with isolated ostium secundum defects are asymptomatic and will be discovered at routine examination. Failure to thrive may occur. There is a little dyspnoea on effort in some patients. About 5% of children will have pulmonary hypertension.

Those who have ostium primum and a mitral valve cleft are more likely to have breathlessness and tiredness and to have congestive cardiac failure. Those with a common arteriovenous canal present in infancy with failure to thrive, heart failure and cyanosis.

PROGNOSIS

- Without treatment, mortality rates are low (0.6 per annum) for ostium secundum defects in the first two decades of life, but rise thereafter. There is a 25% mortality rate by the 27th year, 50% by the 36th year and 75% by the 50th year[1]. Causes of death include congestive cardiac failure, mitral valve disease, atrial fibrillation, or Eisenmenger's syndrome.

- Spontaneous closure of the atrial septal defect can occur[2].

- Without treatment, a large number of those with ostium primum defects will have died by the age of 30. Many of those with common arteriovenous canal will die by the age of 6.

- Hospital mortality for closure of ostium primum defects is about 6%. Mitral insufficiency, which once was a major problem after repair of ostium primum defect, is now rare, but persistent or late postoperative arrhythmias may be a significant problem, occurring in 23% of one series[3].

TREATMENT

Ostium secundum defects

1. A surgical repair (usually 4–5 years) of the defect is indicated if it is of significant size or if there is a significant left-to-right shunt.

Ostium primum defects

1. Those who have isolated ostium primum defects and minimal symptoms normally have elective repair at 4–5 years.
2. Of those with mitral valve defects, 50% will require medical management to control heart failure. If this fails, patch closure and repair of the mitral valve will be necessary.
3. Common arteriovenous canal defects will require repair in infancy.

FOLLOW-UP

Cardiological assessment is required every 2–4 years to detect any arrhythmias. If mitral valve insufficiency is clinically suspected, annual ECG, chest X-ray or echocardiography is required.

[1] Campbell M (1970) *Br. Heart J.*, **32**, 820–6.
[2] Fukazawa M *et al.* (1988) *Am. Heart J.*, **116**, 123–7.
[3] Portman MA *et al.* (1985) *Am. Heart J.*, **110**, 1054–8.

Ventricular Septal Defect

Ventricular septal defect occurs in 1.35–2.5 per 1000 livebirths. In isolation it accounts for 23% of congenital heart disease and is present in a further 26% of cases.

Most children are discovered at routine medical examination with a loud pansystolic murmur at the lower left edge and a thrill; however, large ventricular septal defects may present as congestive cardiac failure in infancy. Often initial ability to exercise is good with little dyspnoea and no cyanosis, but this depends on the size of the defect. Some patients may go on to develop Eisenmenger's syndrome, where progressive vascular resistance reverses the flow of blood across the septum from right to left. As the child gets older, cyanosis, finger-clubbing and reduced exercise tolerance occur.

PROGNOSIS

- Without treatment the defect may get smaller or close (31% in one series)[1].
- The defect may get larger as the child grows and progressive vascular obstruction may occur, either rapidly or slowly. Infundibular narrowing, present at birth, may increase, thus protecting the pulmonary vasculature[2].
- Subacute bacterial endocarditis may occur rarely and aortic incompetence may develop[1].
- Hospital mortality for primary closure of ventricular septal defect in infancy is between 6 and 8%[3,4]. Late mortality is 2.3%[4].
- Mortality is higher in younger infants with pre-existing respiratory problems or a haemodynamically significant lesion preoperatively. Complete primary closure can be achieved in 70%, while 27% may be left with an insignificant shunt.
- In older children with a pulmonary to systemic flow rate of greater than 2 to 1 with low pulmonary resistance, the mortality should be very low (1%); with increasing pulmonary resistance the mortality increases 50–70% in those where resistance reaches systemic levels[2].

TREATMENT

1. No treatment is necessary for those with a small asymptomatic defect.
2. Prophylactic antibiotic therapy is required for those undergoing dental treatment or any surgical procedure.

3. Medical treatment of congestive cardiac failure may be necessary.
4. Infants with failure to thrive, congestive cardiac failure or pulmonary hypertension will normally be treated as a primary repair.
5. Older children with a persistently large shunt (greater than 2 to 1 pulmonary to systemic flow rate) are at risk of developing pulmonary hypertension and will require primary repair by patch closure.

FOLLOW-UP

Once diagnosed, infants should be assessed regularly by a cardiologist. Cardiac catheterization will be necessary to determine pulmonary and systemic flow rates, as well as pulmonary artery pressure and vascular resistance in those with symptoms or where there are ECG abnormalities or cardiac enlargement.

---

[1] Dickinson DF et al. (1981) Ventricular septal defect in children born in Liverpool 1960–1969. Br. Heart J., **46**, 47–54.

[2] Keith JD (1978) Ventricular septal defect. In Heart Disease in Infancy and Childhood, 3rd edn (Keith JD et al. eds), pp. 320–79. New York: Macmillan.

[3] Henze A et al. (1984) Repair of ventricular septal defect in the first year of life. Scand. J. Thor. Cardiovasc. Surg., **18**, 151–4.

[4] Yeager SB et al. (1984) Primary closure of ventricular septal defect in the first year of life: results in 128 infants. J. Am. Coll. Cardiol., **3**, 1269–76.

Patent Ductus Arteriosus

The ductus arteriosus[1], derived from the sixth aortic arch, connects the fetal pulmonary artery to the aorta distal to the left subclavian artery. Closure probably occurs within the first 48 hours of life and is brought about by muscular contraction followed by fibrosis and obliteration. Delay in closure of the duct[2] is associated with maternal rubella infection and in premature infants, especially where there is birth asphyxia or respiratory distress syndrome, but is also associated with other congenital abnormalities, mainly ventricular septal defect, coarctation of the aorta, aortic stenosis, pulmonary stenosis and mitral incompetence.

The incidence in isolation is between 1 in 2500 and 1 in 5000. It amounts to about 12% of all cases of congenital heart disease. The presentation in infancy in about 40% will be congestive cardiac failure, failure to thrive or chest infections, whereas in older children these symptoms are less common.

Clinical examination will reveal a praecordial thrill and a wide pulse pressure of over 45 mmHg. Auscultation will reveal the characteristic machinery murmur in the pulmonary area, starting after the first sound, building to a crescendo by the second sound and then fading again. A noted complication is subacute bacterial endocarditis.

Diagnosis is assisted by X-ray which will show cardiac enlargement, and by ECG which will show left ventricular hypertrophy. Cardiac catheterization will confirm the diagnosis by showing a higher oxygen concentration in the pulmonary artery than in the right ventricle and angiography can define the size of the duct.

PROGNOSIS

- Without treatment, life expectancy is shortened.
- Up to 20% of patients will have died by the age of 30 and 60% by 60 years, unless treatment occurs.

TREATMENT

1. An increased uptake of rubella immunization will decrease the numbers of patent ductus arteriosus caused by fetal rubella syndrome.
2. Treatment of the established case in infancy can be pharmacological or surgical.
3. Indomethacin may aid closure of a patent ductus in the premature infant. In one study[3] of 19 preterm infants the duct initially closed in 58% infants or was constricted in a further 37%, but in 36% and 71% of these the duct reopened and these patients went on to have surgery. In another study, 42% of infants failed to improve with indomethacin and 82% of these required surgery[4].
4. In the same study[4] all infants requiring surgical treatment were successful, and there were no deaths related to the operation. The failure of indomethacin may be related to low birth-weight, the degree of heart failure and the route of administration—the success of the intravenous route is less variable than the oral route[2].
5. In older children the operative mortality is similarly extremely low.

FOLLOW-UP

Follow-up by a cardiologist is advised with assessments of improvement in growth, reduction in heart size, and improvement in cardiographic changes. Recurrences after surgery are rare, but should be considered. Prophylactic antibiotics should be given for dental and other surgical procedures.

[1] Rowe RD (1978) *Heart Disease in Infancy and Childhood*, 3rd edn (Keith JD *et al.* eds) New York: MacMillan, p. 418.
[2] Walters M (1988) *Br. Med. J.*, **297**, 773–4.
[3] Ramsay JM *et al.* (1987) *Am. J. Dis. Child.*, **141**, 294–302.
[4] Palder SB *et al.* (1987) *J. Ped. Surg.*, **22**, 1171–4.

Fallot's Tetralogy

This condition consists of four abnormalities—pulmonary stenosis, right ventricular hypertrophy, ventricular septal defect and over-riding of the aorta. The degree of pulmonary stenosis determines the severity. Cyanosis usually develops in the first 6 months of life, but breathlessness often presents early when the child feeds or cries. Cyanotic episodes with breathlessness are a feature in infancy. Squatting or lying in a curled position is a characteristic feature. This position has the effect of avoiding faintness, and reducing the return of venous blood from the limbs with its very low concentrations of oxygen, thereby effectively increasing the oxygen concentration of the blood in the systemic circulation. Infants with Fallot's often fail to thrive; congenital heart disease may be responsible by a combination of low energy intake and high-energy experiments[1]. Cyanosis tends to worsen after the age of 6 months, but after the age of 2, children seem to adapt, restricting their own activity.

PROGNOSIS

- Without treatment there is progressive decline in health from puberty onwards with increasing cyanosis and dyspnoea leading to death by the age of 20. Some patients however may survive many years. Death is due to hypoxia cerebrovascular accidents, infection, cerebral abscess or SBE (subacute bacterial endocarditis).
- The hospital mortality for palliative Block–Taussig shunt is about 5% and for primary repair about 10%[2].
- The survival at 5 years for those who had repair in infancy is about 98%[3].
- Causes of late death include sudden death due to arrhythmias, complete heartblock, accident, suicide and reoperation[4].

TREATMENT

Medical management of severe cases

The aim is to avoid cerebral damage by:
1. Avoidance of anaemia.
2. Maintenance of a correct fluid balance.
3. Correction of hypoxia and acidosis with oxygen, sodium bicarbonate and by placing the child in knee–chest position.
4. Correction of cyanotic spells with intravenous propranolol or prevention by oral propranolol.

Surgical management

1. *Palliative:* palliative surgery in infants under 3 months may be necessary where there is severe cyanosis, small pulmonary artery size, dyspnoea and feeding difficulties. Palliation allows time for cardiac growth and reduces the risk of complete repair at this age. Palliation is achieved by the Block–Taussig shunt, in which either the subclavian artery is anastomosed directly to the pulmonary artery or a graft is inserted between the two vessels.

2. *Corrective procedures:* infants over 3–6 months with adequate pulmonary artery size, those who require propranolol for hypoxic spells and children over 6 months may undergo primary correction. Intracardiac repair involves patching the ventricular septal defect with dacron mesh and relieving the right ventricular outflow heart obstruction by resection, incision of the fused commissures of the pulmonary artery or, rarely, insertion of a prosthetic valve.

FOLLOW-UP

Once diagnosed the child should be seen regularly by a cardiologist to assess the timing of corrective surgery. After shunt surgery, regular assessments are necessary to time cardiac catheterization prior to correction.

After correction, regular assessments are necessary to assess valvular function and the development of dysrhythmias and heart block.

[1] Menon G et al. (1985) Arch. Dis. Child., **60,** 1134–9.
[2] Kirklin JW et al. (1983) Ann. Surg., **1981,** 251–65.
[3] Walsh EP et al. (1988) Circulation, **77,** 1062–7.
[4] Lillehei CW et al. (1986) Ann. Surg., **204,** 490–501.

Aortic Stenosis

Aortic stenosis may be valvular (83%), subvalvular (9%) or supravalvular.

Obstruction to the outflow tract causes left ventricular hypertrophy. In one series of 128 patients[1] 32% presented in the first year of life, 54% between the ages of 1 and 5, and 13% between 6 and 19 years. In infancy the common presentation is breathlessness or heart failure. Children presenting after infancy commonly present at routine medical examinations with a murmur, while those at older ages of presentation may have breathlessness, syncope or chest pain. Supravalvular aortic stenosis is frequently associated with postnatal feeding problems, slow weight gain in infancy, an elfin facies, mental retardation and hypercalcaemia.

PROGNOSIS

- The overall mortality is 0.03/1000 for males and 0.01/1000 for females.
- In one series treatment of severe aortic stenosis with modern technique carried a mortality of about 10%[2]. There were no deaths in the 2 years after surgery in that series. In another series concerned with those over 2 years requiring surgery, the survival was 93%[3].
- Many patients however remain well, with no symptoms or deterioration in left ventricular hypertrophy.
- Valve replacement may be necessary from 2 to 14 years after valvotomy.
- Sudden death occasionally occurs—1 patient out of 128 (in one series[1]).

TREATMENT

1. Medical management of heart failure.
2. Treatment of the valve lesion depends on the age of the patient and the site of the stenosis. Not all require surgery; in one series[3] surgery was necessary in 36% of cases.
   a. Subvalvular stenosis can be excised simply in some cases but in others the combination of fibrous and muscular tissue makes this impossible.
   b. Supravalvular stenosis usually requires a patch.
   c. In the younger patient valvular stenosis is treated by valvotomy. A second operation may be necessary in about one-third of patients. Primary valve replacement may be possible after the age of 12. Before this age the valve is too small to accommodate the prosthesis.
3. Antibiotic cover is necessary for dental treatment or oral/ear nose throat surgery.

FOLLOW-UP

Follow-up normally requires 6-monthly clinical examination plus two-dimensional echocardiography to assess left ventricular thickness, cavity size and ejection fraction. Increasing left ventricular hypertrophy and a gradient of over 50 mmHg across the valve are indications for operation.

[1] Read JM et al. (1982) *Thorax*, **37**, 902–5.
[2] Messina LM et al. (1984) *J. Thorac. Cardiovasc. Surg.*, **88**, 92–6.
[3] Aukeney JL et al. (1983) *J. Thorac. Cardiovasc. Surg.*, **85**, 41–8.

Pulmonary Stenosis

The age of presentation and severity of pulmonary stenosis depend on the degree of stenosis and the presence of other associated defects. In severe cases there is fusion of the valve cusps; in moderate cases the fusion is peripheral, leaving the central portion patent. Severe forms in infancy present with congestive cardiac failure.

Some 75% of those with severe stenosis will have symptoms; those with right-to-left shunts will have generalized cyanosis, of which the degree depends on the size of the shunt. The degree of shunting and cyanosis may progress as the child gets older. There are usually exercise limitations and exertional dyspnoea.

In milder cases there is lack of cyanosis, and few have exertional dyspnoea. The presentation in these patients is usually by the detection of a systolic murmur.

PROGNOSIS

- Without treatment all infants with severe pulmonary stenosis die within the first month. Balloon valvoplasty gives good immediate and medium-term relief. Long-term results are as yet unknown.
- Mild stenosis carries an excellent prognosis without treatment, with no deaths in one series[4].
- Those requiring surgery have about a 3% hospital mortality[4]. The greatest risk is to infants under 1 week with high right ventricular pressure, and cardiac enlargement. Late death is almost totally confined to infants under 2 whose admission status was deemed to be poor (7 out of 53 in one series[4]).
- Infants with severe pulmonary stenosis having a closed surgical valvotomy often require re-operation 2 years later for complications such as re-stenosis[2].

TREATMENT

1. Infants with severe pulmonary stenosis need treatment urgently. The majority will have right-to-left shunting and can be stabilized before surgery with prostaglandin E$_1$. This ensures pulmonary blood flow by maintaining a patent ductus arteriosus.
2. Surgical treatment involves balloon valvuloplasty or operative valvotomy.
   a. Balloon valvuloplasty via catheter is now being used in all degrees of pulmonary stenosis and in children ranging from infancy to 11 years or older[1], although not all infants are suitable for this procedure. Balloon valvoplasty can result in significant haemodynamic improvement. Repeat catheterization may be necessary in some, with further improvement. Those with least satisfactory initial results may still show continued improvement with time. The techniques may also be useful in those who have poor results after surgical valvotomy.
   b. Closed surgical valvotomy has a lower mortality than open procedures[2].
3. Asymptomatic or minimally symptomatic children[3] who have a right ventricular pressure equal to or greater than systemic pressure should have balloon valvoplasty or surgical valvotomy eventually.

FOLLOW-UP

After treatment regular annual check-ups with clinical assessment, ECG, chest X-ray and echocardiography will be necessary to assess the valve and right ventricle.

Those who have had balloon valvoplasty, surgery in infancy or in whom the degree of unoperated stenosis is thought to be significant should be followed up more regularly.

[1] Sullivan ID et al. (1985) Br. Heart J., 54, 435–41.
[2] Awariefe SO et al. (1983) J. Thorac. Cardiovasc. Surg., 85, 375–87.
[3] Graham TP (1984) Ped. Clin. North Am., 31:6, 1281.
[4] Nugent EW et al. (1977) Circulation, 56 (suppl 1), 1–38.

Transposition of the Great Arteries

In this condition the right ventricle gives rise to the aorta and the left ventricle the pulmonary artery. The condition is 'complete' when there are no connections between the right and left sides of the heart. However, varieties of transposition occur where ventricular septal defect with or without pulmonary stenosis or atrial septal defect can occur.

After birth the ductus arteriosus remains open for a variable period of time. If the septa are complete then closure of the ductus is associated with hypoxia and acidosis. Such babies become cyanosed and distressed shortly after birth.

Those who have transposition with ventricular septal defect and no pulmonary stenosis present a little later, with dyspnoea, heart failure and cyanosis, the latter being variable.

In those who have transposition plus ventricular septal defect and pulmonary stenosis, the obstruction helps to aid mixing of the pulmonary and systemic circulation by encouraging right-to-left flow of blood. These children present later with milder cyanosis; heart failure is rare.

PROGNOSIS

- Without treatment mortality in the first 2 years was 95%[1].
- After balloon atrial septostomy, 82% in one series survived to undergo repair or switch procedure[1]. All deaths occurred within 6 weeks of septostomy. Low birth weight, persistent ductus arteriosus and coarctation were significant risk factors.
- The operative mortality for the Mustard operation in one series[2] was 0.9% with a 10-year survival rate of 93.7%. Causes of late death are dysrhythmias, sudden death, pulmonary venous obstruction and cardiac failure. Some 21% needed to be on treatment for dysrhythmias.
- Treatment of both transposition and ventricular septal defect in one series[3] had a mortality rate at 1 year of 71%.
- Surgery for transposition, ventricular septal defect and pulmonary stenosis has a mortality of 20%. Patients may require medical treatment for dysrhythmias, chest pain or heart failure.

TREATMENT

1. Those with intact atrial and ventricular septa will require balloon atrial septostomy.
2. In those who have had atrial septostomy corrective surgery will be necessary between 3 months and 1 year because of increasing cyanosis.

3. Corrective surgery involves either:
   a. the Mustard operation where a pericardial baffle channels caval blood to the mitral valve and pulmonary venous blood is channelled to the tricuspid valve or
   b. Arterial switch operation creating anatomical correction.
4. Those who have an associated ventricular septal defect are more difficult to treat because to combine the Mustard operation and ventricular septal defect closure is a long procedure. Some surgeons therefore may attempt pulmonary artery banding at the same time as the Mustard operation to avoid ventricular septal defect closure. Arterial switch operation for this group is becoming more popular.
5. Those with transposition, ventricular septal defect and pulmonary stenosis will usually require palliative surgery with a systemic–pulmonary shunt from 6 to 24 months. Repair by the Rastelli procedure will follow at 4–6 years.

FOLLOW-UP

This involves annual clinical assessment, ECG, chest X-ray and echocardiography. Problems to be sought are dysrhythmias, heart failure, baffle leak, caval stenosis, narrowing of the pulmonary venous channel, left ventricular insufficiency and tricuspid incompetence[2].

---

[1] Mok Q et al. (1987) Arch. Dis. Child., 62, 549–53.

[2] Tunster GA *et al.* (1987) *Ann. Surg.*, **206**, 251–9.
[3] Tunster GA *et al.* (1987) *J. Am. Coll. Cardiol.*, **10**, 1061–71.

Coarctation of the Aorta

Coarctation of the aorta accounts for 5–7.5% of cases of congenital heart disease. The lesions are commonly postductal, but may be juxtaductal, preductal or, rarely, at other sites along the aorta.

Other congenital heart defects are found in association with coarctation: patent ductus arteriosus (64% of those presenting in the first year of life), ventricular septal defect (32%), transposition of the great arteries (10%) and atrial septal defect (6.5%). Coarctation of the aorta is twice as common in males as females.

Over 50% of cases present in the first year of life; 8% present suddenly between 10 days and 2 weeks with congenitive cardiac failure associated with closure of the ductus. Others are discovered through the presence of a murmur.

Those who present over 1 year old usually have no symptoms and are discovered at routine examination with the presence of a murmur, hypertension or absent femoral pulses.

PROGNOSIS

- Without any treatment, 60–90% of those children with signs or symptoms died in the first year of life[1].
- The overall mortality in children under 1 year is 0.04 per 1000 livebirths per year.
- In those treated under the age of 2 early mortality is about 12%, while in those over 2 mortality is 1%. Late mortality is <1% per patient year. Morbidity and mortality are determined by associated cardiac malformations and postoperative hypertension. Those with an isolated coarctation who are normotensive postoperatively have an excellent prognosis[2].

TREATMENT

1. *Children under 1 year with congestive cardiac failure*
   a. Correction of cardiac failure.
      i. intravenous frusemide.
      ii. correction of acid–base and electrolyte balance.
      iii. ventilation if required.
   b. Dilatation of ductus arteriosus.
      i. prostaglandin infusion.
   c. Surgical treatment of coarctation.
   d. Repair of associated ventricular septal defect may be performed days or weeks after coarctation repair if congestive failure continues. Some centres perform pulmonary artery banding at the time of coarctation repair, and repair the ventricular septal defect electively later.

2. *Children over 1 year*
   a. Older children should be operated on as soon as diagnosis is confirmed.

3. Children who have minimal symptoms should have treatment delayed until 4–5 years, unless upper extremity hypertension occurs. In these cases repair is carried out earlier.

FOLLOW-UP

Regular cardiological assessment is necessary, with checks on blood pressure, ECG and echocardiography to detect re-coarctation.

[1] Keith JD (1978) *Heart Disease in Infancy and Childhood* (Keith JD *et al.* eds) New York: MacMillan, p. 753.
[2] Koller M *et al.* (1987) *Eur. Heart J.*, **8**, 670–9.

Bronchiolitis

Bronchiolitis is a common lower respiratory tract infection of infancy. It is characteristically an infection of the winter months and mostly affects infants under the age of 1 year. It begins as a coryzal infection which proceeds to cause cough, tachypnoea and expiratory wheeze. There may be intercostal indrawing and subcostal recession with overexpansion of the chest, localized or widespread fine crepitations and localized or widespread expiratory rhonchi. Initial assessment involves the state of hydration, the clinical severity and whether hospital admission is required. The pathogen is usually the respiratory syncytial virus but it may also be caused by parainfluenza virus, adenovirus or *Mycoplasma pneumoniae*.

PROGNOSIS

- The mortality from bronchiolitis is approximately 1%[1].
- Infants under 2 months of age may experience respiratory collapse.
- The illness generally lasts for 7–10 days.
- Complications include secondary bacterial infection demonstrated by a worsening of the respiratory signs, increased fever and increased cough. Otitis media may occur.
- A proportion of children may experience recurrent wheezing after an episode of bronchiolitis. In one series[2] 18 out of 35 children who had had bronchiolitis had experienced subsequent episodes of wheezing compared with a control group. However, the episodes were neither severe nor frequent.
- Parental smoking in the child's first year of life may be associated with increased risk of respiratory syncytial virus bronchiolitis.
- In the above series[2] atopy did not seem to be related to either bronchiolitis or wheezing episodes after bronchiolitis. However, in another study[3] children with acute bronchiolitis had a significantly higher atopic predisposition than controls.

TREATMENT

1. If it is felt the child could be managed at home, regular assessments should be made. Such an assessment involves the ability of the parents to cope and the suitability of the home circumstances. A close watch on the respiratory state is necessary. Worsening of tachypnoea, subcostal recession or indrawing may indicate impending respiratory failure or infection. A temperature of over 38°C will usually indicate secondary infection.
2. Regular small volumes of fluids should be given. A suspicion of early respiratory failure, exhaustion or dehydration makes hospital admission mandatory; respiratory support, fluid therapy, antibiotic treatment and parenteral or tube-feeding may be required.

FOLLOW-UP

Regular follow-up should be made until the child is well. Assessment thereafter is not necessary unless recurrent wheezing occurs. Wheezing may need treatment with bronchodilators.

[1] Forfar JO, Arneil GC (1984) *Textbook of Paediatrics*. 3rd edn. Edinburgh: Churchill Livingstone.
[2] Sims DG *et al.* (1978) *Br. Med. J.*, **1**, 11–14.
[3] Laing I *et al.* (1982) *Br. Med. J.*, **1**, 1070–2.

Gastrointestinal Problems

Coeliac Disease

Coeliac disease is characterized by four features[1]—intestinal malabsorption, histological abnormalities of the duodenal and jejunal mucosa, improvement when the diet is free of gluten and relapse when gluten is reintroduced. Histologically there is loss of the normal villous pattern and lengthening of the crypts in the small bowel; the abnormalities are most obvious proximally. As a result of the loss of villi there is less absorptive surface area and a reduced amount of digestive enzymes, leading to failure to thrive and nutritional deficiencies.

The prevalence of the disease varies—in a study from Edinburgh[2] for boys and girls under the age of 2 at diagnosis the prevalence was 44 and 55/100 000 respectively. The incidence is now reported to be falling[2,3] and this may be due to increased breastfeeding, later introduction of mixed feeds and the increasing trend of processed infant foods to be gluten-free. There is an increased family incidence, and an association with certain histocompatibility antigens. The relationship with dietary gluten and causation of the clinical and intestinal findings is well known, but the exact pathogenesis is yet to be established.

The presentation of the disease is usually between 8 and 9 months with abdominal distension, muscle-wasting (particularly of the gluteal and shoulder areas), hypotonia, malabsorptive-type stools and failure to thrive. Growth which initially was normal starts to decline as soon as mixed feeds are introduced, with the child being miserable and perhaps reluctant to walk. Other children may present later, particularly when the gastrointestinal and growth aspects are less severe. An underlying iron or folic acid anaemia may occur as well as hypoalbuminaemia or hypocalcaemia. The diagnosis is based on clinical grounds, the findings of intestinal biopsy, and response to withdrawal of gluten. Many authorities challenge the need for a diagnostic reintroduction of gluten in straightforward cases.

PROGNOSIS

- The absence of gluten in the diet plus the administration of sufficient calories and supplements where appropriate will improve the clinical picture quickly.
- Mood, mobility and the stools are the first to improve, followed by weight, which may take between 6 and 12 months to reach normal.
- Height and bone age may take up to 2 years to catch up[4].
- The teenage period is a time of danger of dietary relapse. In one study[5] of 102 teenagers, 57 said they were on a strict gluten-free diet, 36 a semi-strict diet and 9 a normal diet. Jejunal biopsy suggested that those who said they were on a gluten-free diet were in fact consuming gluten.
- Lymphoma[6] is a recognized complication of coeliac disease in adulthood, but the number of cases in childhood is very small. Whether strict compliance to a gluten-free diet reduces the risk of lymphoma is not yet known.

TREATMENT

1. Treatment is by gluten-free diet. Patients should be advised by a dietician which foods contain or do not contain gluten. This process has been assisted by the recent introduction of a gluten-free food labelling symbol.
2. Certain gluten-free foods are available on prescription, from a list agreed by the Advisory Committee on Borderline Substances. Most authorities agree that a gluten-free diet should be lifelong and that optimum child growth and health can only be achieved in this way; the mucosa will always relapse if rechallenged with gluten, although deterioration may be slow.
3. Dietary supplements with folic acid and vitamin D may be necessary in the initial period of treatment. Similarly, an adequate calorie intake is essential, particularly for those children who are severely malnourished.

Follow-up of patients should be undertaken by a paediatrician with emphasis on monitoring growth and weight and adherence to a gluten-free diet.

[1] Anderson M (1987) Coeliac disease. In *Paediatric gastroenterology*, 2nd edn (Anderson M *et al.* eds), pp. 375–400. Melbourne: Blackwell.
[2] Logan RFA *et al.* (1986) Prevalence and 'incidence' of coeliac disease in Edinburgh and the Lothian region of Scotland. *Gastroenterology*, **90**, 334–42.
[3] Littlewood JM *et al.* (1980) Childhood coeliac disease is disappearing. *Lancet*, **ii**, 1359.
[4] Barr DGD *et al.* (1971) Pediatr. Res., **6**, 521–7. Catch-up growth in malnutrition studied in coeliac disease after institution of gluten-free diet.
[5] Kumar PJ *et al.* (1988) The teenage coeliac: follow up study of 102 patients. *Arch. Dis. Child.*, **63**, 916–20.
[6] Cooper BT, Read AE (1987) Coeliac disease and lymphoma. *Q. J. Med.*, **63**, 269–74.

Congenital Pyloric Stenosis

This condition presents as non-bilious vomiting usually from the age of 3–4 weeks, but may begin at birth or up to the age of 3 months. It tends to present later in breastfed babies and is due to hypertrophy of the circular smooth muscle of the pylorus. Incidence is about 2.5 per 1000 livebirths and is rising[1]. In Central Scotland the figure is as high as 8.8 per 1000 livebirths[2]. The sex distribution is 4 males:1 female. In about a quarter of cases there may be a positive family history. Vomiting may start gradually and then develop into the classical projectile vomit. The child is hungry and will willingly take another feed after a vomit. Vomiting does not occur after each feed but may be 'saved' for the next feed. Constipation is usual.

Diagnosis is made by a test feed. During a milk feed the child is examined by gently palpating the right hypochondrium. The presence of a small palpable tumour or visible peristalsis points to the diagnosis. The diagnosis however may be difficult to make and may require barium meal or ultrasound examination for confirmation.

Prolonged vomiting may lead to dehydration, hypochloraemia and metabolic alkalosis.

PROGNOSIS

- The operation can carry a significant mortality, varying from 0 to 2.9%. Postoperative vomiting is extremely common and occurs in 46–90% of cases. In one series[3] 15% continued to vomit for more than 3 days. Wound infection may occur in 0.7–11% of cases and reoperation may be necessary in up to 2.1% of cases.

- Duodenal perforation may occur in up to 11.5% of cases, but in most series the figures are much lower.

- In a follow-up study[4] of adults who had had Ramstedt's operation 58% had minor gastrointestinal complaints. Of 34 patients who had a barium meal only 3 had abnormalities, of which 2 were minor. There was no correlation between the severity of the congenital hypertrophic stenosis and later gastrointestinal symptoms.

- Ultrasound examination in infants with hypertrophic pyloric stenosis who had had Ramstedt's operation showed the pylorus returned to normal size 6 months after the operation[5].

TREATMENT

1. Initial hospital assessment involves checking of blood pH, electrolytes, glucose and correction by appropriate i.v. fluids.

2. Vomiting should be controlled by nasogastric tube.

3. Treatment is by the classic Ramstedt operation of pyloromyotomy.

Follow-up should be performed to assess the wound. Assessment of weight gain and feeding should be undertaken until the expected place on the centile chart is reached.

[1] Spicer RD (1982) *Br. J. Surg.*, **69**, 128–35.
[2] Kerr AM (1980) *Br. Med. J.*, **281**, 714–15.
[3] Gray DW *et al.* (1984) *Ann. R. Coll. Surg.*, **66**, 280–2.
[4] Vilmann P *et al.* (1986) *Acta Paediatr. Scand.*, **75**, 156–8.
[5] Bourchier D (1985) *Austr. Paediatr. J.*, **21**, 189–90.

Hirschsprung's Disease

Hirschsprung's disease is a congenital abnormality of the colon in which there is obstruction of the rectum or rectosigmoid and pre-obstruction dilation of the bowel. It is caused by absence of parasympathetic ganglion cells in the affected portion of bowel. The lesions may be confined to the sphincter (14%), extend from sphincter to lower sigmoid (56%), or involve the whole sigmoid (19%). Other types are rare.

Hirschsprung's disease occurs in about one in 5000–8000 livebirths. Eighty per cent of patients are male[1]. There are strong associations with other congenital abnormalities such as Down's syndrome, Waardenberg syndrome, and other neurological abnormalities such as cerebral palsy, mental retardation and developmental delay[2].

The first sign may be the failure to pass meconium within the first 24 hours. If this is missed, the presentation may be that of intestinal obstruction with abdominal distension and bile-stained vomiting. Colonic perforation may also occur. Enterocolitis may occur and present as diarrhoea, dehydration and toxicity.

Later presentations may be mild, and occurring in infancy or even extending to adult life, but with increasing rarity. In infancy there is gradually increasing constipation, abdominal distension, with faecal masses palpable and, unless the abnormality is confined to the sphincter only, an empty rectum. Weaning may exacerbate the presentation[3].

Diagnosis is made by barium enema. This will show the affected portion of colon as normal-calibre bowel, extending on to an area of dilated obstructed colon. The diagnosis should be confirmed by biopsy of the affected segment which will reveal the absence of parasympathetic ganglion cells. Diagnosis has been made easier by histochemical analysis. This will show the presence of acetylcholinesterase which is absent in normal bowel tissue.

PROGNOSIS

- The overall mortality for Hirschsprung's is between 4 and 7%[4,5].
- The highest mortality occurs before definitive surgery, causes of death are enterocolitis, septicaemia or pneumonia. The operative mortality is between 0.5 and 1.5%.
- In one series[5] 55% had minor or major complications after definitive surgery. The commonest were abscess, frequency of stool, stricture, intestinal obstruction, mild faecal soiling or constipation.

TREATMENT

1. An occasional patient can be managed by enema and conservative means to ensure emptying of the bowel. However, he or she is still at risk of developing enterocolitis[2].

2. Initial management is by enterostomy, usually a colostomy.

3. Later, definitive surgery is carried out—excision of the affected portion with end-to-end anastomosis of the proximal colon to the anorectal canal, anastomosis of normal colon side-to-side with the rectum, or a pull-through operation.

Patients should be observed for possible complications: anastomotic strictre, sphincter spasm, rectal sinus, soiling, constipation/diarrhoea. Most important is follow-up assessment of growth as patients very frequently have growth retardation in the neonatal period[6,7]

[1] Blisard KS, Kleinman R (1986) Hirschsprung's disease: a clinical and pathological overview. *Hum. Pathol.*, **17**, 1189–91.

[2] Martin LW, Torres AM (1985) Hirschsprung's disease. *Surg. Clin. North Am.*, **65**, 1171–9.

[3] Burke V, Anderson CM (1975) Hirschsprung's disease. In *Paediatric Gastroenterology*, 1st edn (Anderson C, Burke V eds), pp. 475–80. Oxford: Blackwell.

[4] Harrison MW *et al.* (1986) Diagnosis and management of Hirschsprung's disease. A 25 year perspective. *Am. J. Surg.*, **152**, 49–56.

[5] Joseph VT, Sim CK (1988) Problems and pitfalls in the management of Hirschsprung's disease. *J. Ped. Surg.*, **23**, 398–402.

[6] Sherman JO *et al.* (1989) *J. Pediatr. Surg.* **24**, 833–8.

[7] Bergmeijer JH *et al.* (1989) *J. Pediatr. Surg.* **24**, 282–5.

Intussusception in Childhood

Intussusception is the invagination of one piece of bowel into the lumen of an adjoining piece. The sites may be ileocaecal, ileocolic, or ileoileal. Intussusception occurs most commonly between the ages of 3 months and 2 years, with peak incidence at 6 months, and is commoner in boys. It is generally accepted that a localized patch of lymphoid hyperplasia usually acts as the focus for the intussusception, and half the children may have a history of infection or evidence of adenovirus or rotavirus[1]. There is an association with Henoch–Schönlein purpura and also cystic fibrosis.

Under the age of 4 months there may be no history of pain but rectal bleeding and vomiting are usual[2]. There may be paroxysms of irritability associated with a ghostly pallor.

Above the age of 4 months pain is the commonest symptom. In one series[3] pain was the presenting symptom in 81%, vomiting in 74%, blood was detectable in stool or rectally in 56% and there was an abdominal mass in 56%. Other features were fever, dehydration, diarrhoea or intestinal obstruction. The classic triad was present in only 17%.

On examination a sausage-shaped mass may be felt in the right hypochondrium or epigastrium. If symptoms have been present for over 48 hours the child may be gravely ill with fever and dehydration—the clinical picture resembles meningitis.

PROGNOSIS

- The major complication of barium reduction is perforation, but this is rare.
- Hospital mortality is extremely low. In the above series[5] there was a 10% recurrence rate after barium reduction (at an average of 3 months later, but there was less postprocedure morbidity than in surgically treated patients).
- Hospitalization is shortest for barium enema reduction (1.46 days), longer for intraoperative reduction (9.57 days) and longest where bowel resection was necessary (13.82 days)[4].

TREATMENT

1. *Barium enema*
   a. Treatment is possible in the majority of cases using hydrostatic barium enema. Absolute contraindications are peritonitis and pneumatosis intestinalis, but the method requires an experienced radiologist with modern equipment, a patient who has been adequately resuscitated and the facilities for operation if the reduction fails or if there is a recurrence.
   b. Success varies between centres from 18 to

85%, and is dependent on the time taken to make the diagnosis and refer. In the 55% of failures of this technique in one series[4] symptoms had been present for over 48 hours. In a series of 65 cases, 79% were successfully reduced[5]. The likelihood of success of barium enema reduction was also less if there was shock or rectal bleeding on presentation, or a pronounced degree of intestinal obstruction.

2. *Surgery*

Surgical treatment was necessary after failed or presumed failed hydrostatic reduction; where a Peyer's patch was not thought to be the focus of the intussusception; where there was a previous intussusception, or in the presence of gross bowel obstruction.

FOLLOW-UP

Initial follow-up is necessary to ensure wound healing and a return to a normal feeding pattern.

Although most postoperative recurrences occur while the child is still in hospital, recurrence of symptoms should raise the possibility of further intussusception. Parents should be advised to inform the doctor if symptoms recur.

[1] *Lancet* (1985) II *Editorial* 250–1.
[2] Newman J et al. (1987) *Can. Med. Assoc. J.*, **136**, 266–9.
[3] Sparnon AL et al. (1984) *Aust. N.Z. J. Surg.*, **54**, 353–6.
[4] West KW et al. (1987) *Surgery*, **102**, 704–10.
[5] Liu KW et al. (1986) *Arch. Dis. Child.*, **61**, 75–7.

Infantile Diarrhoea

The most common cause of infantile diarrhoea is the rotavirus[1]. Enteropathic *Escherichia coli*, *Salmonella* and *Shigella* are less common; however, *Campylobacter enteritis* is becoming increasingly recognized as a cause. Rotavirus diarrhoea can be more severe than other forms due to loss of absorptive powers of the small intestine.

Fever and vomiting lasting 1–3 days plus symptoms of upper respiratory tract infection may precede the diarrhoea; stools are watery and of large volume. The faeces rarely contain blood or mucus and the volume loss may lead to dehydration. The illness can last 4–7 days but the stool may not return to normal for several weeks. Virus is shed from the third to the eighth day, but can survive for weeks on environmental surfaces[2]. Secondary lactose intolerance may prolong the diarrhoea.

PROGNOSIS

- Intestinal infectious disease still has a significant mortality, but it is falling. In 1985 24 infants and 4 1–4 year-olds died in England and Wales[3].
- Most children recover quickly from gastroenteritis; a common example is rotavirus infections which may last up to 7 days.
- Lactose intolerance may occur in up to 18.5% of cases[4]. In one study 53% became lactose-tolerant after 2 weeks, and 81% were lactose-tolerant by 4 weeks after taking a lactose-free diet. However, 6% were still lactose-intolerant when rechallenged at 20 weeks[4].

TREATMENT

1. The mainstay of treatment is oral rehydration therapy (ORT). Recent guidelines have been published[5]. ORT should be given for the first 24 hours. If the child is vomiting, ORT should be given as frequent small volumes: 200 ml/kg (more if the child is thirsty) should be offered in the first 24 hours. The World Health Organization recommendation for ORT includes 90 mmol/l sodium ions, but many authorities favour a lower sodium content of 35–50 mmol/l.

2. Persistent vomiting, abdominal distension, hypothermia, altered conscious levels and oliguria are indications for hospital admission.

3. If the child is being breastfed then this should continue. If the child is bottlefed, milk should be withheld for 24 hours, and replaced with ORT as above.
4. The majority of children will have recovered sufficiently in 24 hours for normal feeds to be reintroduced. Children over 6 months who have mild diarrhoea after ORT may return immediately to their normal feeds. Children under 6 months should progress to regrading after 24 hours' ORT. The child's infant formula is diluted with ORT solution, firstly as one-quarter, 3 parts ORT to 1 part made-up formula, then half strength, then three-quarter strength and finally full strength. The intervals between changes may be 12 to 24 hours depending on the clinical condition.
5. If important symptoms return then the child should be managed with regrading (see above).
6. A return of vomiting or diarrhoea may be caused by lactose intolerance. This is usually brief and may be managed by a return to regrading.
7. A return of diarrhoea may also indicate a new pathogen or other gastrointestinal cause. If these are excluded then a nutritionally complete formula based on oligopeptides or amino acids should be used. If this fails further investigation is necessary. Once an infant has been placed on a special feed it should be continued until the expected weight is achieved. A challenge with regular formula may then be attempted and if successful, gradual reintroduction may be instituted.

FOLLOW-UP

Once the child has recovered no follow-up is necessary. If lactose intolerance occurs then the child should be monitored until cow's milk has been completely reintroduced. Failure to respond to regrading or recurrence of diarrhoea should be investigated by a paediatrician.

[1] Davidson GP (1986) *Clin. Gastroenterol.*, **15**, 39–53.
[2] Senturia YD (1986) *J. Epidemiol. Commun. Health*, **40**, 236–9.
[3] Mortality Statistics—Childhood. Office of Public Consuses and Surveys, 1985.
[4] Davidson GP *et al.* (1984) *J. Paed.*, **105**, 587–90.
[5] Wharton BA *et al.* (1988) *Br. Med. J.*, **296**, 450–2.

Neonatal Jaundice

Clinical jaundice is visible when the serum bilirubin is greater than 85 mmol/l. It is detectable in about 50% of all infants. In the vast majority, it is considered physiological, reflecting the slower metabolism and excretion of bilirubin in the neonate. Physiological jaundice appears after 24 hours of age in a well infant. It is not severe (maximum serum bilirubin is 200 mmol/l, with less than 15% of the bilirubin being direct, i.e. conjugated). It is gone by 10 days of age in the mature infant and by 20 days in the preterm infant.

Jaundice not fulfilling these criteria should have its cause elucidated. Early unconjugated hyperbilirubinaemia may be due to haemolytic disorders—blood group incompatibility, such as Rhesus or ABO G6PD deficiency; red cell membrane or enzyme disorder; polycythaemia; birth trauma with excessive bruising; dehydration; infection, or high intestinal obstruction, classically pyloric stenosis. Some metabolic disorders are associated with increasing jaundice in addition to other clinical features in the first or second week of life, such as galactosaemia or fructosaemia. Protracted jaundice is most commonly associated with breastfeeding (it occurs in 2% of breastfed infants) and in this situation the infant will be well and thriving with no abnormal physical signs, the bilirubin will be >85% unconjugated, liver function tests will be normal, and the urine will not contain bilirubin. Other causes of protracted jaundice include Down's syndrome, congenital hypothyroidism, infection, cystic fibrosis, the various forms of neonatal hepatitis, and biliary tract anomalies causing obstruction to the excretion of bile.

PROGNOSIS

- Kernicterus is now extremely rare. Classically in the acute stage the infant becomes lethargic and irritable, progressing to opisthotonos, hypertonia, a high pitched cry and seizures. These symptoms resolve as the bilirubin level falls, leading to a period of apparent normality. Development then becomes abnormal in infancy with choreoathetotic cerebral palsy, high-frequency nerve deafness, paralysis of upward gaze, mental retardation, and staining of the teeth.

- The prognosis of bile duct obstruction depends on the age at diagnosis and the presence of a surgically correctable lesion. Biliary atresia is thought to be a progressive obliterative disorder. The longer it has been present, the likelier it is that intrahepatic ducts will be obliterated and portoenterostomy will be unsuccessful. The critical age for surgery is thought to be 8 weeks, before which up to 90% of patients may have good bile drainage established. The 5-year survival of this group is currently 36%, but paediatric liver transplantation is now a viable treatment option.

- Breast milk jaundice has no long-term sequelae but may occur in 25% of siblings. The jaundice peaks in the second or third week then slowly declines to normal by 4–6 weeks of age.

TREATMENT

Early jaundice

1. Physiological jaundice requires no treatment.
2. Pathological jaundice first requires a diagnosis to be made. If serum bilirubin is > 300 mmol/l on day 3–4, investigations should include: total and direct bilirubin; haemoglobin and haematocrit determination with blood film and reticulocyte count; direct Coombs' test on the infant's red blood cells; blood grouping of mother and child; assessment of maternal antibodies, together with urine microscopy and culture.
3. Phototherapy in hospital is required if the unconjugated bilirubin is greater than 280 mmol/l in a full-term infant, or less in a preterm infant. If there is haemolysis, it will be required at an earlier stage. Phototherapy is continued until the bilirubin level is stable or starts to fall, and is primarily used to prevent the serum bilirubin reaching values at which exchange transfusion is mandatory.

4. Fluid balance and fluid intake should be monitored. Weight loss of $>8\%$ of birth weight may indicate dehydration and fluid supplements (5% dextrose or water) should be given. In all jaundiced infants, adequate fluid intake is important, although the value of routinely supplementing feeds with water is dubious.

5. Exchange transfusion is indicated if the serum unconjugated bilirubin is likely to reach a level at which neurological damage (kernicterus deafness) might occur. This would usually be performed at about 400 µmol/l in a well full-term infant without haemolytic disease, but at 340 µmol/l in the presence of haemolysis and at much lower levels in an ill or preterm infant.

6. In haemolytic jaundice the haemoglobin level must be monitored. Late anaemia is uncommon in ABO incompatibility but common in Rhesus disease, especially if exchange transfusion has been avoided. Haemoglobin should be checked at least fortnightly for the first 6 weeks.

7. Exchange transfusion is sometimes performed on the first day of life in the baby with severe blood group incompatibility as a primary treatment for anaemia and to promote removal of maternal antibodies.

Prolonged jaundice

1. Any full-term baby with jaundice after 2 weeks or a premature infant with jaundice after 3 weeks needs investigation.

2. If screening has not already been performed then hypothyroidism, galactosaemia and fructosaemia must be excluded by blood and urine testing.

3. Liver function testing, total and direct bilirubin, and urinalysis for bilirubin should be performed. If liver function tests are abnormal or there is bilirubinuria or pale stools, urgent referral is required for exclusion of the neonatal hepatitis syndrome. This is also true if the infant is ill, or there are skin lesions, cataracts, congenital abnormalities, hepatomegaly, or palpable abdominal masses.

4. Treatment will be that of the underlying condition.

5. Prolonged unconjugated hyperbilirubinaemia may be due to Crigler–Najjar syndrome. This is the only condition in which long-term phototherapy is indicated.

FOLLOW-UP

No follow-up is required after physiological or breast milk jaundice. Other causes will need specialist paediatric review.

Enuresis

Enuresis is the involuntary discharge of urine at least once a week at an age when voluntary control of the bladder is to be expected. Wetting at night (nocturnal enuresis) is more common in boys, while diurnal enuresis is more common in girls and may be associated with infection. The incidence of wetting at least once a month is 10–15% at 5 years and 7% at 10 years[1]. Enuresis is greater in lower social classes, firstborns and when either or both parents or a sibling were enuretic. Enuresis may be primary where control was never achieved, or secondary where a relapse occurs after being dry for at least a year. Primary enuresis is thought to be due to a delay in maturation of the central nervous system. It may also be due to a structural abnormality such as spina bifida.

Secondary enuresis can be caused by emotional stress—moving house, starting a new school, death of a parent, parental divorce or physical abuse. Urinary tract infection and diabetes may also cause enuresis. Constipation may be a predisposing factor[2], as well as any condition causing perineal irritation.

PROGNOSIS

- Untreated enuresis improves, with 10–20% remitting per annum.
- Only 1% of adults continue to have enuresis.
- Some 50% of enuretic children become dry without specific therapy[1].
- Treatment with imipramine produces an effect in approximately 50% of children, often in the first week of treatment; the cure rate is between 30 and 60%[1].
- Children with problems in the family, or who have personality problems themselves or in the family members, do less well with treatment[3].

TREATMENT

1. Treatment revolves around sympathetic handling. Stress should be placed on the good prognosis and careful explanation of the causes. Chastisement and anxiety within the family only serve to slow natural recovery.
2. A full history and examination and urinalysis should be carried out to exclude any of the organic causes.
3. Investigation of the renal tract is probably only appropriate in those with a history of urinary tract infection, and a positive mid-stream specimen of urine at the time of examination or symptoms of bladder outlet obstruction.
4. Treatments such as restricting fluids prior to going to bed, lifting the child and taking him or her to the toilet at parental bedtime may help.

5. The use of a star chart may help some children. A dry night merits a silver star and four dry nights in a row a gold star. A gold star means a reward.
6. The anticholinergic effects of the tricyclic antidepressant imipramine may be of help. This drug is often used along with a star chart.
   a. For children aged 6–7 years (20–25 kg) the dose is 25 mg at night just before bedtime.
   b. For children 8–11 years (25–35 kg) the dose is 25–50 mg at night just before bedtime.
   c. For children over 11 years (35–54 kg) the dose is 50–75 mg at night just before bedtime.

   The maximum period of treatment should not exceed 3 months, and withdrawal should be gradual.
7. Electric buzzer alarms designed to wake the child as soon as the contact pad is soaked with urine can be helpful. Two-thirds of children in one study became dry, but 23% had relapsed after 2 years[4].

FOLLOW-UP

Regular follow-up is necessary to support both the child and parents until cure is achieved; the frequency of follow-up depends on the severity of the problem and its effect on the family.

If after imipramine therapy a relapse occurs, a further course of treatment should not be started until a full physical examination has been made.

[1] Novello AC, Novello JR (1987) *Ped. Clin. North Am.,* **34,** 719–33.
[2] O'Regan S *et al.* (1986) *Am. J. Dis. Child.,* **140,** 260–1.
[3] Polak H (1987) *Public Health,* **101,** 185–90.
[4] Halliday S *et al.* (1987) *Arch. Dis. Child.,* **62,** 132–7.

Urinary Tract Infection in Children

Bacteriuria is more common in males than in females in the neonatal period but thereafter females have a greater incidence by a ratio of 50:1 at 5 years. Diagnosis is based on the culture of significant numbers of pathogenic bacteria. This can be difficult because of the problems of contamination and the problems in general practice of obtaining a sample and getting it to the laboratory in time.

Many doctors allow girls to have one urinary infection before the renal tract is investigated but renal scarring may occur with the first infection. Clinical suspicion of urinary tract infection as a cause of symptoms is paramount and a high index of suspicion must be present when dealing with the unwell infant, particularly in those under 5 who are vulnerable to further renal damage. It is important to consider that vulvitis and constipation may mimic the symptoms of urinary tract infection.

PROGNOSIS

- Those with a normal urinary tract are not at risk of renal damage.
- Those with vesicoureteric reflux and no scarring who reach adulthood do not appear to be at greater risk of renal damage than those without reflux.
- Renal scarring seems to occur before the age of 5; very few scars develop after the age of 7.
- Patients with unilateral reflux and scarring may have compensatory hypertrophy of the opposite kidney and no overall loss of glomerular filtration rate.
- Those with reflux and scarring who have severe bilateral reflux or proteinuria are at greatest risk of developing chronic renal impairment.

TREATMENT

1. Prior to starting treatment samples must be taken to confirm the diagnosis. Treatment involves the use of an appropriate antibiotic and liberal fluids.
2. All those with a significant culture should be referred for assessment, looking for obstruction, calculi, renal screening and vesicoureteric reflux.
3. One author[1] performs intravenous urography in children under 3 years old. In older children or those under 3 where the diagnosis of urinary tract infection is in doubt ultrasonography is performed. If abnormalities are found on ultrasound then the next investigation is intravenous urography. Following this, in children under 5, micturating cystourethrography is carried out.
4. Low-dose chemoprophylaxis is used in those with renal tract obstruction awaiting surgery; in those with significant reflux, and in the group of girls who are prone to recurrent urinary tract infections but have a normal renal tract.
5. Where vecisoureteric reflux occurs the debate is whether to treat with low-dose prophylaxis or surgical correction.

   A study over 5 years comparing operative with non-operative treatment of severe reflux showed no significant difference in renal function, breakthrough urinary infection, renal growth, the development of new scars or progression of new scars between the two groups[2]. However, the non-operated group had the advantage of not having surgery.

FOLLOW-UP

Those with urinary tract infection who have normal renal tracts can be managed by the general practitioner. Those with reflux and no scarring should be followed up by a paediatric nephrologist until adulthood.

Those with reflux and scarring should also be monitored by a paediatric nephrologist until renal and body growth has ceased and a final assessment of severity is made. Thereafter a periodic check on blood pressure and urine should be performed. The former is designed to discover hypertension which will impair renal function, the latter proteinuria which may indicate glomerulosclerosis. Those with proteinuria, extensive reflux and scarring or signs of impaired renal function should be monitored by an adult renal physician.

[1] White RHR (1987) *Arch. Dis. Child.*, **62**, 421–7.
[2] Birmingham Reflux Study Group (1987) *Br. Med. J.*, **295**, 237–41.

Prematurity

About 7% of infants in the UK weigh less than 2.5 kg at birth (they are considered of low birthweight); most of these babies are premature, i.e. born before 37 weeks' gestation. Low-birthweight infants have a mortality about 30 times higher than infants weighing more than 2.5 kg. Perinatal mortality in this group has fallen rapidly and steadily over the past 50 years, due to improved social conditions, improved neonatal care and the development of neonatal intensive care. Also important have been changes in obstetric practice to encourage intervention for the sake of the fetus at an earlier stage, together with steady improvement in the ability to monitor fetal wellbeing.

The extremely premature infant (less than 30 weeks' gestation) is likely to require intensive care. In the UK regionalization of facilities has allowed development of expertise in the care of this group, and in particular of infants from 24 weeks' gestation onwards. If a high-risk delivery can be predicted, the mother should be transferred antenatally to such a specialized regional or subregional centre in anticipation of care for her infant, which may include ventilation, parenteral nutrition and surgery. The infant will be transferred back to the district hospital when intensive care is no longer required. Postnatal transfer of such infants is also common, when delivery or need for intensive care has not been anticipated.

Neonatal mortality in most centres is currently about 70% at 25 weeks and less (not all such infants will be offered intensive care). With more mature infants, mortality rates improve to 50% at 26–27 weeks, 20% at 28–30 weeks, and 10% above this.

Many deaths result from prenatal or perinatal complications, particularly those resulting in cerebral haemorrhage or infarction. The fatal complications of postnatal origin are predominantly the respiratory complications of surfactant deficiency, intraventricular haemorrhage, infection, and necrotizing enterocolitis.

PROGNOSIS

- Increasing survival of premature infants has not led to a decrease in the percentage of handicapped survivors. Most major neurological handicap relates to periventricular leucomalacia, a condition of white matter infarction related to cerebral hypoperfusion. This may be pre- or perinatal or postnatal in origin and may be predictable in the neonatal period by cerebral ultrasound. Visual handicap from retinopathy of prematurity is rare. Deafness is also uncommon and usually part of a multihandicap picture.

  Spastic diplegia, however, occurs predominantly in neonates who have not required intensive care, and in small-for-gestation infants.

- Major handicap rates are approximately 20% for survivors of <1000 g birthweight, and 5–8% for survivors weighing 1000–1500 g. Approximately a further 10% of survivors in each group have more minor neurological or behavioural defects[1].

- Minor learning difficulties, behavioural and attentional problems, and even minor degrees of cerebral palsy may not become evident until school age.

TREATMENT

1. Most premature infants who do not require intensive care will develop normally. Immunizations should be given at 3 months of age, without regard to immaturity. Growth in most who are initially less than the third centile for gestation will catch up within the first 6 months, including head growth. If it does not, these individuals, who have had significant intrauterine growth retardation, will be permanently small and slender.

2. Infants who have required intensive care have a 30% incidence of rehospitalization during infancy. This is predominantly for upper and lower respiratory tract infection, otitis media or croup. There may also be subglottic stenosis after protracted neonatal intubation causing later stridor, or failure to thrive in the infant who has had a very prolonged oxygen requirement and has residual tachypnoea, chest deformity and wheeze due to bronchopulmonary dysplasia. All these complications are greatly reduced after infancy.

3. Other complications in infancy may be inguinal hernia, which requires urgent assessment regarding surgery; late complications of a persistently patent ductus arteriosus, which will require surgery if it causes cardiac failure or is still present at 1 year; gastroenterological problems related to malabsorption following neonatal necrotizing enterocolitis, and, rarely, late development of hydrocephalus following neonatal intraventricular haemmorhage, which requires insertion of a ventriculoperitoneal or ventriculoatrial shunt. Squint due to delayed establishment of binocular vision also occurs.

4. Neurodevelopmental handicap is commoner in premature infants than in the general population. Surveillance of high-risk infants is undertaken by every unit performing neonatal intensive care. Growth, general health, neurological examination and development are monitored at intervals to 2 years of age and sometimes beyond. Specific screening of vision, hearing and language is necessary, because of increased incidence of squint, eye abnormalities (retinopathy of prematurity), visual disturbance (cortical), nerve deafness and middle ear disease, and language delay.

5. Laser treatment can now be offered for retinopathy of prematurity of major degree.

---

[1] Stewart AL (1986) Follow up studies. In *Text book of Neonatology* (Roberton NRC ed.). Edinburgh: Churchill Livingstone.

Cerebral Palsy

The cerebral palsies are disorders of movement of posture, caused by non-progressive damage to the immature brain. The origin may be pre-, peri- or postnatal; 50% of cases have no history of birth asphyxia.

Several patterns of handicap exist, with differing origins, and can be defined with relation to muscle tone change (spastic, flaccid) and to distribution. Accompanying problems vary from minimal to profound.

Transient tone changes in the first 6 months of life may mimick developing cerebral palsy, but recover completely, especially in premature infants.

PROGNOSIS

Hemiplegia

- In mild cases sitting is little delayed but walking is 2–3 months later than normal. Some 'bottom shufflers' walk even later.
- The mean IQ is about 80 but in many cases IQ is average or above. Specific learning difficulties are more common than in the general population.
- Speech and language difficulties are rarely a problem.
- Hearing and vision should be checked but are usually normal.
- For children with IQ above 70, education should be within the normal system.

Diplegia and quadriplegia

- The early development of spasticity is associated with better outcome than those in whom hypotonia and delayed postural reflexes persist for many years.
- Recognition of upper limb involvement, which may be asymmetrical, is often delayed in diplegia.
- Severity of motor disorder usually reflects the extent of cerebral damage, and is associated with profound mental handicap, sometimes cortical blindness, and myoclonic-type seizures (50% of quadriplegics).
- The prognosis for ambulation may be predicted from the motor stage (in months) at age 3 years. If > 12, free ambulation by age 7 can be expected. If < 10, free ambulation is rarely achieved.
- Squint is common due to refractive error, cortical blindness or optic atrophy.

Dyskinesia and athetosis

- The IQ does not correlate with the degree of physical disability.
- Speech may be impossible for about 30% and alternative communications systems are necessary. Eye movement control may be preserved and permit some degree of response.
- Severe motor disability and involuntary movement will necessitate mobility by electric wheelchair.

TREATMENT

1. Regular assessment of all areas of development by a multidisciplinary 'handicap team' is an important element of care.
2. *Hemiplegia:* physiotherapy should start as soon as asymmetry is detected, usually at 3–6 months, to encourage two-handed activities, awareness of the affected arm and later, effective weight-bearing. Foot and ankle supportive bracing may help the tendency to equinus; Achilles tendon surgery will be necessary if passive stretching fails to prevent tendon tightening to the extent that the foot cannot be placed plantigrade. Assessment to exclude associated cortical sensory less or visual attention defect is important.
3. *Diplegia:* this is the characteristic handicap of premature infants, and of small-for-dates term infants, often without a particular history of neonatal difficulty. Arm involvement is variable, and there is sometimes difficulty in delineating diplegia (affecting legs only) from quadriplegia (affecting all four limbs, but with leg function more affected than arm function).

   Early physiotherapy will help permit logical chronological progression towards walking, avoiding mistaken early promotion of attempted weight-bearing and extension posturing. Prone positioning and correct seating precede structured crawling, weight-bearing and mobilization. Surgical treatment is needed if hip adductor tightening, knee or ankle contractures limit movement or comfortable handling.

4. *Quadriplegia:* the underlying lesion has affected a wide area of brain, and therefore accompanying mental defects are almost inevitable to some extent. There may also be associated visual or hearing handicap.

There is spasticity of both legs and, to a lesser functional extent, of both arms, though distinction from double hemiplegia can be difficult.

Pseudobulbarpalsy may lead to tongue protrusion, gagging, inco-ordination of swallowing, and speech difficulties. Speech therapy advice may help management of all these areas. Physiotherapy aims to suppress primitive reflexes and promote useful functional postures, e.g. supported sitting to promote eye–hand co-ordination. Regular home-based programmes of posture changes using slopes and boards may help prevent secondary fixed deformity and scoliosis. Surgery will be required to relieve painful deformations such as dislocating hips due to adductor hyperaction. Surgery to the salivary glands may help severe drooling. Drugs to relieve painful spasms, e.g. baclofen, may improve function. Multidisciplinary help to assess visual and auditory handicap and develop means of alternative communication is invaluable. Usually all these treatments can be offered, based at the child's school, by a combined team.

5. *Dyskinesia:* this includes disorders with sudden extreme tone fluctuation and involuntary movement, particularly athetosis (snakelike sinuous distal limb involuntary movements) and chorea (jerking mass movements of limb or body). It is almost invariably caused by perinatal anoxia or by kernicterus.

Physiotherapy to suppress unwanted reflexes, promote head control and, with appropriate aids, promoting sitting posture is the mainstay of treatment. Ataxia is often superimposed on the athetosis and may mean that standing and walking development take years.

Speech is affected by lack of orofacial muscle control but may improve as late as the early teens. Severely affected children, however, will require an electric wheelchair and an alternative communication system.

6. *Hypotonia:* there is some doubt that this is a separate entity, as hypotonia, the 'floppy baby syndrome', often accompanies mental handicap of a wide variety of origins. Delayed intellectual, communicative, and social development accompany the extreme motor delay.

Management problems

a. Tongue-thrusting, gagging or choking occur, particularly in children with severe bilateral damage, and make feeding difficult. Speech therapists or physiotherapists may suggest helpful feeding positions or techniques, including desensitization of mouth reflexes.

b. Vomiting and oesophageal reflux are common. Small frequent feeds, or feed thickeners may reduce reflux. Rarely, surgery may be necessary.

c. Dribbling can be intractable and distressing. Salivary duct transplantation has been tried. Barrier cream or 1% hydrocortisone cream will help soreness and inflammation of chin and neck.

d. Constipation has multiple origins. Glycerine suppositories may suffice, but regular lactulose may be required if the diet is small-volume and refined.

e. Sleep and screaming problems: physical pain, e.g. from dislocating hip or reflux oesophagitis, and ordinary paediatric problems such as otitis media or urinary tract infection should be excluded before these problems are presumed to have a neurogenic basis.

f. Chilblains and cold injury result from poor circulation and immobility. Socks and gloves help prevent them.

FOLLOW-UP

All children with cerebral palsy require 6-monthly multidisciplinary assessment of development, physical disability, locomotor status, vision, hearing, and social, educational and family situation[1].

It is important that families of the more handicapped children are supported. Mother-and-toddler groups at the local assessment centre, and respite care by local grannies or in a ward on a regular basis are invaluable. Most such families are entitled to and should receive full attendance allowance and mobility allowance from the time the child is 2 years, plus necessary aids to care as needed.

¹ Hall DMB *The Child with a Handicap*. Blackwell Scientific Publications.

Child Abuse

Child abuse is defined as harm inflicted on children by adults. It may consist of different types, such as physical injury, neglect, emotional deprivation or sexual abuse.

Physical abuse may present as a range of injuries from minor to major trauma. Certain injuries are more common: burns, facial bruises, a torn fraenum of the lip, finger-shaped bruises, subconjunctival or retinal haemorrhages, subdural haematoma or skin bruises of different ages. The child may show failure to thrive and signs of neglect. X-rays may show unsuspected fractures or fractures of different ages.

Positive points in the history involve a delay in presentation, an implausible explanation, other injuries or a previous history of abuse in the child or sibling. The children are usually younger than 3 years[1]. Risk factors include male sex, illegitimacy, low birthweight, previous injuries and parental emotional stress[2].

Sexual abuse can present early and continue into adolescence. The incidence has been hard to define, partly because of differences in surveys. Some surveys, for example, include experiences of exhibitionism; others have different age cut-offs, and the number of patients reporting abuse depends on the interview method. A recent review[3] showed that in the USA the figures for women ranged from 8 to 22% or from 12 to 38%, and for men from 5 to 9% or 3 to 6%. In the UK for women the figures can vary from 16% to 54%. The majority of abusers are male and are usually known to the child—relatives, friends or stepfathers especially.

Abuse may take the form of genital fondling, orogenital contact or viewing the genitalia. Other forms are perineal masturbation, violent rape and buggery and non-violent intercourse, the latter tending to occur in pre-adolescent and adolescent children[4]. First presentation may occur when the child informs an adult; but inappropriate sexual play, behavioural disturbances, sleep disturbance or physical abuse may also be clues[5]. Many cases present as psychological problems in adulthood.

PROGNOSIS

- Deaths from subsequent physical injury range from 2 to 2.5%, re-injury rates vary from 10 to 20%. Failure to thrive and failure of neurological development may occur.
- Emotional problems may occur and school performance may suffer[6].
- Sexual abuse has lasting effects. In a study[7] of 152 women, almost all had been upset by their experiences; 50% had sustained lasting effects. The effect on their lives involved negative feelings about sex, men or themselves. Other feelings involved anxiety and mistrust, difficulties in forming or maintaining intimate relationships, and sexual problems. The worst prognosis involves those relationships in which force or physical abuse takes place over a long time with older men, particularly fathers or stepfathers.

TREATMENT

1. Doctors must constantly be aware of the possibility of child abuse, particularly if injuries do not match the history. Any child giving a history of sexual abuse must be taken seriously,

for example using anatomically correct dolls to confirm the diagnosis.

2. If physical or sexual abuse is suspected the child should be fully but gently examined and notes taken of all injuries. If physical abuse is suspected, clinical photographs must be taken, a skeletal survey ordered and blood taken for clotting factors.

3. Cases of sexual abuse need very gentle handling, particularly when examining the genitalia and anus. Bacterial and forensic samples should be taken. The presence of a relative at the examination will help; examination should ideally be performed by a doctor with experience in this problem.

4. The child in all cases should be admitted to a paediatric ward for assessment. Care should be taken not to accuse any party. If the parents refuse, a Place of Safety order can be sought by the Social Services, National Society for Prevention of Cruelty to Children or police. A case conference will then take into considera-tion the medical, social and psychological aspects before forming a plan of action.

FOLLOW-UP

Follow-up of all cases is arranged at the time of the case conference. Where a child is returned to the family, continual assessment of the child should be performed by a specific social worker and by those professionals involved with the child—the teacher, school nurse, health visitor and general practitioner, for example, should be alerted to the signs of further abuse.

[1] Kempe CH et al. (1962) J.A.M.A., 181, 17–24.
[2] Hensey OJ et al. (1983) Dev. Med. Child. Neurol., 25, 606–11.
[3] Kelly L (1988) Surviving Sexual Violence, pp. 59–60. Polity Press.
[4] Kempe CH (1978) Pediatrics, 62, 382–9.
[5] Hobbs CJ et al. (1986) Lancet, 792–6.
[6] Rosenbloom L et al. (1985) Arch. Dis. Child, 60, 191–2.
[7] Heiman J et al. (1986) Am. J. Psychiatry, 143, 1293–6.

Conduct Disorders

The main feature of a conduct disorder is antisocial behaviour[1] which interferes with the rights of others. By contrast, in 'oppositional defiant' disorders, there is hostile and defiant behaviour without the violation of others' rights. Conduct disorders may involve stealing, aggression, truancy, vandalism, arson and drug abuse. The child with a conduct disorder may be solitary in behaviour, showing the characteristics of bullying, stealing, violent behaviour and disobedience. Alternatively he or she may perform these actions in a group or gang.

Causes may be genetic with a family disposition to deviant behaviour, chromosomal (such as XXX karyotype), brain damage (prenatal, intrapartum or postnatal), or related to isolated physical or educational handicaps. Personality factors may be important, and environmental factors can contribute, for example, where a child is brought up in a family without a loving environment. In an unstable environment, such as a disharmonious marriage[1], father absence, bereavement, large family size or frequent hospitalization, a conduct disorder may occur. The absence of a consistent school environment with clear rules and fair teaching may contribute to the development of problems. Children with conduct disorders may have an associated reading disability, depression or a hyperactivity disorder.

PROGNOSIS

- Most highly antisocial children recover.
- Minor problems may clear without specific treatment.

- Short-term hospital admission for behaviour modification can be highly successful for carefully selected children[2].
- Psychoeducational day-school programmes can

produce improvements in behavioural, academic and family functioning but continued intervention is usually necessary[3].

- The immediate and long-term effects of family therapy are variable. This may reflect the different presenting problems and the different techniques employed. There is evidence that in the long term, children treated with family therapy show better results than those treated in other ways. Positive changes in the attitudes of parents can be achieved by these techniques.
- The number of different childhood antisocial behaviours that a child exhibits is a better predictor of severe adult antisocial behaviour than specific behaviours or family variables[4].

TREATMENT

1. Treatment must initially involve:
   a. Assessment of the family including a review of family history and observation of family functioning.
   b. Assessment of the child including developmental, physical, psychological and educational attainment.
   c. Assessment of the school and wider environment in which the child plays or interacts.
2. Treatment is directed to correct the failure to learn or abide by rules for acceptable social behaviour, and will involve:
   a. Explanation to parents of the role of chromosomal abnormalities or genetic factors so that a more favourable environment is created for the child.
   b. Explanation to parents of the role of physical handicap in conduct disorder.
   c. Assessment and treatment of physical problems—hearing, vision, speech and physical deformity.

   d. Treatment of temperamental factors in the child by counselling the parents and arranging a programme to deal with the important features.
   e. Treatment of family factors and development of clearly defined family rules for all activities. Parents need to understand the importance to the child of their involvement in the child's activities and their appreciation of the child's feelings on important issues. This can be achieved through parental counselling, family therapy[5], and psychotherapy.
   f. A plan should be agreed on how to deal with family problems before they become serious and what to do when problems occur.
3. Changes may also be necessary in the schooling, possibly with a change of school, class or teacher. Group therapy, day treatment or residential treatment[4] may be necessary.
4. Reading and writing disabilities, depression and hyperactivity may need to be treated separately.

FOLLOW-UP

Regular assessment should be carried out at intervals determined by the nature of the problem, the family's abilities and progress. Long-term follow-up with booster sessions is probably required for many families.

[1] Jouriles EN (1988) *J. Abnorm. Child Psychol.*, **16**, 197–206.
[2] Raemer JC (1986) *Am. J. Dis. Child.*, **140**, 242–4.
[3] Baenen RS *et al.* (1986) *Am. J. Orthopsychiatry*, **56**, 263–70.
[4] Robins LN (1978) *Psychol. Med.*, **8**, 611–22.
[5] McCauley R (1982) *J. Child Psychol. Psychiatry*, **23**, 335–42.

9

Infectious Diseases

F. M. Hull

Measles

Measles[1] is a virus disease which occurs classically in epidemics every second year as new non-immune populations of children occur[2]. After an incubation period of 10–14 days the disease begins with coryzal symptoms. At this stage the child is only slightly ill but there may be diagnostic Koplik's spots appearing as granular white macules on the buccal mucosa. The rash begins on the second or third coryzal day, spreading from the face to the trunk and peripherally down the limbs. At this stage there will be a violent irritant cough. Complications include bacterial infections of the respiratory tract ranging from otitis media to pneumonia, conjunctivitis and mild encephalitis. The fatal condition of subacute sclerosing panencephalitis (SSPE)[3] complicates measles occurring in children under the age of 2.

PROGNOSIS

- In most cases speedy recovery follows the full development of the exanthema but there is a small mortality rate of 0.02% and hospital admission is required in 1%.
- Secondary infection especially in ears (5%), eyes (2%), central nervous system (CNS) (0.6%) and lower respiratory tract (4%) may complicate measles. Long-term prognosis may be affected because of permanent pulmonary damage leading to bronchiectasis.
- Neurological complications include febrile convulsions and more serious postinfective encephalitis, which occurs in 0.1% and may lead to permanent brain damage in 25% of cases with a mortality rate of 15%. The very rare, invariably fatal 'slow virus' condition SSPE[3] develops in a small and variable proportion of children when the original attack of measles occurs before the age of 2. In England and Wales the annual death rate has varied[4] between 3 and 11 between 1979 and 1985. Altogether 170 cases have been reported[5] in the whole of the UK between 1970 and 1981. Though the incidence of SSPE is of the order of 6–22 per million cases of measles, this is much higher in France[6] where 35 cases were recorded in 1980. The disease develops 4–7 years after an episode of measles, it progresses quicker in girls but is 2–4 times more common in boys[7,8].
- In severely malnourished children, in populations who have not been exposed to the virus and in immunosuppression, the mortality rate may be much higher. Measles is rare in the elderly but may be fatal.

TREATMENT

1. Measles is an unpleasant and preventable disease with rare but potentially serious neurological and respiratory complications. Some 100 000 cases are notified annually in the UK[5]. Measles vaccine is a live attenuated virus vaccine grown on chick embryo. Its use may produce an acute febrile reaction in children and should be covered by measles specific immunoglobulin if there is a history of convulsions. The vaccine is given in a dose of 0.5 ml subcutaneously; in most European countries this is administered between the ages of 9 months and 2 years. In Sweden and Czechoslovakia measles vaccination is given twice and these countries have almost eliminated the disease. Elimination of the disease in Europe would be attainable if 96% of children of one year of age were vaccinated.

2. This target has been reached in the USA where there has been an abrupt fall in the incidence of encephalitis and SSPE.

3. The treatment of measles is largely symptomatic with care to maintain fluid balance in febrile, miserable children. Antibiotics are rarely required but may be indicated for secondary chest infection or otitis media.

4. Approximately one in 1000 cases of measles develop postinfectious encephalitis in which there is general congestion of the brain associated with demyelination. Clinically the disease may vary from transient drowsiness to deep unconsciousness leading to death or severe motor and mental retardation. Irritability occurring at the time the child should be

improving, some 3–4 days after the appearance of the rash, especially when accompanied by convulsions should alert the general practitioner to the possibility of encephalitis which may be confirmed by EEG.

FOLLOW-UP

Measles is a notifiable disease. Patients should be nursed at home, but since infectivity is greatest in the early coryzal stage most cross infection occurs before diagnosis. The possibility of long-term complications such as SSPE should be borne in mind.

[1] Pickles WN (1939) *Epidemiology in Country Practice*. Bristol: John Wright.

[2] Velimvoric B, Greco D, Piergentili P *et al.* (1984) Figures and trends for Measles in Europe 1950–1980. In *Infectious Diseases in Europe* (Velimvoric B ed.), pp. 79–82. Copenhagen: World Health Organisation.
[3] Haase AT (1986) The pathogenesis of slow virus infections. *The Journal of Infective Disease*, **153**, 441–7.
[4] OPCS Communicable Disease Statistics (1985) London: HMSO.
[5] Miller CL (1983) Current impact of measles in UK. *Rev. Inf. Dis.*, **5**, 427–32.
[6] Rey M, Celus J, Monton Y *et al.* (1983) Impact of Measles in France. *Rev. Inf. Dis.*, **5**, 433–8.
[7] Aaby P, Buckle J, Lisse IM *et al.* (1984) Risk factors in subacute sclerosing panencephalitis. *Rev. Inf. Dis.*, **6**, 239–50.
[8] Sever JL (1983) Persistent measles infection of the central nervous system: subacute sclerosing panencephalitis. *Rev. Inf. Dis.*, **5**, 467–72.

Mumps

Mumps is a common disease of childhood occurring in 5.6 per 1000 at risk[1] and is caused by a paramyxovirus. The disease is showing a slow but steady decline in Europe possibly due to increased immunization[2]. The disease affects rapidly dividing glandular tissue particularly the parotids, gonads and pancreas. Rarely (in less than 0.5%) there may be a transient arthritis[3]. Like many other viral exanthemata, mumps may involve the CNS. Mumps meningitis is quite common especially in adults where as many as 10% develop meningism; a rare and much more severe encephalitis may give rise to permanent brain damage or death. Mumps may occur in the fetus without evidence of teratogenicity when delivery may be complicated by hugely swollen parotid glands in an infant.

PROGNOSIS

- Almost invariably good, especially in children who show only mild constitutional upset.
- Orchitis occurs in 25% of adult males but rarely leads to testicular atrophy or permanent sterility although there may be impaired fertility in 13%. Oophoritis occurs in 7% of post-pubertal females.
- CNS involvement is rarely serious or permanent.

TREATMENT

1. Symptomatic treatment is all that is required in children.
2. Analgesia may be necessary for the headache of mumps meningitis but any suspicion of alteration of consciousness should raise the possibility of encephalitis when hospital admission is required for reduction of cerebral oedema and maintenance of the airway.
3. Testicular pain may be severe requiring scrotal support and analgesia. Pain may be relieved by injecting 10–20 ml of 1% lignocaine into the spermatic cord at the external inguinal ring. Where there is severe scrotal swelling referral for incision of the tunica may be indicated to relieve pain and prevent permanent sterility.
4. A live attenuated vaccine prepared on chick embryo is available for immunization of pre-pubertal susceptible individuals especially males.

FOLLOW-UP

Consider a check on male fertility in post-pubertal mumps.

[1] *Morbidity statistics from General Practice. Third National Study* (1986) London: HMSO.
[2] Velimvoric B, Greco D, Piergentili P *et al.* (1984) *Figures and trends for selected infectious diseases in Europe.* In *Infectious Diseases in Europe* (Velimvoric B, ed.), p. 86. Copenhagen: World Health Organisation.
[3] Gordon SC, Lanter CB. (1984) *Rev. Inf. Dis.,* **6,** 338–43.

Rubella

Rubella is a common and ubiquitous viral disease; it is reported in 3.2 per 1000 individuals at risk but, since it may often be mild and transient it is often under-reported[1]. It is best considered as postnatal and antenatal rubella.

Postnatal rubella

The disease occurs in recurring epidemics with an interval of 6–8 years. After an incubation period of 2–3 weeks from infection by inhaled droplet a very variable picture develops: in some individuals there may be little or no sign of illness except for a change in antibodies, in others especially adults there may be an acute illness for fever, sore throat, a generalized red, macular rash and arthralgia. There is commonly shotty occipital lymphadenopathy. The diagnosis of rubella may be quite difficult but is important because of risk to the fetus[2].

Antenatal rubella

The virus crosses the placenta to infect the fetus at any time in pregnancy. Concurrent maternal rubella may be florid or unnoticed but 15–20% of fetuses may develop severe abnormality. Maximum risk to the fetus occurs at eight weeks, 80% of fetuses exposed to rubella before the twelfth week of gestation show evidence of congenital rubella (mostly involving the heart and ears); by 13–14 weeks the incidence of abnormality has fallen to 54% (involving the ears) and has virtually gone by the age of 16 weeks[3,4].

PROGNOSIS

- In postnatal rubella the prognosis is invariably good though there may be transient arthritis affecting 60% of adults, especially women. As with other exanthemata, encephalitis occurs very rarely in adults when its mortality may be as high as 20%.
- In antenatal rubella there may be intrauterine death, gross mental retardation, severe cardiac abnormalities, nerve deafness or blindness due to cataract, retinopathy or glaucoma. Abnormalities may occur in the brain, ear, eye, heart and rarely in the liver and long bones. There may be abortion or stillbirth but many fetuses survive to be brain damaged, blind, deaf or have heart defects.

TREATMENT

1. Treatment of postnatal rubella is symptomatic.
2. The only treatment of antenatal rubella lies in prevention. Rubella vaccines are available, they are all live virus vaccine grown on chick embryo. Though vaccination should be avoided in pregnancy there is no evidence that Rubella vaccine is teratogenic.
3. There are two preventive options open:
   a. Reduction of rubella incidence by vaccinating all children
   b. Pubertal vaccination of all girls
   Epidemiologists argue about the relative merits of these schemes, the first is adopted in the USA and the latter in Britain. WHO aim to eradicate rubella in Europe by the end of the century but point out that this will require more than 90% of the population to be immune[2]. If congenital rubella defects are to be eliminated vaccination of girls is insufficient because it appears that antenatal rubella is related to the uncontrolled circulation of

rubella in children with some apparently immune mothers having affected babies.

4. There are several live vaccines available, some are grown on chick embryo and may be contra-indicated in allergic individuals. Vaccination against rubella should be avoided in pregnancy though there is no evidence that the vaccine is teratogenic.

FOLLOW-UP

This depends on management of the permanent sequelae of antenatal rubella which may include the long-term care of grossly handicapped children with eye, ear, heart and other congenital defects. Sero-negative women should be vaccinated against rubella.

[1] *Morbidity statistics from General Practice. Third National Study* (1986) London: HMSO.
[2] Velimvoric B, Greco D, Piergentili P (1984) In *Infectious Diseases in Europe*, pp. 96–101. Figures and trends for selected infectious diseases in Europe. (Velimvoric B., ed.) Copenhagen: World Health Organisation.
[3] Miller CL, Miller E, Waight PA (1987) *Br. Med. J.*, **294**, 1277.
[4] Miller E, Craddock-Jones JE, Pollock TM (1982) *Lancet* **ii**, 781–4.

Chickenpox

Varicella or chickenpox is a highly infectious disease of children caused by the herpes varicella/zoster virus. It occurs in 3.5 per 1000 at risk but is a disease predominantly of young children, occurring in 15.7 per 1000 children in the first four years of life[1]. It is characterized by a cropping rash of lesions distributed over the trunk and proximal parts of the limbs which progress from macule through papule and vesicle to pustule in the course of a few days such that lesions at all stages of maturity coexist[2]. The disease is highly infectious and occurs in epidemics. In adults the disease runs a more severe course with systemic upset and often a florid rash affecting mucous membranes of mouth, respiratory tract, conjunctiva and vagina. In adults with herpes zoster (*vide infra*) careful search will often reveal the co-existence of a sparse chickenpox rash.

PROGNOSIS

- The prognosis of chickenpox is excellent apart from rare ocular or CNS complications but may be severe even fatal in the immuno-suppressed.
- Abnormalities in chest X-rays due to miliary calcification are common following adult chickenpox but rarely important. More serious is the extremely rare varicella pneumonia which may be fatal in 30% of adults.
- Encephalitis is rare, affects children more than adults, and is characterized by cerebellar signs. Eighty per cent recover spontaneously but 5% may die and 15% have residual CNS defects.
- There is a possible link between chickenpox and Reye's syndrome but this may be related to aspirin taken to relieve symptoms rather than to the varicella virus itself[3].

TREATMENT

1. Varicella requires symptomatic treatment; calamine to the rash or starch baths will relieve skin irritation.
2. Occasional secondary infection of pocks may require antibiotics.
3. A vaccine is being developed in Japan and trials of this in 1981–2 have shown excellent tolerance[3].

FOLLOW-UP

Adult patients having had chickenpox may develop diffuse pulmonary calcification apparent on chest X-ray.

[1] *Morbidity statistics from General Practice. Third National Study* (1986) London: HMSO.

[2] Emond RTD (1974) *A Colour Atlas of Infectious Disease.* London: Wolfe Medical Publications.
[3] Velimvoric B, Greco D, Piergentili P (1984) In *Infectious Diseases in Europe*, p. 86. Figures and trends for selected infectious diseases in Europe. (Velimvoric B., ed.) Copenhagen: World Health Organisation.

Herpes Zoster (Shingles)

Herpes zoster[1], caused by the same virus as chickenpox, produces an extremely painful vesicular rash distributed in one or more dermatomes. The precise epidemiology of zoster is unknown but it may follow epidemics of varicella, suggesting a direct infection, or the virus may lie dormant in the sensory root ganglia of the spinal cord or of the trigeminal nerve awaiting some stimulus to trigger off a typical episode of herpes zoster or shingles. Such a stimulus may be due to altered immune state (florid zoster occurs in AIDS) due to carcinomatosis or lymphoma but may equally be started off by intercurrent infection or emotional upsets such as bereavement.

PROGNOSIS

- In 50% of cases of herpes ophthalmicus the eye is affected. Of these, 52% suffer iritis leading to permanent damage to the iris in 12%. Ophthalmoplegia may develop in a third of cases and slowly recovers over about 2–3 months. Optic neuritis occurs in 1% leading to permanent loss of sight in the eye[2].
- Zoster often gives rise to the intractable pain of post-herpetic neuralgia which is often difficult to treat and may be so severe as to drive elderly patients to suicide.
- Post herpetic neuralgia is unlikely if there is a normal skin flare in response to 0.1 ml of 1:100 000 histamine injected into the affected dermatome.

TREATMENT

1. Zoster has many treatments and as usual in such circumstances nothing is very effective in shortening the course of the disease or limiting complications.
2. Pain should be relieved with appropriately strong analgesics.
3. Secondary infections, particularly of the eye in trigeminal herpes, may require topical antibiotics and in severe cases, referral to an ophthalmologist.
4. Many therapies have been tried such as radiotherapy and steroids to lessen the chance of post-herpetic neuralgia. Local painting with idoxuridine is said to minimize post-herpetic neuralgia but this is expensive and it is not known how effective it is.
5. Acyclovir is active against the varicella/zoster virus. It is expensive and to be effective must be given very early in the illness. With immuno-suppressed individuals with herpes zoster intravenous acyclovir should be considered.
6. Post herpetic neuralgia may be relieved by intercostal and sympathetic ganglion nerve blocks. Some relief may be gained by adding amitriptyline to simple analgesia.

FOLLOW-UP

Long-term follow-up of elderly patients who have had shingles may be necessary since the severe pain of post-herpetic neuralgia may be life threateningly depressing. Since the disease occurs in the presence of reduced immunity, the possibility of some underlying immuno-deficiency should be considered.

[1] Hull R (1987) *Infective Disease in Primary Care.* London: Chapman and Hall.
[2] Banatvsala JE, Welch JM (1986) Viral diseases. In *Treatment and Prognosis: Medicine* (Hawkins R ed.) Oxford: Heinemann.

Infectious Mononucleosis[1,2,3]

This is an infectious, highly variable disease caused by the Epstein–Barr virus. This virus is ubiquitous but in developed countries with a high standard of living it causes the frequent affliction of infectious mononucleosis whereas in developing countries it plays a part in the aetiology of Burkitt's lymphoma and undifferentiated nasal carcinoma. Formerly infectious mononucleosis was known as glandular fever which is now recognized as consisting of a collection of indeterminate illnesses with many causes (e.g. cytomegalovirus and toxoplasmosis) whose clinical picture mimics and may be clinically indistinguishable from mononucleosis. True infectious mononucleosis occurs in three forms:
1) anginose, characterized by pharyngitis and lymphadenopathy;
2) hepatic, which may resemble mild hepatitis, and
3) the febrile form is a non specific feverish illness with or without rash.
Many symptoms and signs may accompany mononucleosis including fever, jaundice, widespread lymph gland enlargement, hepatomegaly, pharyngitis, transient neurological signs and a rash which may be quite marked on the palate. The diagnosis is supported by the presence of mononuclear cells and tests for heterophile antibodies (Paul Bunnell, Monospot) are commonly but not universally positive.

PROGNOSIS

- This is good but in some very acute forms of infectious mononucleosis symptoms can be quite alarming, particularly if faucial swelling causes incipient respiratory obstruction.
- Very occasionally there may be associated auto-immune problems, such as thrombocytopaenia.
- Rupture of the spleen has been reported following heavy handed palpation.

TREATMENT

1. This is largely expectant but where there is a threat of respiratory obstruction steroids (200 mg hydrocortisone) will reduce faucial swelling.
2. The unwary prescription of ampicillin may precipitate a severe exfoliative dermatitis. (The Medical Defence Union consider the administration of ampicillin for sore throats indefensible because of this.)

FOLLOW-UP

This is rarely needed, but peak incidence at times of school leaving exams may have marked educational implications.

[1] Editorial (1982) *Lancet*, **2**, 1253–5.
[2] Hull R (1987) *Infective Disease in Primary Care*. London: Chapman and Hall.
[3] Banatsvala JE, Welch JM (1986) Viral diseases. In *Treatment and Prognosis* (Hawkins R ed.). Oxford: Heinemann.

Cytomegalovirus Infections

This virus causes a variety of infections including the glandular fever syndrome, atypical pneumonia (particularly in immuno-suppressed individuals), encephalitis and pyrexia of undetermined origin[1,2]. Even more than rubella, cytomegalovirus causes abnormalities in the fetus[3]. The virus may be transmitted in utero, at birth or by breast milk. It occurs in 1% of live births (range 0.5–4%) when the virus may be detected in the urine of the neonate.

PROGNOSIS

- Most adult cytomegalovirus infections are shortlived and self-limiting.
- Damage caused to developing fetal organs is often fatal or may cause permanent disability.
- Less than 5% of infected embryos show congenital cytomegalovirus disease but as many as 20% may suffer long-term sequelae[4]. When infection occurs early in pregnancy the fetus may show major CNS developmental defects with a high mortality rate. Of those infected, but apparently normal or with minimal abnormality, 10–15% will subsequently be shown to have intellectual or hearing deficits in later life. The incidence of deafness due to cytomegalovirus (CMV) is estimated at 0.5–1 per 1000 live births. Recently defects of the development of tooth enamel which may predispose to severe caries has been demonstrated in 40% of children who survive congenital CMV infection. Infection late in pregnancy causes cytomegalovirus inclusion disease in which there may be hepato-splenomegaly, thrombocytopaenia, jaundice, and abnormalities of lung and eye. Most cytomegalovirus inclusion disease is, however, mild and frequently undiagnosed. The organism may be isolated from throat, nose, urine, breast milk and blood.

TREATMENT

1. Vaccines have been developed but their safety and effectiveness is not certain.
2. Antiviral therapy with iodoxuridine and interferon have been tried on infected infants with little success.

[1] Hull R (1987) *Infective Disease in Primary Care*. London: Chapman and Hall.

[2] Banatvsala JE, Welch JM (1986) Viral Diseases. In *Treatment and Prognosis: Medicine* (Hawkins R ed.). Oxford: Heinemann.

[3] Grist NR (1984) The future of viral pathology. In *Infectious diseases in Europe*. Copenhagen: World Health Organisation.

[4] Gilbert GL (1985) Congenital and perinatal cytomegalovirus infections. *Australian & New Zealand Journal of Obstetrics and Gynaecology*, **25(3)**, 169–71.

Poliomyelitis

This disease, formerly known as infantile paralysis, is a severe viral disease of world wide distribution[1,2]. Though largely eradicated in developed countries (its incidence has fallen from 16 000 in 1950 to 12 in the years 1978–83 in the USA[3,4]. However it still occurs in developed countries. Between 1982 and 1986 six cases were reported from Scotland[5] and Finland suffered a small epidemic in 1985. The disease should always be considered as a possibility in travellers for it is still endemic in the Third World.

The virus occurs in three strains (Brunlhild, Lansing and Leon) without cross immunity. The disease is spread by faecal contamination of food and water. Following an incubation period of 7–14 days a variety of forms may develop. In the first there is simply a mild 'flu-like' illness with slight fever and possibly diarrhoea. In subclinical poliomyelitis symptoms are more pronounced and there may be myalgia, some meningeal irritation and gastro-intestinal symptoms. In paralytic poliomyelitis the virus attacks the anterior horn cells of the spinal cord producing at first severe muscle pain and later paralysis of muscle groups anywhere in the body depending on which anterior horn cells are affected. Milder forms of the disease can be transmuted to paralytic poliomyelitis forms by fatigue, violent exercise or intra-muscular injections. Bulbar poliomyelitis and polioencephalitis may cause ophthalmoplegia, dysphagia or respiratory failure.

PROGNOSIS

- In the milder forms the prognosis is good, indeed the disease may pass unnoticed.
- The degree of paralysis may be affected by the patient's general health and state of muscle fatigue at the time of infection.
- The immediate threat to life is through respiratory failure, and provided this is properly managed there is little threat to life.
- The degree of permanent paralysis is very variable and this can be improved with skilled physiotherapy and prostheses.

TREATMENT

1. Though poliomyelitis is entirely preventable it still occurs.
2. Prevention is by means of live oral vaccine (Sabin) or killed vaccine given by injection (Salk) and boosted every 5–10 years.
3. Travellers to Third World countries should be protected against poliomyelitis. In developed countries Sabin vaccine is commonly used but this may be less effective in the tropics where Salk vaccine provides a better immunity.
4. In paralytic polio there is no specific treatment. Management aims at preserving vital functions, until spontaneous recovery occurs.
5. Permanent disabilities then require physiotherapy and prosthetic aids.

FOLLOW-UP

Most patients with paralytic poliomyelitis will be left with permanent neuro-muscular deficits which may lead to complex problems requiring lifelong physical and psychosocial supportive measures.

[1] Hull R (1987) *Infective Disease in Primary Care.* London: Chapman and Hall.
[2] Lucas AO, Gilles HM (1984) *Preventive Medicine for the Tropics,* 2nd edn. London: Hodder and Stoughton.
[3] Velimvoric B, Greco D, Piergentili P *et al.* (1984) Figures and trends for selected infectious diseases in Europe 1950–1980. In *Infectious Diseases in Europe.* Copenhagen: World Health Organisation.
[4] Grist NR ibid *The future of viral pathology*
[5] Bell EJ, Riding MH, Grist NR (1986) *British Medical Journal,* **293,** 193–4.

Diphtheria

Diphtheria is an acute, dangerous but now rare infectious disease caused by *Corynebacterium diphtheriae*. In 1980, 1200 cases were reported in Europe[1], but the disease is much commoner in the Third World[20]. Recent reduction of immunization, due to scares about whooping cough vaccine, have rendered the possibility of the return of diphtheria more likely[3,4]. In addition immunity slowly wanes after primary immunization; 19% of individuals may be susceptible to diphtheria 20–30 years after childhood immunization. Commonly the disease affects the pharynx but it may also occur as 'surgical diphtheria' through infection of a wound or ulcer. There is usually a short (1–3 day) incubation period but this may be extended to as long as a week allowing time for patients infected abroad to return home. Typically diphtheria begins with a sore throat sometimes with gross lymphadenopathy giving rise to 'bull neck'. There is a spreading membranous exudate which, in the larynx, may lead to life-threatening respiratory obstruction. The organism produces a powerful exotoxin which may lead to cardiac or neurological complications. Surgical diphtheria is particularly common in developing countries.

PROGNOSIS

- This is very variable since diphtheria may be relatively mild.
- Death may occur through asphyxia or due to acute heart failure.
- Neurological lesions may lead to loss of normal laryngeal reflexes which render respiratory obstruction the more likely.

TREATMENT

1. Attention should be paid to ensuring a high rate of diphtheria immunization in children as this has proved a reliable measure for the control of the disease. It is administered usually in combination with pertussis vaccine and tetanus toxoid for the immunization of infants starting from 2–3 months old. Immunity should be boosted at school entry[2].
2. As soon as diagnosis is suspected the patient should be isolated preferably where life supporting measures are immediately available.
3. Patients should be given immediate antitoxin (30–60 000 units according to the severity and threat of respiratory obstruction) and either penicillin (250 000 six hourly) or erythromycin (250 mg six hourly).
4. Since most cases of diphtheria are seen in travellers to Third World countries, care should be taken to check patients' immunity to diphtheria before they set out.

FOLLOW-UP

Patients should be isolated until throat cultures (or, in surgical diphtheria, wound cultures) are negative for *C. diphtheriae*.

[1] Kwantes W (1984) Diphtheria in Europe. *Journal of Hygiene*, **93**, 433–7.
[2] Lucas AO, Gilles HM (1984) *Preventive Medicine for the Tropics*, 2nd edn, pp. 253–6. London: Hodder and Stoughton.
[3] Editorial (1985) Diphtheria and tetanus boosters. *Lancet*, **1**, 1081–7.
[4] Kjeldsen K, Simonsen O, Heron I (1955) *Lancet*, **1**, 900–2.

Pertussis (whooping cough)

Whooping cough is caused by *Bordatella pertussis* and *B. parapertussis*. It is an acute, sometimes fatal, respiratory infection of childhood and especially dangerous under the age of two[1]. The disease has become more prevalent since scares with regard to extremely rare neurological complications following immunization occurred in the late 1970s[2]. These led to a thirtyfold increase in notifications of pertussis with a fourfold increase in deaths between 1972 and 1978. The safety of whooping cough vaccine is still not completely accepted but the risk is infinitely less than that of the disease it prevents[3]. Whooping cough is spread by droplet infection and has a variable incubation period (5–17 days). The disease starts as a cold with mild malaise. Some ten days later the typical paroxysmal cough develops, it is worse at night and produces a series of violent expiratory unproductive coughing bouts eventually ending in a forced inspiration (the whoop). Fits of coughing may be triggered by exercise, fright, eating and drinking or change in atmosphere and may culminate in vomiting.

PROGNOSIS

- In children over the age of 2 and in adults whooping cough is rarely serious, though it can persist and be very troublesome.
- Under the age of 2 it may lead to sudden death due to respiratory or cardiac failure.
- In 1985 there were 4 deaths from whooping cough among 22 046 notified cases of the disease[4] whereas the risk of vaccination resulting in permanent brain damage has been estimated at about 1 in 300 000 vaccinations[5].
- The cough may be so violent as to inflict structural damage to lung parenchyma or bronchi and there may be sublingual, subconjunctural, nasal or intracranial haemorrhage.
- Inhaled vomit may lead to sudden death.
- It is important to realize that early diagnosis may be difficult particularly for inexperienced doctors to whom the disease appears to be just another upper respiratory infection (there are few if any physical signs). The diagnosis is often made by grandparents who have heard the noise before and the question 'is it whooping cough?' should never be ignored.
- There may be neurological damage or death due to intracranial haemorrhage caused by extreme vascular congestion during a paroxysm.
- Long-term complications may include chronic lung conditions, particularly bronchiectasis.

TREATMENT

1. This is largely supportive.

2. Conditions likely to precipitate a paroxysm should be discussed with parents. A stable humid atmosphere should be maintained and children should be encouraged to eat and drink slowly.
3. Though antibiotics do not influence paroxysmal whooping cough erythromycin given early in the disease may reduce both its severity and duration. Given at a dose of 50 mg/kg it will render the child non-infectious after 10 days.
4. The most important aspect of whooping cough is its prevention by immunization usually given in combination with diphtheria vaccine and tetanus toxoid as triple antigen at 2, 3 and 4 months with a booster of dual antigen (diphtheria and tetanus at 4 years[6]. Vaccination should not be carried out in children who have a history of any severe local or general reaction, including a neurological reaction, to a preceding dose or a history of cerebral irritation or damage in the neonatal period, or who have suffered from fits or convulsions[5].
5. In epidemics children under the age of 2, or when at risk because of pre-existing respiratory disease, may be given some protection with erythromycin and hyperimmune globulin.

FOLLOW-UP

Recovery from whooping cough may be very slow. Often the paroxysmal cough returns with each subsequent upper respiratory tract infection after the disease itself has disappeared. This has given rise to the belief that autumn whooping cough was not cured until the following spring. Children recovering from severe whooping cough should be watched carefully for signs of bronchiectasis.

[1] Hull R (1987) *Infective Disease in Primary Care.* London: Chapman and Hall.

[2] Miller D *et al.* (1981) Pertussis immunization and serious neurological illness in childhood. *British Medical Journal,* **282,** 1595–9.
[3] Stewart G (1981) Whooping cough in relation to other childhood infections in 1977–79 in the United Kingdom. *J. Epidemiol. Community Health* **35**(2), 139–45.
[4] OPCS (1980) *Statistics for infectious disease 1978.* London: HMSO.
[5] *British National Formulary No 12* (1986) pp. 392–3.
[6] Velimvoric B. (1984) Infectious diseases in Europe, p. 312. Copenhagen: World Health Organisation.

Tetanus

Tetanus is caused by the neuropathic exotoxin produced by *Clostridium tetani.* This is a common soil organism, particularly when contaminated with animal faeces, and is a spore bearing anaerobe which may lie dormant for many years. Dormant tetanus bacilli sometimes contaminate old war wounds; surgical disturbances of foreign bodies such as shell splinters may give rise to tetanus. The commonest means of infection is through a dirty wound. Road and agricultural accidents and animal bites are particularly likely to be infected[1]. Tetanus is not uncommon—there were 2500 cases in Europe in 1980 and it is commoner still in developing countries. Tetanus may result from trivial injury[2,3] for example four deaths were reported in England and Wales in 1978 of which three were attributed to 'cut finger gutting fish', 'stubbed shin on bamboo in garden' and 'diabetic gangrene of toe'. Neonatal tetanus occurs in the Third World due to umbilical infection. There were 52 cases of tetanus in England and Wales between 1981 and 1983 of which half were associated with gardening injuries[4]. Two cases followed routine cholecystectomy and a similar case has been reported from Belgium[5] suggesting the need for immunization before surgery.

The toxin gains entrance to the nervous system via nerve sheaths and there may be a variable incubation period from a few days to several weeks (in the case of old war wounds even years or decades). Signs of tonic contractures of striated muscle begin in the jaws (hence 'lockjaw') with trismus and the development of the classical 'risus sardonicus'. There will be neck stiffness and increased (especially extensor muscle) tone. Throughout the illness the patient may be fully and distressingly aware of what is happening.

PROGNOSIS

- Overall mortality is about 40% (though in England and Wales in 1981–3 it was 10%).
- Mortality is highest where:
  a. The patient is a child or very old
  b. There is a short incubation period
  c. There is a short interval between the onset of symptoms and convulsions
  d. Treatment is delayed
  e. The infected wound is on the head or neck
  f. If trismus develops early
- Death is frequently due to cardiac or respiratory failure.
- Where patients survive they make a complete recovery.
- In Third World countries the mortality from neonatal tetanus ranges from 5 to 60 deaths per 1000 live births (amounting to 25–72% of all neonatal deaths). Tetanus neonatorum presents with failure to suck in a previously healthy infant[6]. Death rates for tetanus among the newborn are particularly high in rural India.
- There are recent reports from the USA of increased deaths from tetanus among drug abusers, especially female cocaine addicts.

TREATMENT

1. Tetanus is entirely preventable by primary immunization usually given in combination with diphtheria vaccine and tetanus toxoid as triple antigen at 2, 3 and 4 months with a booster of dual antigen (diphtheria and tetanus) at 4 years[7] followed by regular re-immunization every ten years.
2. Tetanus immunity should be reviewed before elective surgery.
3. Early diagnosis is essential and the patient should be given human tetanus immunoglobulin (HTIG) and admitted to hospital.
4. In the absence of HTIG antitetanus serum (ATS) may be used but this is derived from horse serum and may cause anaphylaxis.
5. During the phase of acute spasms the patient will require neuro-muscular blockade and maintenance on a respirator.

FOLLOW-UP

Survivors of tetanus will have life-long immunity. There is no danger of cross infection from infected individuals. Follow-up may be necessary if there is permanent neurological deficit but this is rare.

[1] Edmondson RS, Flowers MW (1979) Intensive care in tetanus: management, complications and mortality in 100 cases. *British Medical Journal*, **1**, 1401.
[2] Editorial (1985) Diphtheria and tetanus boosters. *Lancet*, **1**, 1081–2.
[3] OPCS (1978) Statistics of Infectious Disease.
[4] Public Health Lab. Services (1985) CDSC Report. *B.M.J.*, **290**, 696–7.
[5] Stanfield JP, Galazka A, (1984) Bulletin WHO **62(4)**, 647–69.
[6] Lucas AO, Gilles HM (1984) *Preventive Medicine for the Tropics*, 2nd edn, pp. 253–6. London: Hodder and Stoughton.
[7] Velimvoric B (1984) Infectious diseases in Europe, p. 312. Copenhagen: World Health Organisation.

Scarlet Fever

This disease is caused by erythrogenic strains of the *β-haemolytic streptococcus* (*Strep. pyogenes* Lancefield group A) and occasionally a similar disease may be produced by strains of *staphylococci* which produce erythrotoxic and exfoliative enzymes[1]. The organism gains entry through the throat (but may occasionally infect a wound giving rise to surgical scarlet fever). After 1–2 days incubation there is an acute febrile illness with sore throat, and the typical 'strawberry' appearance of the tongue. The rash appears on the face sparing the circumoral area and is a punctate erythema. Pastia's sign, of staining in the limb flexures may be present. After 4–5 days there is the so called branny desquamation.

PROGNOSIS

- The *β-haemolytic streptococcus* has undergone many changes in virulence throughout history. Though now a relatively benign disease, in 1881 scarlet fever was described as 'an angel of Death with an irreperable warrant to destroy' especially children. Diseases caused by the *β-haemolytic streptococcus*, particularly scarlet fever and rheumatic fever, have waxed and waned in severity following changes in the virulence of the organism.
- Early this century scarlet fever was a severe life-threatening disease either during the acute phase or due to secondary glomerulo-nephritis or rheumatic fever, its mortality rate is now assessed at less than 0.5% in the USA.
- Later complications include renal (secondary to glomerulo-nephritis) and cardiac failure due to stenosis of the mitral or aortic valves following rheumatic fever. The latter occurs particularly in the Third World[2].
- The World Health Organisation report a pan-European increase in the incidence of scarlet fever in the five years up to 1984; this is not associated with increased late sequalae of the disease.
- Steptococcal disease not only undergoes periodic changes in severity but is also seen at its

more severe in conditions of poverty, malnutrition, overcrowding and poor hygiene. Thus scarlet fever, rheumatic fever, puerpural fever and erysipelas are all more severe in developing rather than in developed countries.

TREATMENT

1. Often the disease is so mild as to be unrecognized and self-limiting.
2. The risk of rheumatic fever and glomerulonephritis is still present. When scarlet fever is diagnosed the drug of choice is penicillin.
3. Patients who have suffered rheumatic fever should be protected against recurrence with phenoxymethyl penicillin 500 mg daily for 5 years in adults and 250 mg daily throughout the school years in children. Prophylactic amoxycillin in a dose of 3 g should be given 1 hour before dental procedures in patients with cardiac prostheses or damaged heart valves[4].
4. Staphylococcal scarlet fever will require specific antibiotics following culture of the organism and its sensitivity.

5. A practical point is to be aware of grandmaternal anxiety from the days when scarlet fever was serious. The name can easily give rise to alarm so the synonym of scarlatina may be much less frightening.

FOLLOW-UP

Because of the possibility of renal involvement the urine of all children with diagnosed scarlet fever should be examined for protein ten days or more after recovery from the disease.

[1] Hull R (1987) *Infective Disease in Primary Care*. London: Chapman and Hall.
[2] Lucas AO, Gilles HM (1984) *Preventive Medicine for the Tropics*, 2nd edn, pp. 253–6. London: Hodder and Stoughton.
[3] Velimvoric B, Greco D, Piergentili P *et al.* (1984) Figures and trends for selected infectious diseases in Europe 1950–1980. In *Infectious Diseases in Europe*. Copenhagen: World Health Organisation.
[4] British National Formulary No 12 (1986) p. 188.

The Meningitides

Infection of the CNS may effect the meninges (meningitis) the brain (encephalitis) or the spinal cord (myelitis). In fact infection is rarely limited to one or other structure, however there may be a predominance of meningeal as opposed to brain or cord inflammation in bacterial infections whereas viral infections are often more encephalitic or encephalomyelitic. For this reason bacterial disease is listed in this section and viral disease under encephalitis (see p. 225). This distinction is more of convenience than reality[1].

Bacterial causes of meningitis include:
- *Haemophilus influenzae*
- *Neisseria meningitidis* (the meningococcus)
- *Streptococcus pneumoniae* (the pneumococcus)
(these three organisms account for approximately 60%, 20% and 10% of all cases of meningitis respectively)
- *Mycobacterium tuberculosis*
- rarely *Escherichia Coli, Pseudomonas spp, Klebsiella spp, Listeria monocytogenes* and many others.

Meningococcal meningitis (spotted fever)

This disease is declining in Europe[2] but there has been an epidemic[3,4] in Gloucestershire in 1984–8 and similar epidemics in Belgium, Finland and Norway occurred[5] in the 1970s. About 20% of bacterial meningitis is caused by the meningococcus which chiefly affects young adults. The organism enters through the throat causing bacteraemia during which constitutional upset may vary from minimal to profound suprarenal failure (the Waterhouse Friedrichsen syndrome). In about half the cases there is a sparse rose or purplish macular rash but this is easily overlooked. Later the patient develops symptoms and signs of meningeal irritation; headache, vomiting and neck stiffness.

PROGNOSIS

- During the bacteraemic phase the bacteria may concentrate in the suprarenal giving rise to haemorrhage and life threatening and cataclysmic shock.
- Death may occur in the acute phase, particularly if diagnosis is delayed. In the Icelandic epidemic of 1975–7 the mortality rate was 16 out of 168 cases (9.5%).
- Recovery may be associated with long-term neurological disorders including hydrocephalus and mental impairment.
- There may be cranial nerve damage (particularly to sixth and eighth nerves) giving rise to squint and deafness and there may be iridochoroiditis leading to loss of sight.
- There may also be associated arthritis and extravasation of blood into the skin leading to necrosis of large areas of skin[6].

TREATMENT

1. Prompt diagnosis and admission to hospital may be life saving when intravenous penicillin is effective.
2. In the Waterhouse Friedrichsen syndrome immediate steroid replacement is required. Intravenous hydrocortisone in large dose (e.g. 500 mg) may maintain life until the patient can be admitted to an intensive care unit but critical evidence of the value of such treatment is lacking[7].

FOLLOW-UP

There is often complete recovery but long-term neurological deficit, deafness or ophthalmoplegia may require life-long management.

Where meningococcal meningitis occurs in epidemics (e.g. in Gloucestershire during 1984–8) conditions leading to overcrowding, such as schools, barracks etc., should be avoided. Rifampicin 600 mg should be given twice daily for two days (5–10 mg/kg for children) to close contacts who must be observed for early signs of the disease.

Polysaccharide vaccines are available against many strains of meningococci and provide the most effective means of controlling an epidemic.

Pneumococcal meningitis

Pneumococcal meningitis is less common but clinically similar to meningococcal meningitis. It tends to affect adults, particularly alcoholics. The infection is blood borne usually from a focus in the sinuses, middle ear or lower respiratory tract. Patients who suffer from sickle cell disease or who have been splenectomized are particularly prone to pneumococcal infections[8].

PROGNOSIS

- The mortality rate of meningitis due to the pneumococcus is greater than that of meningococcal meningitis but there is no risk of suprarenal failure.
- Permanent neurological deficit may occur.
- Individuals who have undergone splenectomy are susceptible to overwhelming postsplenectomy infection (OPSI) which is due to pneumococcal infection in 50–90% of cases[8].

TREATMENT

1. The pneumococcus responds to intravenous penicillin (10–20 mg/kg up to 24 mg daily).
2. Patients at risk due to sickle cell disease or splenectomy should be protected by immunization with polyvalent pneumococcal vaccine (e.g. Pneumovax (Morson) 0.5 ml s/c) it should not be given to children under 2 years old who should be treated with oral phenoxymethylpenicillin 250 mg daily.

FOLLOW-UP

Often there is complete recovery but long-term neurological deficit, deafness or ophthalmoplegia may require life-long management.

Haemophilus meningitis

Meningitis caused by *H. influenzae* is common in

children under the age of six and can be quite undramatic in its early stages but increasing fever, drowsiness, headache, photophobia and vomiting are suggestive. Later neck stiffness develops but this may be less severe than in pneumococcal or meningococcal meningitis.

PROGNOSIS

The mortality from haemophilus meningitis is much less than coccal variants of the disease. There may however be long-term CNS damage with mental impairment.

TREATMENT

- In addition to general supportive treatment, ampicillin (200–400mg/(kg·d)) is the usual antibiotic.
- Since up to 35% of strains of haemophilus are resistant, chloramphenicol (100 mg/(kg·d)) is now recommended in addition.

FOLLOW-UP

Often there is complete recovery but long-term neurological deficit, deafness or ophthalmoplegia may require life-long management.

Other acute bacterial meningitides

Meningitis due to infections with *Escherichia, Pseudomonas, Klebsiella* or *Listeria* may occur in neonates or immuno-suppressed adults. Treatment is with ampicillin and an aminoglycoside such as gentamicin.

Tuberculous meningitis

This chronic form of meningitis is usually part of disseminated tuberculosis and occurs in children and young adults.

PROGNOSIS

- With prompt diagnosis and treatment the condition now has a good prognosis.

TREATMENT

1. Treatment depends on regimens consisting of isoniazid combined with streptomycin, rifampicin or ethambutol.

[1] Hull R (1987) *Infective Disease in Primary Care*. London: Chapman and Hall.

[2] Velimrovic B, Greco D, Piergentili P *et al.* (1984) Figures and trends for selected infectious diseases in Europe, 1950–1980. In *Infectious Diseases in Europe* (Velimvoric B ed.). Copenhagen: WHO.

[3] News (1986) *Nature*, **324,** 97.

[4] Davey PG, Cruikshank JK, McManus IC *et al.* (1982) Bacterial menigitis diagnosis and initial antibiotic therapy. *J. Hygiene*, **88,** 383–401.

[5] Dagbjartsson A, Ludvigsson P (1987) Bacterial meningitis—ten *Paediatric Clinics of North America*, **34, 1,** 219–30.

[6] Emond RTD (1974) *A Colour Atlas of Infectious Diseases*. London: Wolfe Medical Books.

[7] *The British National Formulary*. No 12 (1986).

[8] Reid D, Pinkerton IW (1986) *Treatment and Prognosis: Medicine*. (Hawkins R ed.) Oxford: Heinemann.

Encephalitis

A very wide range of organisms including viruses, possibly slow viruses (as in Kuru, Creutzfeldt-Jakob, subacute sclerosing panencephalitis and perhaps encephalitis lethargica), fungi (*candida, cryptococcus*), spirochaetes (syphilis, leptospirosis), protozoa (amoebae, malaria, toxoplasmosis) and helminths (*Taenia echinococcus, Toxacara spp.*) may give rise to brain inflammation[1].

There are many viral causes of encephalitis which are listed[1,2] in Table 9.1. Encephalitis is frequently quite a trivial disease complicating influenza and other viral illnesses and so its true incidence is unknown. Some of the viral encephalitides are life threatening or cause serious neurological handicap[3]. A large number of arboviruses may give rise to geographically localized zoonotic encephalitides which are transmitted to man by arthropod vectors. These diseases include equine encephalitis (in the Americas) and tick borne encephalitis (TBE) which is the most important of these diseases in Europe[4]. TBE is seen with increasing frequency from Southern Siberia to Britain and it exists in a reservoir of small mammals from whom it is transmitted to man by tick bite.

Table 9.1
Classification of Viral Encephalitides

Arboviruses (arthropod transmitted zoonosis)

Virus	Animal host	Arthropod vector
Western equine encephalitis	Horse	Mosquito
Eastern equine encephalitis	Horse	Mosquito
Venezuelan equine encephalitis	Horse	Mosquito
St Louis encephalitis	Rodents and birds	Mosquito
Japanese B encephalitis	Pigs and birds	Mosquito
Murray Valley	Birds	Mosquito
Yellow fever	Monkeys	Mosquito
Dengue		Mosquito
Tick-borne encephalitis (TBE)	Rodents, birds Sheep/cattle/goats	Tick

Other viruses

Rabies	Herpes simplex	Lymphocytic choriomeningitis
Poliomyelitis	Herpes zoster	Encephalomyocarditis
Coxsackie A and B	Influenza	Cytomegalovirus
Mumps	Psittacosis	*Mycoplasma pneumoniae*
Measles	Infectious hepatitis	
ECHO	Infectious mononucleosis	

Encephalitis may occur after many of the exanthematous diseases of childhood and may complicate some forms of immunization. The encephalitis caused by Herpes simplex is particularly dangerous with a high mortality.

The slow virus diseases, such as Russian spring–summer, Kuru and subacute sclerosing panencephalitis, are attracting interest because similarities with other diseases suggest that there may be a slow viral cause of multiple sclerosis and Alzheimer's disease.

Encephalitis lethargica was a presumed viral disease which erupted with a worldwide pandemic in the 1920s. Many people died in the acute phase and others passed into the strange twilight state of post-encephalitic Parkinsonism[5].

Syphilis is now a rare cause of neurological disease (general paralysis of the insane, Tabes dorsalis). Cryptococcosis and candidiasis may cause encephalitis, as may some protozoa in cases of impaired immunity, especially AIDS. The Human Immune Virus also causes encephalitis.

PROGNOSIS

- The mortality of TBE varies from 1–20% suggesting that the clinical picture may comprise more than one disease.
- The prognosis in the various forms of encephalitis is immensely variable between diseases and between individuals with the same disease.
- All may be comparatively trivial and all may lead to death, or permanent neurological deficit.
- Herpes simplex encephalitis has a mortality of 80%.

TREATMENT

1. This is largely supportive. Severely ill patients, especially those with Herpes simplex infections, should be nursed in an intensive care unit. Epilepsy will require control with phenytoin or i.v. diazepam and treatment with steroids, such as dexamethasone 20 mg daily, should be started. Antiviral agents are of no proven value but where they are used acyclovir or intravenous adenine arabinoside should be tried.

FOLLOW-UP

This may be required for long-term neurological difficulties.

[1] Hull R (1987) *Infective Disease in Primary Care*. London: Chapman and Hall.
[2] Gilroy J, Stirling Meyer J (1979) *Medical Neurology*, 3rd edn. New York: Macmillan.
[3] Ashworth B, Saunders M (1985) *Management of Neurological Disorders*. London: Butterworth.
[4] Velimrovic B (1984) The challenge of tropical, unusual and 'new' diseases in Europe. In *Infectious Diseases in Europe* (Velimvoric B ed.). Copenhagen: World Health Organisation.
[5] Sacks O (1982) *Awakenings*. London: Picador.

Herpes Simplex

This virus occurs as two types; type I gives rise to common circumoral or gingivo-stomal vesicles or shallow ulcers. Ocular manifestations include dendritic ulcers, whose diagnosis is important because of risks of perforation of the globe following treatment with steroids. Type II gives rise to herpes genitalis[1] (*see* p. 321).

Type I oro-pharyngeal lesions are activated after upper respiratory infections or trauma. Rarely herpes simplex I causes severe encephalitis especially in neonates. The possibility should be considered in any febrile child with focal seizures and neurological signs. Both herpes simplex viruses cause widespread problems in the immuno-suppressed and as such are of growing importance in AIDS[2].

PROGNOSIS

- Apart from encephalitis (vide supra) is uniformly good.
- Herpes encephalitis has an overall mortality of 80%, may be fatal in the acute stage or may leave permanent neurological lesions.
- Recurrence of the oral lesions are to be expected. Possible triggers include bright sunlight, cold or viral upper respiratory tract infections.

TREATMENT

1. Symptomatic treatment or oral lesions is sufficient.
2. Ocular lesions must *never* be treated with steroids or severe panophthalmitis or perforation may occur. Eye lesions require urgent referral and treatment with acyclovir eye drops.
3. Severe herpetic infections may be treated with adenine arabinoside (vidarabine) which may also be used intravenously in herpes encephalitis.

4. Recurrent oral lesions may be avoided by the use of complete sunscreens before sun exposure.
5. Topical acyclovir cream will shorten duration of oral lesions, especially if used at the onset of parastresiae and before the ulcers have appeared. Cream should be applied 4 hourly for 5 days.

FOLLOW-UP

The herpes viruses are extremely infectious and patients should be warned of the risk of kissing, and cross infection from towels, cutlery and drinking vessels.

[1] Brett EM (1986) Herpes simplex virus encephalitis in children. *British Medical Journal*, **293,** 1388–9.
[2] Greenspan D, Greenspan JS, Pindborg JJ *et al.* (1986) *AIDS and the Dental Team.* Copenhagen: Munksgaard.
[3] Whitley RJ, Seng-Jaw S, Hirsch M (1981) Herpes simplex encephalitis: vidarabine therapy and diagnostic problems. *N. Engl. J. Med.*, **304,** 313–18.

Influenza

Influenza is an acute epidemic disease whose explosive nature throughout history has produced recurring pandemics. The disease is caused by a group of rapidly mutating myxoviruses leading to epidemics of different character of which some are fairly trivial but others such as that in 1918 killed more than the war which preceded it. Though the disease is rarely so serious it accounts for a huge amount of morbidity.

PROGNOSIS

- Uncomplicated influenza lasts a few days or a week and recovery is usually complete and spontaneous.
- Secondary chest infection may complicate the disease especially in the elderly or debilitated.
- Death rates vary with epidemics and are usually due to secondary infection of which acute staphylococcal pneumonia is the most serious.
- A rare complication of influenza in children is Reye's Syndrome occurring in 7 per million children under 16 with a mortality of over 40% and characterized by liver failure and encephalopathy. The association with influenza and other virus diseases is not clear but a relationship with treatment by aspirin has been confirmed.

TREATMENT

1. Influenza rarely requires anything more than rest and symptomatic therapy.

2. Secondary chest infection may require antibiotics.
3. The great antigenic variability of the disease makes vaccination programmes difficult: one tends to be vaccinating against strains that have gone rather than those that are coming. However vaccination of people in closed communities; schools, barracks, old persons' homes may limit epidemics and reduce morbidity and perhaps mortality.

FOLLOW-UP

Patients recovering from influenza may be particularly prone to depressive illnesses.

Hull R (1987) *Infective Disease in Primary Care*. London: Chapman and Hall.

Typhoid (enteric fever)

Typhoid fever is caused by *Salmonella typhi*. Shortly after ingestion of the organism in water or contaminated food there may be transient, slight diarrhoea which is followed by constipation. About a week after infection the patient develops vague rather influenzal symptoms, fever, cough, malaise and myalgia. The temperature climbs daily in a step-like chart and at this stage the picture is one of pyrexia of undetermined origin. In the second week the temperature is less swinging but the patient is more severely ill with ileitis due to concentration of the salmonella in Peyers patches which are acutely inflamed, ulcerated and may perforate. At this stage there may be diarrhoea and the classical 'rose spots' of typhoid. Early diagnosis which depends on being aware of the possibility and on culture of the salmonellae from blood is essential. Typhoid has been declining in Britain by 50% every 10 years[1] and is now most commonly seen (90%) in patients returning from travel outside Europe especially the Indian subcontinent[2].

PROGNOSIS

- The mortality in well treated cases is about 2%.
- The course in children is often mild but elderly and debilitated patients do badly.
- Complications worsen prognosis: towards the end of the second week there may be haemorrhage into the gut in up to 8% and death may occur from perforation (which causes about 25% of deaths), toxaemia, pneumonia or meningitis.
- Up to 15% of patients may relapse.
- Residual carrier states occur frequently and convalescent patients need to be investigated by urine and faecal culture. Persistent carriers will need counselling about their work and exclusion from food handling. There may be a focus of infection in the gall bladder and cholecystectomy should be considered.

TREATMENT

1. The drug of choice is still chloramphenicol in a dose of 500 mg six hourly. The patient's white count should be monitored to exclude lecopaenia, thrombocytopaenia or aplastic anaemia which complicate the use of chloramphenicol.
2. Some strains of *S. typhi* are not sensitive to chloramphenicol when ampicillin or co-trimoxazole may be used.

FOLLOW-UP

Typhoid is a notifiable disease. Where possible it should be prevented and travellers, particularly in Third World tropical countries should be given hygienic advice not to eat green salads, damaged or unpeeled fruit. Care should also be taken with local water supplies and where their use is unavoidable boiling or sterilization with hypochlorite tablets should be advised. Immunization with a suspension of killed *Salmonella typhi* organisms confers partial immunity but is no substitute for good food hygiene.

[1] Cvjetanovic B (1978) Bulletin, WHO, **56** (suppl), 45–65.
[2] *Public Health Laboratory Service Communicable Diseases Surveillance Centre* (1983). *Br. Med. J.* **287**, 1205.

Cholera

Cholera is a waterborne enteritic disease caused by a vibrio. Classical cholera, caused by *Vibrio cholerae*, has been responsible for untold millions of deaths throughout the world. A 1987 pandemic caused by the strain known as El Tor (named after a quarantine centre in Egypt where the strain was identified in 1920) spread throughout the Mediterranean, Asia, North Africa and the Middle East[1]. Cholera last occurred as an epidemic in London in 1854. In 1832 an epidemic in Yorkshire gave rise to 1347 cases with 400 deaths. Another allied organism *V. parahaemolyticus* occurs in sea and estuarine water and may give rise to a profuse but self-limiting diarrhoea. Cholera is characterized by profuse hypersecretion of electrolytes and fluid from the gut (so called 'rice and water stools') which may lead to death from dehydration.

PROGNOSIS

- Classical cholera was very frequently fatal due to dehydration and shock.
- In untreated cholera the mortality ranges from 20–80%.
- The El Tor strain is less severe.
- With good management mortality is reduced to 2%.

TREATMENT

1. Treatment of both classical and El Tor strains depends on replacement of the enormous fluid and electrolyte loss.
2. The organism is sensitive to tetracycline which should be prescribed in a dose of 500 mg six hourly for 48 hours, if the organism is sensitive then chloramphenicol 500 mg six hourly may be added.
3. Vaccines for cholera offer only partial protection against the classical and El Tor strains. Adults may be given two injections of 0.5 ml i.m. at least one week and preferably four weeks apart. Children require smaller dose according to age. Booster doses are required at six month intervals.

FOLLOW-UP

Strict control of infected material is required to contain epidemics.

[1] Velimrovic B (1984) Epidemiology and control of foodborne diseases in Europe. In *Infectious diseases in Europe*. Copenhagen: World Health Organisation.

Malaria

Malaria is the commonest infective disease in the world after dental caries. It occurs naturally between latitudes 60° North and 40° South but is increasingly seen outside these areas due to air transport of infected mosquitoes or individuals already in the pro-dromal stages of infection. Malaria is caused by protozoa of the genus *Plasmodium* notably *P. falciparum, vivax, malariae* and *ovale*. Of these the first two, causing malignant and benign tertian malaria, are the most important. The plasmodia are transferred by the Anopheles mosquito. Malaria presents with protean symptoms and should be considered in all febrile travellers no matter what their symptoms. Suspicion of malaria demands examination of thick blood films[1]. Malaria notifications in Britain vary between 750 and 2000 per year[2].

PROGNOSIS

- Malignant malaria due to *P. falciparum* is fatal in over 10% of cases due to cerebral, renal or gastrointestinal complications.
- Though most life threatening, falciparum malaria may be cured when correctly treated.
- Less virulent forms, e.g. vivax and ovale may be more difficult to eradicate and may lead to recurring bouts of malaria for up to 5 years following original infection.

TREATMENT

1. This depends on the organism and its particular strain especially in regions of SE Asia and parts of Latin America where malarial parasites are frequently chloroquine resistant.
2. Updated information or special advice may be needed about these areas of chloroquine resistance from experts in tropical medicine. Where parasites are still sensitive to chloroquine this should be used in dosage of 600 mg, followed by 300 mg after 6 hours followed by 300 mg on each of the next 2–4 days. Where chloroquine resistant parasites occur the drug combination of pyremethamine and dapsone or pyremathamine and sulphadoxine are usually recommended.
3. In chloroquine-sensitive malarial zones the choice of prophylaxis rests between proguanil (100–200 mg daily) pyremethamine (25 mg weekly) or chloroquine (300 mg weekly). A daily dose is often easier to remember. Pyremethamine and Dapsone (Maloprim) one tablet or proguanil 100 mg should be taken in addition if there is any doubt about the presence of resistant parasites.
4. The commonest reason for consultation about malaria concerns chemoprophylaxis. Increasingly people are visiting malarial zones on holiday and at the same time malarial protozoa are evolving resistance to treatment. Rules of malaria prophylaxis:
   a. Avoidance of exposure to mosquitoes by use of protective clothing, mosquito nets and insect repellents is sensible but not always feasible.
   b. Antimalarials must be taken from the day before until 6 weeks after returning. *Even when taken properly they do not confer absolute immunity but markedly reduce risk.*
   c. Never believe local accounts that a zone is malaria free.
   d. An open aircraft door in a malaria zone may allow in a mosquito: such stopovers, however short, require proper chemoprophylaxis.
   e. Great care must be taken in certain malaria zones where resistant forms of malaria change very rapidly.

FOLLOW-UP

Malaria is a notifiable disease in the UK and is under surveillance by WHO which is promoting a world wide eradication programme.

[1] Hull R (1987) *Infective Disease in Primary Care*. London: Chapman & Hall.
[2] Velimrovic B (1984) *Infectious Diseases in Europe*. Copenhagen: WHO.

10

Dermatology

V. W. M. Drury

Acne Vulgaris

Teenage acne is an endocrine disease of pilosebaceous glands. The relationship between the condition and the levels of androgen is however unclear. Up to 80% of adolescents will have some degree of acne and the lesions occur on the areas with most sebaceous glands. Comedones (blackheads) are a mixture of keratin and sebum; excessive production of these materials blocking the openings are the essential lesion, which may then progress to pustules, cysts and scarring.

PROGNOSIS

- Acne usually lasts from puberty to late teens or early 20s but occasionally (in 1–2%) it may persist to middle age[1].
- About 3–4% of boys and 0.5% of girls suffer severe acne with scarring[2].
- Treatment is effective in most cases.

TREATMENT

1. A sympathetic response from the general practitioner to requests for treatment is important as the psychological disturbance may be out of proportion to the degree of disfigurement.
2. There is little evidence that diet or frequent washing of the area helps. Advice to wash may be taken as implying a lack of personal cleanliness and will add to the patient's embarrassment.
3. Ultraviolet light may be helpful to some patients, probably as it causes the skin to peel. However, some patients' acne is made worse by it.
4. Removal of comedones by an extractor after bathing the area with hot water may help but too much squeezing and manipulation may encourage pustule formation. Local preparations, such as 1–5% sulphur in a cream base, may help as a keratolytic but benzoyl peroxide 5 or 10% (Panoxyl, Benoxyl, Acetoxyl) may be more effective. If the skin becomes sore, treatment should be withheld for a day or two, or a non-alcohol base for the benzoyl peroxide should be used (e.g. Panoxyl aquagel).

5. Oxytetracycline 250 mg b.d. for at least 2 to 4 months is the mainstay of oral treatment. It should be gradually tailed off and not stopped suddenly. It must not be taken with milk or alkalis. Erythromycin 250 mg b.d. is an alternative.
6. Initial doses may be doubled in severe cases or during bad flare-ups.
7. Antiandrogens will suppress sebum formation and can be used in women. A contraceptive pill with ethinyloestradiol and cyproterone acetate (Dianette) is available, but feminization of the male fetus has occurred when taken mistakenly during early pregnancy.
8. In severe acne with scarring a synthetic retinoid, 13-cis-retinoic acid has proved effective. The patients should be referred to a dermatologist for supervision. This drug is teratogenic.
9. Surgery is sometimes required for large cysts or to deal with extensive scarring. Dermabrasion is the commonest employed surgical technique.

FOLLOW-UP

Patients should be seen regularly until the control of the condition satisfies them. They may then be encouraged to return if the acne recurs.

[1] Cumliffe WJ, Cotterill W (1975) The Acnes—Clinical Features, Pathogenesis and Treatment. London: WB Saunders/Lloyd Luke.
[2] Kligman AM (1974) J. Invest. Dermatol., **62**, 268.

Acne Rosacea

Acne rosacea is a disorder of the blood vessels of the face affecting mainly middle-aged females. It produces pustules, papules and telangiectases on the cheeks, chin and nose primarily. Stress plays some part in its production but the cause is unknown. It may affect all or part of the face, and tends to wax and wane in severity. Rhinophyma, a condition with hypertrophy of the nose, is a complication, as are keratitis and ulceration of the cornea. The main problem produced by the condition is a cosmetic one.

PROGNOSIS

- Rosacea tends to be a relapsing condition persisting for several years. Because of the psychological effect, patients suffering from the condition need especially sympathetic handling.
- Control can usually be effected by careful treatment.

TREATMENT

1. Careful reassurance and explanation of the nature of the condition is an important first step. Attention to causes of stress is important.
2. Reduction of foodstuffs which promote vasodilatation is advisable. These include alcohol, highly spiced foods, strong tea and coffee.
3. Oral oxytetracycline is the most effective treatment. It should be given in a dose of 250 mg twice daily and continued for several weeks. It should not be taken with milk or alkalis which hinder absorption or within 1 hour of food. Metronidazole 200 mg daily for 6 weeks is an alternative if this fails.
4. Local treatment with 1–2% sulphur in a cream base may help but topical steroids are not advised.
5. Eye complications or rhinophyma need referral for specialist advice.

FOLLOW-UP

Follow-up should be continued monthly until the condition is under control. The patient should be encouraged to return to the general practitioner if there is a relapse.

Eczema

Eczema is an inflammatory condition of the skin. Features include redness, swelling, blistering, scaling, thickening and fissuring, depending upon the severity of the condition and the part of the body involved. Eczema is currently classified as either *exogenous*, when an external factor acts as an irritant or allergen, or *endogenous*, when there are no specific external causes but such factors as immunological deficiency, abnormality of sebum secretion or venous stasis may precipitate the various types of eczema. The morphological features are the same whatever the cause.

Exogenous eczema is subdivided into allergic eczema and irritant eczema; endogenous eczema encompasses atopic, seborrhoeic, pompholyx, discoid and varicose eczema.

Allergic eczema

Allergic reactions to ingested substances, food additives or drugs may manifest themselves dermatologically in a variety of ways, ranging from anaphylactic purpura to blistering, erythemata and urticaria. Penicillin accounts for more than 50% of drug reactions[1], and salicylates make up the largest part of the remainder. Rashes are usually of sudden onset, widespread and itchy. They occur 1–6 weeks after starting the drug.

PROGNOSIS

- Once established, a true allergic response will occur whenever the patient is exposed to the allergen.
- Acute urticaria occurs within a few hours and may last from minutes to a few days. Chronic urticaria may last from months to many years and can be very difficult to treat.
- Infrequent ingestion of the allergen does not protect and is more likely to aggravate allergy than to produce tolerance.
- In general, drug rashes do not persist after the withdrawal of the drug[2].

TREATMENT

1. The best treatment is the identification of the allergen and its avoidance. This may be easy with an acute urticaria or rash but is otherwise difficult.
2. Skin testing is unprofitable because of false negatives, difficulty in interpretation of positives and risk of anaphylaxis.
3. Antihistamines in adequate dose—terfenadine (Triludan) 10 mg twice daily or astemizole (Hismanal) 10 mg three times daily—should be used for 2 or 3 days.
4. If the urticaria is painful or persistent, oral prednisolone 15 mg daily for 2 or 3 days is effective.
5. Anaphylaxis or angio-oedema of the upper respiratory tract requires adrenaline 1/1000 0.5 ml subcutaneously, consideration of intubation or tracheostomy and hydrocortisone 100 mg intravenously.

FOLLOW-UP

Those patients who have had an allergen identified need no special follow-up beyond emphasizing the need to avoid the allergen. Those in whom no allergen has been identified may require regular follow-up to provide symptomatic relief.

Contact eczema

Contact eczema shows itself as severe itching, swelling, tenderness, reddening or a weeping exudation. It most commonly affects the hands but for reasons not understood may spread to distant parts of the body. It may be caused by the irritating nature of the substance itself or may be directly allergenic. When it is due to a constituent of the ointment being used for the treatment of endogenous eczema it may be exceedingly difficult to diagnose.

PROGNOSIS

- Removal of the offending substance invariably leads to a cure but in the case of housewives' hands where it is due to detergents, constant wetting and cold, drying winds it may be difficult to eradicate.

● Patch-testing can be helpful in establishing the cause.

TREATMENT

1. If further exposure to the causative agent is avoided no further treatment is necessary. If this is not achieved no treatment will avail.
2. Rubber gloves with cotton linings should be worn, since sensitivity to the rubber can occur.
3. Topical antihistamines or anaesthetics must be avoided.
4. In the acute stages a weeping lesion should be treated with compresses or soaks. Potassium permanganate 1:8000 solution soaks for hands and feet should be used for 15 minutes three times a day, although this will stain skin and clothing. Physiological saline compresses are suitable for other parts and produce no staining.
5. When the lesion is dry, 1% hydrocortisone cream can be applied three times daily. Stronger steroids should be used only in resistant cases.
6. A cream containing sodium fusidate should be used if secondary infection occurs.
7. A sedative antihistamine such as promethazine 10–25 mg can be used at night if irritation keeps the patient awake.

FOLLOW-UP

No follow-up is needed once the condition has cleared.

Atopic eczema

Atopic eczema is the result of a genetic disposition and is associated with asthma, hayfever, a tendency towards migraine, allergy to insect bites and urticaria. It occurs in up to 10% of all children, although in most of these it is very mild. In 70% of cases there is a positive family history of atopy. Atopic eczema is not present at birth and rarely appears before 3 months of age[4].

PROGNOSIS

● In 90% of children with atopic eczema the eczema will clear by 15 years of age[5].
● Where eczema persists it will occur most commonly in the flexures and on the hands and the condition will become less severe with the passage of time.
● Skin dryness, anxiety, heat, local irritation and perhaps food are trigger factors.

TREATMENT

1. Time spent in careful explanation to the parents is most important. They should feel able to consult the general practitioner whenever they are worried. Nails should be kept short and cool, loose cotton clothing worn.
2. Bland emollients such as aqueous cream and emulsifying ointment should be used on the skin and as a soap substitute. Bath additives, like oilatum emollient, should be used. Bathing in tepid water (preferably soaking for 10 minutes) should be encouraged daily.
3. Topical steroids are the main standby though it should be made clear to parents that they are suppressive and not curative. Usually 1% hydrocortisone ointment is sufficiently strong. It should be used on the face rarely and sparely. Occasionally a stronger steroid (group 2 or group 3) is needed for short periods (2 or 3 weeks) in older children for a local flare-up. It is better to use a strong steroid for a short period than a moderate steroid for a longer time.
4. Substitution of soya milk for cow's milk may be helpful in children who are not responding. Complete avoidance of cow's milk for the first 6 months of life for children of atopic parents may be helpful. Advice from a dietician may also be helpful.
5. A sedative antihistamine such as promethazine hydrochloride 1 hour before bedtime will be helpful in those children who cannot sleep because of the irritation.

FOLLOW-UP

Severely affected children need regular follow-up. Steroids should not be available on repeat prescriptions. Counselling may be required for school-leavers about reconsidering the choice of a career such as hairdressing or nursing in which contact with irritants is likely.

Discoid eczema

Discoid eczema is endogenous in origin but can follow an insect bite. It is commonest in young adults and consists of coin-shaped lesions symmetrically distributed and mainly on limbs and the back of the trunk. The face is rarely affected. The lesions are often very itchy and bathing in hot water aggravates.

PROGNOSIS

- The condition usually runs a course of one to two years before becoming quiescent[6].
- Despite a good response to treatment, relapses tend to occur[7].

TREATMENT

1. Lesions usually improve on moderate strength steroids applied twice daily though occasionally more potent varieties are needed short term.
2. Antihistamines may be helpful to control pruritus.
3. Proprietary coal-tar preparations are preferred by some patients.

FOLLOW-UP

Patients should be seen regularly until the condition clears. No patient on strong steroids should be allowed to use them without regular review.

Varicose eczema

This term, used synonomously with hypostatic eczema, describes the skin changes resulting from venous stasis due to high pressure in the superficial veins draining the leg. This may be due to congenital weakness or absence of venous valves or damage from phlebitis. It is seen most commonly over the inner shin.

PROGNOSIS

- Eczema may precede an ulcer but may be present for many years without the skin breaking down.
- Topical treatment will not produce a cure unless the underlying venous stasis is dealt with.

TREATMENT

1. Stasis is helped by raising the foot of the bed and elevating the limbs when sitting down.
2. Whilst walking is helpful, prolonged standing is harmful.
3. Supporting external pressure should be applied until the eczema is healed. It can consist of crêpe bandage, blueline bandage or viscopaste bandages left on for 2–3 weeks.
4. Topical treatment with wet dressings of either 1% silver nitrate solution or 1:10 000 potassium permanganate should be applied to wet eczema or ulcers. The important part of the treatment is proper support bandaging and elevation of the limb where possible. Regular dressing of ulcers by an experienced nurse is usually needed.
5. Referral to a surgeon should be considered for permanent cure of venous stasis, particularly for minor varices below the mid-thigh[8]. This gives good results in two-thirds of patients, although one-third develop recurrences[9].

FOLLOW-UP

Patients should be advised to return to the general practitioner if recurrence occurs or if support hose needs replacing.

Infantile seborrhoeic eczema

Infantile seborrhoeic eczema occurs in infants between the age of 6 weeks and 18 months. The aetiology is unknown. It presents as cradle cap, nappy rash or occasionally a more generalized form.

PROGNOSIS

- All these varieties of eczema will clear with simple treatment. In children the eczema usually resolves spontaneously after about 18 months of age.

TREATMENT

1. Cradle cap will respond to 1% sulphur and 1% salicylic acid in aqueous cream applied at night and removed with a gentle shampoo in the morning. Occasionally very piled-up lesions will require a stronger cream.
2. Nappy rash will respond to exposure of the affected part to the air, but this is not easily done. Keeping the area as dry as possible is the next best solution, and using 1% hydrocortisone cream. If a secondary infection with thrush occurs the steroid cream can be combined with nystatin.
3. Generalized seborrhoeic eczema may follow a nappy rash. The prognosis is excellent and the rash disappears when the infant is out of nappies.

FOLLOW-UP

No follow-up is necessary.

Adult seborrhoeic eczema

The adult variety of seborrhoeic eczema involves those areas of the skin containing most sebaceous glands, such as the scalp, the face—particularly the nasolabial folds—the exterior ear canals and the axillae, groins, submammary folds and the front of the chest. The cause is unknown but there is often a positive family history. Tension and anxiety seem to make the condition worse.

PROGNOSIS

● The condition is incurable. It may be persistent or episodic.
● With proper treatment it can be kept under control.

TREATMENT

1. Mild scalp disease needs frequent shampooing only. Tar-containing shampoos may be helpful in resistant cases. More severe cases will be helped by steroid-containing scalp lotions or

by local ketoconazote (Nizoral shampoo). Where there is thickened scaling on the scalp, 2% sulphur and 2% salicyclic acid in aqueous cream applied two or three times a week and shampooed in the morning will remove the plaques.
2. On the face 1% hydrocortisone cream used sparingly is the most effective treatment.
3. Trunk lesions also respond to topical steroids but these often have to be stronger (group 2 or 3) and intertrigo is frequently secondarily infected with thrush, especially where satellite lesions are present.

FOLLOW-UP

These patients are frequently on a repeat prescribing system. Arrangements should be made to ensure that they are seen periodically to check that the condition is under control.

Pompholyx eczema

This condition affects the sides of digits and the palms or soles of the feet. Characteristically sterile pustules occur.

PROGNOSIS

● The condition occurs in attacks lasting 2 or 3 weeks. It is worse in hot weather or in times of emotional tension.
● There may be periods of several years of freedom.

TREATMENT

1. In the weeping phase soaks of 1:8000 potassium permanganate help.
2. When lesions are dry 1% hydrocortisone cream will speed resolution.

FOLLOW-UP

Patients will need regular follow-up while the lesions are present. During remissions follow-up is not necessary.

[1] Fellner MJ (1976) Penicillin allergy. *Int. J. Dermatol.*, **15,** 497.
[2] Baker H (1980) Drug reactions. In *Textbook of Derma-*

tology, 3rd edn. Oxford: Blackwell Scientific Publications.
3 Atherton DJ (1981) Allergy and atopic eczema. *Clin. Exp. Dermatol.*, **6**, 317.
4 Harper J (1985) *Handbook of Paediatric Dermatology*. London: Butterworths.
5 Atherton DJ (1981) Allergy and atopic eczema. *Clin. Exp. Dermatol.*, **6**, 317.
6 Burrows D (1985) Eczema and associated conditions. In *Dermatology*, 3rd edn. (Hall-Smith R and Cairns RJ eds.) London: Butterworths & Co.
7 Fry L, Cornell MNP (1985) *Eczema in Dermatology*. Lancaster: MTP Press Limited.
8 Hobbs JT (1968) *Br. J. Surg.*, **55**, 777.
9 Lofgren KA (1978) In *Venous Problems* (Bergan JJ, Tao JST eds). Chicago: Year Book.

Psoriasis

Psoriasis affects 2% of the population in northern climates. Inheritance plays a part in its occurrence, but it may be that it only increases the susceptibility under certain conditions as there is a family history in only 30% of patients[1]. Psoriasis most commonly affects knees, elbows and scalp and is characterized by a 10-fold increase in speed of epidermal cell proliferation. Psoriasis can be aggravated by worry, trauma, certain drugs and streptococcal infection. It has a peak onset in young adults.

PROGNOSIS

- Once present, psoriasis tends to wax and wane throughout life.
- Remission, whether spontaneous or as a result of treatment, varies greatly in length but 40% of patients show remissions lasting a year or more[2].
- Guttate psoriasis carries a much better prognosis than other forms, especially in the absence of a family history.
- Arthritis occurs in 7% of patients[3].

TREATMENT

1. A sympathetic listening doctor is an important part of treatment, especially as cosmetic appearance is the major disability and may profoundly affect the patient's life.
2. No treatment at all may be needed for guttate psoriasis except for careful explanation. Irritation can be helped by a group II steroid.
3. If the disease is not widespread it can often be controlled by the use of group I or II steroid for 2 weeks. It is essential to avoid long-term use as tachyphylaxis occurs commonly.
4. Short-course dithranol can be used on limited lesions. Start with 0.1% dithranol and increase the strength if necessary. Proprietary brands such as Psoradrate, Psoriderm or Dithrol a can

be left in contact with the lesion for 1 hour daily and then washed off. It usually takes 3–4 weeks to clear the condition. Dithranol should not be used on the face, genitalia or intertriginous areas where steroid creams help.

5. It may be necessary to refer a patient to hospital for reassurance, admission for rest, or further treatment. Methotrexate, an antimetabolite, is used for severe unresponsive psoriasis. Psoralen and ultraviolet A (PUVA) therapy or oral retinoids are other forms of treatment that may be given.

FOLLOW-UP

Patients require the ability to consult and discuss their problems whenever they feel the need. Those receiving treatment with topical steroids or dithranol should be seen fortnightly until remission occurs.

The Psoriasis Association (7 Milton Street, Northampton; telephone 0604-711129) can be very supportive.

1 Abele DC (1963) *Arch. Dermatol.*, **88**, 38.
2 Baker H, Wilkinson DS (1974) Psoriasis. In *Textbook of Dermatology*, 3rd edn. Oxford: Blackwell Scientific Publications.
3 Ingram JT (1954) *Br. Med. J.*, **ii**, 823.

Bacterial Infections of the Skin

Commonly occurring bacterial infections are impetigo, folliculitis, boils and carbuncles. The commonest organism is *Staphylococcus aureus*, although *Streptococcus pyogenes* may be involved in impetigo, where there is a characteristically thick crust. Folliculitis is most common in the beard region (sycosis barbae). If the subcutaneous tissue is involved then a boil or carbuncle will occur. Boils of the nose and upper lip are particularly dangerous because of their ability to cause cavernous sinus thrombosis. The urine should be tested for glucose for all patients presenting with a boil. Cellulitis is most frequently caused by the streptococcus.

PROGNOSIS

- Unless the infection spreads resolution will be complete with appropriate treatment.
- A carbuncle may lead to an indented scar.

TREATMENT

1. Impetigo is highly contagious and measures to prevent spread such as avoiding direct contact, using separate towels etc. are required.
2. Crusts should be removed from impetiginous lesions by gentle bathing with cotton wool and warm water and then chlortetracycline (Aureomycin) cream applied four times a day.
3. Drainage of pus is the best treatment for boils. Local heat may encourage this but incision is sometimes required. Antibiotics are only required if infection seems to be spreading or a lesion persists. Flucloxacillin 250 mg four times daily is appropriate. Boils on the face should always be treated with flucloxacillin.
4. Cellulitis is usually due to the streptococcus. It is best treated with penicillin (e.g. Triplopen) by intramuscular injection every 3 days until resolution has occurred. Erythromycin 250 mg 6-hourly is an alternative in a penicillin-sensitive individual.
5. Recurrent boils can be treated by attempting to reduce the bacterial skin count using daily baths containing chlorhexidine 0.05%. Use of topical or oral antibiotics should be avoided since these will not prevent recurrences. Identification of carriers of the staphylococcus in the family using nasal swabs followed by treatment with an antiseptic cream in the nose, such as Naseptin, may help.

FOLLOW-UP

Patients should be seen regularly until resolution has occurred.

Fungal Infections of the Skin

Fungal infections of the skin, hair and nails are reported to general practitioners by about 1% of the population each year[1]. The fungus generally lives in the keratin of the skin and it is important to confirm the diagnosis by laboratory examination of skin scrapings, nail clippings or hairs. As different species have a predilection for different parts of the body this is used as a classification.

Tinea pedis

This accounts for more than half the cases of fungal infection of the skin. It is commonest in young and middle-aged males and is uncommon in children. Host susceptibility is the most important factor in spread and some people obviously have a high protection against the disease. The disease mainly occurs in the second to fourth interdigital spaces.

PROGNOSIS

- Fungal infection between the toes tends to be persistent and although it is possible to suppress the symptoms, recurrence usually occurs.
- Fungal infection elsewhere on the foot may recur in hot weather but the prognosis is better.
- Most patients develop resistance in middle age and the problem resolves.

TREATMENT

1. Only topical treatment is required for interdigital infection. Whitfield's ointment (benzoic acid 6%, salicyclic acid 3%), miconazole or clotrimazole should be applied daily after bathing for 6 weeks.
2. Wet or macerated areas may respond more rapidly to magenta paint.
3. Acute and blistering lesions are best treated with 1:8000 soaks of potassium permanganate four times daily or normal saline followed by 1% hydrocortisone cream.
4. Recurrence may be lessened by frequent washing followed by careful drying and foot powder and by wearing cool socks and sandals or shoes with ventilation.

FOLLOW-UP

No follow-up is necessary once symptoms have settled.

Tinea cruris

This is seen in young adults and the male:female incidence ratio is 4:1[2]. The infection starts in the groin and may spread to the thigh or buttock. It is most common in tropical countries and may be spread from foot to groin by towels.

PROGNOSIS

- Tinea cruris usually responds well to treatment without recurrence, except in sportsmen and women who are more exposed to the infection from communal changing rooms.

TREATMENT

1. Griseofulvin 500 mg daily for 1 month should be taken. Local treatment is less effective but magenta paint may help wet or macerated areas.

FOLLOW-UP

Follow-up is as for tinea pedis.

Tinea capitis

Tinea capitis is a disease of children. Specimens of hair and skin should be taken to distinguish it from alopecia areata.

PROGNOSIS

- Untreated, the condition may eventually be cured by the degree of inflammation but this may lead to scarring and permanent hair loss.
- If treated, hair will always regrow.

TREATMENT

1. Griseofulvin 125 mg three times daily should be taken for 6 weeks.

2. No other treatment is worth considering.

Tinea unguium

Ringworm infection of the nails is a disease of adults. It most frequently affects the toes in middle age and is most common in men. The diagnosis should be confirmed by nail and skin specimens but these may have to be taken on several occasions. The infection starts at the side of the nail, causing yellowish discoloration and later spreads to the nailbed, causing hyperkeratosis. It is not known why some people have tinea between the toes and never have nail infection, whereas in others both sites are involved.

PROGNOSIS

- Untreated, the infection may spread to all the nails on the affected foot or hand.
- Treatment of fingernails gives a high cure rate, although it may take 6 months for normal nails to appear.
- Treatment of toenail infection is more difficult and it may be 2 years before resolution is achieved.
- The relapse rate of toenail infection is very high, so many authorities feel treatment is not worth embarking upon[3].

TREATMENT

1. Griseofulvin 500 mg daily is standard treatment for fingernail infections. It has to be taken for 6 months, so the diagnosis must be confirmed before treatment is started.
2. Local treatment of nail infection is unsatisfactory.
3. Griseofulvin treatment (500 mg daily for 1 year) may occasionally be required for toenail infection if the nail is painful or in women who are disturbed by the appearance. An alternative for the latter situation is to give 1 month of treatment before removing the nail, continuing until the new nail has grown. Nevertheless recurrence is still common.

FOLLOW-UP

Follow-up is as for tinea pedis.

Tinea versicolor

Tinea versicolor is caused by the fungus *Pityrosporum obiculare* and produces fawn-coloured patches over the upper trunk, neck and upper limbs. It is often diagnosed because affected patches do not suntan.

PROGNOSIS

- Tinea versicolor responds well to treatment but there is a high incidence of reinfection.

TREATMENT

1. Half-strength Whitfield's ointment applied nightly to the whole upper trunk for 1 month will usually cure the condition.
2. Selenium sulphide (Selsun, Lenium shampoo) applied to the whole body—avoiding the face—and left on overnight is more acceptable but less effective. It can be repeated once after a week.
3. Miconazole nitrate 2% cream (Dermonistat) or Ketoconazole 2% cream (Nizoral) applied twice daily until 10 days after lesions have disappeared is also effective.

FOLLOW-UP

Examination of hair, nail clippings or skin scrapings may be required after treatment is finished in order to demonstrate cure.

[1] Hodgkin K (1973) *Towards Earlier Diagnosis*. London: Churchill Livingstone.
[2] Fry L, Wojnarowska F, Shahrad P (1985) *Illustrated Encyclopaedia of Dermatology*. 2nd edn. Lancaster: MTP Press.
[3] Roberts SOB *et al.* (1984) *A Clinician's Guide to Fungal Disease*. New York: Marcel Dekkar.
[4] Roberts SOB (1969) Pitygriasis versicolor. *Br. J. Dermatol.*, **81,** 315–26.

Warts

Warts are caused by the various papavoviruses, each of which is associated with a particular type of wart. There is a prolonged incubation period after the wart has entered the skin through a small abrasion. Some individuals seem to have a high incidence of infection whilst others are resistant. Children between the age of 10 and 16 years are the most frequently affected. Pox virus causes molluscum contagiosum.

PROGNOSIS

- Some 20% of warts disappear spontaneously within 6 months and 65% clear in 2 years[1].
- Whatever the form of treatment, it will usually take 3 months to cure a wart.

TREATMENT

1. Treatment is only required for warts that are painful or cosmetically unacceptable.
2. Salicylic acid is the best local treatment, usually in the form of Salactol or Duofilm paint applied after removal of excessive keratin daily.
3. Patients with genital warts should be considered for referral to an STD clinic. They may be treated with podophyllin paint for 2–6 hours daily and counselling is required (see p. 312).
4. Formalin 10% soaks can be used for multiple warts on the soles of the feet.
5. Liquid nitrogen application for 5–20 seconds can be used for warts on the face or those resistant to paints.
6. Molluscum contagiosum can be treated by puncture of the lesion with an orangestick dipped in 1% phenol.

FOLLOW-UP

None is required.

---

[1] Bunney MH (1980) Viral warts. *Medicine*, **31**, 1593–6.

Hair Problems

Baldness, sometimes called alopecia, is most commonly due to physiological sexual maturation. It may be due to local disease of the scalp such as seborrhoeic eczema, tinea capitis or hair-pulling. Alopecia areata has no known cause but occurs in about 3/1000 people per year[1]. The cause of total alopecia is also unknown.

Hirsutism occurs commonly in postmenopausal women but if excessive, another endocrine cause should be sought.

Male-pattern baldness occurs in 90% of men and 80% of women and a familial history usually exists.

PROGNOSIS

- Treatment of local disease of the scalp (see p. 239) will normally result in hair regrowth.
- Physiological balding is unlikely to respond to treatment. However, topical minoxidil has been reported to be of some value in 8% of men after 4 months of treatment and 40% after 12 months[2].
- Alopecia areata occurring on the vertex in children will recover in more than 90%[3]. Hair loss at temples or the occipital area is more likely to be permanent. New growth is often initially white.
- Hirsutism, if due to an endocrinological cause, such as pituitary tumour or adrenal tumour, responds to treatment of the underlying lesion.

TREATMENT

1. Wigs or hair transplants may be required for people having to make public appearances.
2. Alopecia areata that causes severe disturbance or is persistent in adults may be worth referring to a dermatologist. Treatment options include triamcinolone injections[4] and photochemotherapy.
3. Normal hirsutism in postmenopausal females can be treated by bleaching with 20 volume hydrogen peroxide, wax applications or electrolysis.
4. The possibility of an endocrine disturbance should be considered if hirsutism develops before the menopause or is gross in postmenopausal patients.
5. Male-pattern baldness may respond to topical minoxidil. Applied twice daily, this effect only occurs with continuous drug use and any regrown hairs fall out within 3 months of stopping treatment.

FOLLOW-UP

None is required.

[1] Hodgkin K (1973) *Towards Earlier Diagnosis*. London: Churchill Livingstone.

[2] Editorial (1988) *Pharm. J.*, **240**, 534.

[3] Mitchell AJ, Krull EA (1984) Alopeciata areata: pathogenesis and treatment. *J. Am. Acad. Dermatol.*, **11**, 763–75.

[4] Abell E *et al.* (1973) *Br. J. Dermatol.*, **88**, 55.

Erythema Multiforme

Erythema multiforme can persist in a wide variety of ways. Lesions are usually coin-shaped or target-shaped, affect hands and feet more than the trunk and are symmetrically distributed. The mucosa, mouth, genitalia and eyes are commonly involved and a severe form associated with fever and toxicity is called the Stevens–Johnson syndrome. In 50% of cases the cause is unknown but in others it is thought to be hypersensitivity to a drug (most commonly sulphonamides) or a virus (herpes simplex most commonly). The latent period after drug exposure is 1–3 weeks.

PROGNOSIS

- If mucosal lesions are not present the condition is usually mild and resolves in about 2 weeks; however, recurrences are common.
- In the presence of mucosal lesions the patient is more ill and the condition may take up to 6 weeks to resolve.
- Pneumonia may complicate up to 30% of the more severe cases and conjunctival scarring may result.
- Mortality in the Stevens–Johnson syndrome is 5–15%[1].

TREATMENT

1. Precipitating causes should be removed if identified.
2. Patients with minor lesions may require no treatment apart from observation and reassurance. Those with fever and arthralgia need bedrest and oral antihistamines such as promethazine hydrochloride (Phenergan) 25 mg twice daily if the rash is very irritating.
3. Patients with mucosal involvement who are ill should be admitted to hospital where treatment usually consists of steroid therapy and, if appropriate, antibacterial or antiviral therapy.
4. Mucous membrane lesions may respond to topical triamcinolone (Orabase).

FOLLOW-UP

Patients should be seen at weekly intervals until resolution has occurred.

[1] Chanda JJ (1981) Erythema multiforme. In *Cutaneous Aspects of Interval Disease* (Callen JP ed), pp. 121–30. Chicago: Yearbook.

Lichen Planus

Lichen planus is a highly irritating rash afflicting both sexes equally and occurring mainly in young and middle-aged adults. The condition probably has an immunological base and the typical lesion is flat-topped, purplish in colour with small white lines (Wickham striae) and most commonly occurs on the front of wrists, the shins and the lumbar region. It may involve mucous membranes (the mouth in 50% of cases), the genitalia including the glans penis and may produce hyperkeratotic plaques on the palms and soles.

PROGNOSIS

- The onset may be very sudden or gradual. Most cases clear slowly in about 1 year. A total of 85% clear within 18 months[1].
- Some 20% of patients will have a relapse after a first episode.
- Ulcerating forms on the genitalia, in the mouth and hypertropic forms tend to be long-lasting.

TREATMENT

1. If the condition is limited probably no treatment is required.
2. Group II or III steroid ointments (Betnovate, Eumovate, Locoid, Synalar etc.) as an ointment or cream can be used if irritation is troublesome.
3. If the disease is widespread or persistent, referral to a dermatologist for consideration of PUVA or systemic or intralesional steroids is indicated but 25% of cases will relapse when this treatment is stopped.

FOLLOW-UP

During systemic steroid therapy initial follow-up is necessary weekly or fortnightly. Subsequently no follow-up may be necessary if the condition settles. However, if active treatment continues regular follow-up monthly or two-monthly may be necessary.

[1] Ryan TJ (1986) Lichen Planus 20.42. In *Oxford Textbook of Medicine* (Weatherall DJ *et al.* eds). Oxford: Oxford University Press.

Pityriasis Rosea

Pityriasis rosea usually starts as a single scaly reddish-brown patch on the trunk. Other smaller patches appear on the rest of the trunk between 1 and 2 weeks later and characteristically lie in a slightly linear fashion along the lines of skin tension. These patches tend to develop an annular appearance. They do not involve the face and only occasionally the limbs below the elbow or knee.

Pityriasis affects young adults most commonly in the spring and because of its limitation to one attack in individuals it is thought to be viral in origin. The only symptom is itching, which may be intense.

PROGNOSIS

- The condition resolves within 8–10 weeks.
- Lymphadenopathy, malaise and fever may accompany the onset of the attack.

TREATMENT

1. Once the patient has been reassured about the non-infectious nature of the condition and its ultimate resolution, no further treatment is usually required.
2. If pruritus is intense then an antihistamine (such as Phenergan 25 mm at bedtime) and the use of a group II steroid (Betnovate, Locoid) on the lesions twice daily will help.
3. A non-sedative antihistamine such as terfenadine 60–120 mg daily or astemizole 10–20 mg daily can be used in the daytime.

FOLLOW-UP

None is required.

Urticaria

Urticaria is a condition characterized by swelling and reddening of the skin due to accumulated fluid and vasodilation. There is a wide variety of causes including contact (such as jellyfish sting, sun exposure and some ointment bases); cholinergic urticaria in young adults brought on by heat, emotion or exercise; cold urticaria; heat urticaria; oedema of the mouth due to eggwhite, milk products, shellfish, tomatoes etc. and serum sickness from beestings, penicillin and so on. In some cases, particularly chronic urticaria, it is very difficult to determine the exact cause, though familial urticaria is recognized[1].

PROGNOSIS

- Providing the precipitating factor can be identified and removed the condition will normally resolve and not recur.
- The urticaria of serum sickness, penicillin reaction or that accompanying some infectious diseases may persist for several days or weeks.
- Angioneurotic oedema involving the upper respiratory tract is rare but can be life-threatening.
- Candidiasis is an occasional cause—eradication may cure.

TREATMENT

1. Urticaria due to physical factors, sunlight, cold or heat will often respond to subthreshold exposure over a period of time[2].
2. Acute upper respiratory obstruction is treated with 0.5 ml of 1:1000 adrenaline subcutaneously and 100 mg hydrocortisone intravenously. Intubation and oxygen administration may be required.
3. Antihistamines should be given in adequate dosage. Astemizole (Hismanal) 30 mg daily for

up to 7 days or terfenadine (Triludan) 60 mg b.d. are suitable drugs.

4. The addition of an H_2-blocker, cimetidine or ranitidine, may help a small number of cases.
5. In patients with urticaria secondary to presumed dietary allergen or other identifiable precipitating factors, avoidance of these agents is important.
6. Bedrest may be helpful for some patients.
7. Chronic urticaria suggests that a search for underlying infection, parasitic disease or malignant disease should be started.

FOLLOW-UP

Follow-up is unnecessary once the condition has resolved.

[1] Czarnetz MB *et al.* (1984) Clinical, pharmacological and immunological aspects of delayed urticaria. *Br. J. Dermatol.*, **111,** 315–23.
[2] Warin RP, Champion RH (1975) Urticaria. In *Major Problems in Dermatology* (Root A ed), p. 171. London: Lloyd Luke.

Sun-induced Skin Conditions

Sunlight produces a range of effects upon the skin. Sunburn is due to overexposure to longwave ultraviolet rays and production of prostaglandins in the erythematous area. It develops 4–8 hours after exposure. Protection is achieved by the use of screening creams which filter out ultraviolet rays but allow gradual tanning. Health education about sun damage is important. Chronic sun exposure may also cause loss of elasticity and encourage telangiectases and prominent sebaceous glands, but more serious is the increasing incidence of keratoses. These are yellowish-brown hyperkeratotic lesions on a red telangiectatic background in which the scale is difficult and painful to remove and bleeds if it is scraped off. They occur on any exposed part of the body and are most common in fair-haired and fair-skinned individuals. Basal cell and squamous carcinomas and malignant melanoma are also features of sun exposure.

Solar keratosis

PROGNOSIS

- Some 10–25% of keratoses will eventually develop into squamous cell carcinomas but malignancy is local and rarely metastasizes.

TREATMENT

1. Referral for specialist advice is indicated.
2. Cryosurgery is the most usual form of treatment, using liquid nitrogen. The thawing of intracellular ice crystals destroys the cells. Scarring afterwards is usually minimal.

Basal cell carcinoma

Basal cell carcinomas have a central erosion and telangiectasia run over the edge.

PROGNOSIS

- Basal cell carcinomas rarely metastasize. If they do so (in <1:1000 cases[1]), metastasis is usually to local lymph glands.
- For lesions less than 1 cm in diameter there is a 90% cure rate from cautery and curettage[2]. Surgery or radiotherapy has an even lower recurrence rate but the cosmetic effects are less acceptable.

TREATMENT

1. Early referral is indicated.
2. Young people are usually treated by curettage; radiotherapy is preferred for older persons.

Squamous cell epithelioma

Squamous cell epitheliomas appear most commonly in exposed places such as hands, ears and lips. They start as a small lump which may ulcerate, fissure and bleed. They are most common in men and the average age of onset is 60 years.

PROGNOSIS

- Lesions arising in sun-damaged skin are slow-growing and have a reported incidence of metastasis of 0.5–3%[3].
- Mucocutaneous lesions are much more aggressive and spread more widely.

TREATMENT

1. Early referral of any suspicious lesion is important.
2. Small skin lesions may be treated with curettage and cautery; others may be excised and closed primarily or grafted.
3. Lesions on eyelids, nose or lips are frequently treated by X-ray.

Malignant melanoma

There has been a steady increase in the incidence of malignant melanoma, especially amongst younger women. For example, the incidence in Scotland has doubled in the last few years[4]. Malignant melanomas occur most commonly in fair or red-haired and fair-skinned people with blue eyes, in people who have already had one primary melanoma and in those with a family history. It is believed that sun exposure is a cause and the incidence is highest in Australia. The lesion is irregular, variably pigmented and grows rapidly. Ulceration is common.

PROGNOSIS

- Prognosis is difficult to determine accurately. It is probably dependent on the thickness of the lesion[5]. Prognosis is better in women than in men, in young rather than older patients, and lesions on the trunk, particularly the upper back, neck and shoulders have a worse prognosis than those on the limbs. Malignant melanoma is curable if treated early but fatal once it disseminates.

TREATMENT

1. Urgent referral of any slightly suspicious lesion is essential.
2. Wide excision and graft is the usual primary treatment with excision of glands if involved but superficial melanomas are now treated less aggressively.
3. Radiotherapy is sometimes used in elderly patients.

FOLLOW-UP

Follow-up of all malignant lesions is usually carried out at a specialist centre. Patients should be seen at frequent intervals in the first year and then for 5 years after therapy.

---

[1] Costanza ME et al. (1974) Cancer, **34,** 230.
[2] Fry L, Cornell M (1985) Dermatology. Lancaster: MTP.
[3] Moller R et al. (1979) Metastases in dermatological patients with squamous cell carcinoma. Arch. Dermatol., **115,** 703–5.
[4] Mackie RM et al. (1985) Lancet, II 859–62.
[5] Breslow A (1970) Ann. Surg., **192,** 902.

11

Rheumatology

V. W. M. Drury and F. D. R. Hobbs

Osteoarthritis

Osteoarthritis is the commonest cause of joint disability. It is a degenerative condition of joints, with breakdown of articular cartilage and remodelling of subchondral bone. Prevalence of radiological osteoarthritis increases with age and affects 67% of males and 61% of females at 45–54 years but 97% of people over 65[1]. However, less than 50% of people with radiological evidence actually get symptoms. Primary (idiopathic) osteoarthritis commonly affects middle-aged women.

The commonest joints affected are the distal interphalangeal joints (86%), carpometacarpal joint of thumb (60%), proximal interphalangeal joints (41%), metatarsophalangeal joint of big toe (33%), knee (53%, usually bilateral), spine (48%), and hips (30%)[2]. Symptoms include pain, stiffness (after inactivity) and loss of function. Progression is usually slow. Effusions, joint deformity and crepitus can occur. Heberden's nodes may develop as inflamed, painful swelling of the distal interphalangeal joints. There are no diagnostic tests available although x-rays show joint deformity, bony sclerosis, osteophyte formation and cysts.

PROGNOSIS

- Sport has not been shown to increase the prevalence of osteoarthritis[3].
- Repetitive occupational joint usage increases the risk of osteoarthritis[4,5].
- Obesity can exacerbate established osteoarthritis but does not significantly contribute to the development[6].
- Disease progression is normally slow, especially in primary osteoarthritis.
- Time between onset of hip or knee symptoms and severe joint disease is usually around 10 years.
- Osteoarthritis of the knee has the worst joint prognosis.

TREATMENT

1. Treatment is aimed at relief of symptoms and preservation of joint function. It is important that the patient understands the chronic nature of the condition and does not seek a non-existent cure.
2. Drug therapy is principally aimed at adequate analgesia. Many doctors will prescribe non-steroidal anti-inflammatory drugs (NSAIDs), although these have no disease-modifying effect and are frequently weak analgesics. If used, drugs chosen should be cheap, preferably taken once or twice daily and minimally gastrotoxic (such as ibuprofen). In elderly patients NSAIDs are frequently not well tolerated and can cause fatal gastric erosion or renal failure. The CSM reports that although NSAIDs only constitute 5% of all prescriptions, they produce 25% of all adverse reactions.
3. Analgesics that can be tried include paracetamol 500 mg–1 g q.d.s., co-dydramol 2 tablets q.d.s. or co-proxamol 2 tablets q.d.s. in ascending order of strength.
4. Once osteoarthritis has developed, weight reduction and avoidance of joint overuse is important. Walking aids, using chairs with arms and avoiding stairs may all help to reduce the load on joints.
5. Physiotherapy should be aimed at reducing joint deformity, correcting abnormal posture and building up muscle power to counteract the wasting effect of reduced mobility. Hydrotherapy and isometric (rather than isotonic) exercises are particularly beneficial.
6. Joint injection of a corticosteroid can significantly improve pain and mobility, but has a short-lived effect.
7. Surgical treatment may be considered in severe cases. This will remove the pain but has less influence on joint mobility. Joint replacement is well proven in hips and knees (over 90% of Charnley hips are still successful at 9 years[7]). The main long-term complications include loosening and infection of the prosthesis.

FOLLOW-UP

Patients should be seen at regular intervals so that

the progress and effects of the disease can be monitored and adjustments to treatment made. Patients on NSAID therapy require regular review to detect adverse affects.

[1] Lawrence JS et al. (1966) Ann. Rheum. Dis., 25, 1–24.
[2] Kellgren JH, Moore R (1952) Br. Med. J., 1, 181–7.

[3] Puranen J et al. (1975) Br. Med. J., 2, 424–5.
[4] Mintz G, Fraga A (1973) Arch. Environ. Health, 27, 78–84.
[5] Hadler NM (1981) In Epidemiology of Osteoarthritis (Peyran JG ed). Rueil-Malmaison: Ciba-Geigy.
[6] Danielsson LG (1964) Acta Orthop. Scand., 66 (suppl), 1–61.
[7] Charnley J, Cupic F (1973) Clin. Orthop., 95, 9–25.

Rheumatoid Arthritis

Rheumatoid arthritis is a chronic inflammatory disease which primarily affects the synovium of joints. Aetiology is unknown although slow viral infections are suspected. Genetic factors also play a role (possession of human leukocyte antigen DW4 and SRW4 is significantly more frequent in rheumatoid arthritis patients). Prevalence is about 1% of adult population but shows racial and geographical variation. The female to male ratio is 3:1. Peak age of onset is 35–55 years (if onset is before 16 years the condition is termed juvenile arthritis; see p. 255). Polyarticular rheumatoid arthritis occurs in 80% of patients—usually in the proximal interphalangeal, metacarpaphalangeal and metatarsophalangeal joints and wrists. Onset is monoarticular in 20% of patients—in the knee or wrist.

Rheumatoid arthritis has a variable course; 75–80% of disease is persistent while 20–25% is episodic. Symptoms include morning stiffness, pain, tenderness, swelling, reduced muscle power, malaise and depression. Signs include swelling and warmth of joints and wasting of muscles. Non-articular manifestations include nodules (25%), anaemia, lymphadenopathy (30%), splenomegaly (5%), vasculitis, carpal tunnel syndrome (50%), keratoconjunctivitis (10–30%), episcleritis, diffuse lung and cardiac involvement.

Rheumatoid factor is positive in 80% of patients as shown by Latex or 20% by Rose Waaler. These are not specific to rheumatoid arthritis but high titres are unusual in other conditions. Antinuclear antibodies appear in 20–40% (particularly in Sjögren's syndrome) and lupus erythematosus cells occur in 10% of patients.

PROGNOSIS

● Prognosis is worse in patients with:
1. Young age at onset.
2. Insidious onset and persistent disease activity[1].
3. Seropositivity at diagnosis with high RF titre[2].
4. Early erosive changes[2].
5. Marked systemic changes.
● Episodic arthritis generally lasts about 6–12 months, with remissions of months or years.
● Persistent activity of over 3 years is unlikely to remit.
● Some 40% of monoarticular sufferers become polyarticular within 10 years.
● After 10 years, the outcome of treated patients

is as follows: 30% are symptom-free; 37% are mildly incapacitated; 21% are severely incapacitated and 12% are housebound[3].
● The adverse reaction rate to treatment is high, and 50% of patients stop treatment within 12 months of starting. Of the remainder, only 20% will continue to benefit for more than 3–4 years[4].

TREATMENT

1. In acute flare-ups initial short-term bedrest is important to reduce joint damage. However, graded physiotherapy is a mainstay for promoting joint mobility and muscle power. Physiotherapy might include exercises, hydrotherapy, splintage or wax treatments.

2. NSAIDs, such as ibuprofen 400–600 mg t.d.s. and naproxen 250–500 mg t.d.s. reduce the pain and swelling but effects are short-lived. They have no modifying effect on the long-term course of the disease.

3. Aspirin is an effective symptomatic remedy in doses of 4–6 g daily. However, this will frequently produce unacceptable gastric side-effects, including haemorrhage.

4. Intramuscular gold can modify disease although the action is unknown. It has no anti-inflammatory effect.
   a. Usual dosage is 1 mg i.m. testdose followed by 20–50 mg weekly to 1 g, then 20–50 mg every 4 weeks.
   b. A third of patients will achieve remission, but spontaneous remission occurs in 9–11.5%[5]. Any improvement is likely to persist for at least 6 months, but usually disappears by 30 months[6].
   c. Side-effects occur in 40%[4] and include rash, proteinurea (25%) and an aplastic marrow. Although side-effects respond to withdrawal, gold therapy carries a greater risk of death than any other single drug[7].
   d. Patients must be monitored by urinalysis and blood count every 4–6 weeks.
   e. Auranofin (Ridaura) 3 mg b.d. orally is now an alternative to the above. It has the same range of contraindications and side-effects and may produce dose-related gastric intolerance. It should be stopped after 6 months if there is no response.

5. Penicillamine is another slow-acting disease modifier.
   a. Usual dose is 500–750 mg daily as a single dose, starting with 125 mg, and titrating upwards against response every 2–4 weeks. Several studies have shown that 125 g daily has no benefits compared to placebo.
   b. Remission rates are similar to gold.
   c. Side-effects are very common (58% of patients) and include rashes (44%), altered taste (20%), gastrointestinal upset (18%), mouth ulcers (10%), and proteinurea (7%). Thrombocytopenia is an uncommon but serious risk. In all, 27% of patients stop the drug because of adverse effects[8].

6. Immunosuppressive drugs are third-line treatments.
   a. These drugs modify the immunological response and possess anti-inflammatory activity.
   b. Drugs include azathioprine 1.3–2.5 mg/kg/day, cyclophosphamide 75–150 mg/day, methotrexate 5–20 mg/week or chlorambucil 0.1–0.2 mg/kg/day.
   c. Because of toxicity they are reserved for life-threatening states, vasculitis, severe progressive joint disease or extra-articular complications.
   d. Adverse effects include leukopenia, gastrointestinal upset, rashes, hair loss and sexual dysfunction.

7. Oral steroids are also a third-line treatment due to the risk of severe rebound flare-ups on withdrawal of therapy. Prednisolone 7.5 mg daily reduces this risk. Oral steroids (5–10 mg daily) however can be a reasonable option in the elderly to improve quality of life.

8. Antimalarial therapy such as chloroquine 200 mg daily can have an effect as a disease modifier. Toxicity is unlikely at this dose.

9. Intra-articular steroid injections (such as methylprednisolone 40–80 mg per joint) are frequently beneficial in relieving pain and stiffness. These can be repeated for long-term benefits. The risk of local osteoporosis is an unsubstantiated concern.

10. Surgical treatments are available for severe disabling rheumatoid arthritis. These include joint replacement (phalanges, knees, hips), joint fusion, tendon repair and removal of bursae.

FOLLOW-UP

Depression and anxiety are common in sufferers and may require specific treatment. Anaemia is common and may require iron therapy. The primary care team will need to assess requirements for aids. These might include special cutlery, keyholders, items of furniture and conveniently located grab-handles. Advice may also be needed on financial assistance from social services for mobility, disability and attendance allowance.

[1] Duthie J et al. (1964) Ann. Rheum. Dis., 23, 193–203.
[2] Fleming A et al. (1976) Br. Med. J., II 1243–5.
[3] Scott DL et al. (1983) J. R. Coll. Phys. Lond., 17, 79–85.
[4] Shrinivasan R et al. (1979) Arthritis Rheum., 22, 105–10.
[5] Butler R (1984) Gold in the treatment of rheumatoid

arthritis. In *Rheumatoid Arthritis*. (Goddard D, Butter R. eds.) London: Macmillan.
[6] Empire Rheumatism Council (1961) *Ann. Rheum. Dis.*, **20**, 315–34.

[7] Girwood RH (1974) *Br. Med. J.*, **1**, 501–5.
[8] Stein HB *et al.* (1980) *Ann. Intern. Med.*, **92**, 24–9.

Juvenile Chronic Arthritis (Still's Disease)

Chronic juvenile arthritis (Still's disease) is defined as persistent arthritis in one or more joints in a patient under 16 with no other obviously causative disease. It affects 1 in 1000 children per year[1]. There are three different presentations, including *systemic* onset (the least common), with persistent high fever and rash leading to widespread arthritis; *polyarticular*, with five or more joints affected, and *pauciarticular* (the largest group), with less than four joints affected.

Systemic onset affects more boys than girls, usually under 5 years old. Arthritis will develop in 50% within 3 months of onset of the systemic signs.

Seropositive polyarticular disease (juvenile rheumatoid) is found in 6% of children with juvenile arthritis. Girls (usually around puberty) are predominantly affected. Arthritis is often severe and progressive. Antinuclear antibodies are positive. Rheumatoid factor is positive (60–75%). Seronegative polyarticular disease is common. It affects mainly girls (female to male ratio 9:1) and occurs throughout childhood, with a peak at 6–7 years old. Rheumatoid factor is negative, but antinuclear antibodies are positive in up to 25%.

Pauciarticular arthritis predominantly affects girls around 3 years or adolescent boys. It is the commonest form—70% of arthritic children have this type. Rheumatoid factor is negative, but antinuclear antibodies are positive in 50–90%.

PROGNOSIS

- Overall 70–80% of children make a satisfactory recovery without serious functional impairment[2].
- Some 10% will have severe disability by adulthood.
- In all, 2–4% will die due to renal failure or amyloidosis[3].

Systemic onset

- 50% will get gradual remission over 2–3 years.
- 50% will get recurrent exacerbations of polyarticular arthritis.
- 25% will end up with severe disease with systemic complications, including amyloidosis.
- Death may occur through early infection or amyloidosis, leading to renal failure.

Seronegative polyarticular arthritis

- Prognosis is good.
- Remission is likely, even after years of disease activity, without residual joint disability.
- Systemic complications are rare, but include chronic uveitis in 5%[2].

Seropositive polyarticular arthritis

- This resembles adult rheumatoid arthritis with early development of joint erosions and nodules.
- Systemic complications, including pulmonary fibrosis and vasculitis, occur.
- Long-term prognosis is poor.

Pauciarticular arthritis

- Young girls are very likely to develop chronic

uveitis, particularly if antinuclear antibodies are positive.

- Older boys will frequently develop sacroileitis (50%), uveitis (20–25%), and arthritic hips.

TREATMENT

1. Treatment is principally aimed at avoiding contraction deformities since in the majority of children the disease settles after months or years of activity.
2. Exercises at home and the avoidance of bed-rest (unless there is serious systemic illness) are essential.
3. Contact sports should be avoided, but swimming can be encouraged.
4. Rest splints at night are used to maintain the best joint position.
5. NSAIDs are the usual first-line treatment; for example, ibuprofen 30–40 mg/kg/day or naproxen 10–15 mg/kg/day.
6. Aspirin (80–100 mg/kg/day) is used in non-responders or to control fever.
7. Gold or D-penicillamine are used as second-line therapy or as soon as erosions develop in seropositive polyarthritis.
8. Oral steroids are only indicated in life-threatening disease. Suppression of growth occurs rapidly and they should be withdrawn as soon as possible.
9. Intra-articular steroid injections are beneficial for isolated joint disease.
10. Chronic iridocyclitis usually responds to mydriatics at night and topical corticosteroids.
11. Surgical treatment may be required, including tendon release. Joint replacement should be delayed where possible until growth is completed.

FOLLOW-UP

Follow-up should be frequent to prevent development of contractures or spread of disease. Care will be shared between the general practitioner, paediatrician, rheumatologist and physiotherapist. Children on second-line therapy require monthly blood counts and urine tests. Children with uveitis require regular checks for glaucoma, keratopathy or cataracts.

[1] Sullivan DB et al. (1975) Arthritis Rheum., **18,** 251.
[2] Edmonds J, Hughes G (1985) Lecture Notes on Rheumatology. Oxford: Blackwell Scientific Publications.
[3] Bywaters EGL (1977) Arthritis Rheum., **20,** 256.
[4] Ansell B (1986) Practitioner, **230,** 343–50.

Gout

Gout has a diagnostic incidence of about 1.5 per 1000 patients in general practice. It is three times as common in men as in women[1]. It is characterized by hyperuricaemia due to increased purine intake or turnover or decreased elimination, with tissue deposit of crystals. Some 19 out of 20 hyperuricaemic people remain asymptomatic[2]; of those who do have symptoms, 25% have one attack of renal colic before getting joint symptoms. Gout should be considered in any patient with monoarticular arthritis, bursitis or tenosynovitis. Diuretic treatment is the commonest cause of gout.

PROGNOSIS

- The first attack of gouty arthritis usually occurs in men between 30 and 60 years and in 70% of cases involves the great toe[2]. If untreated it will last 3–4 weeks.
- Some patients have only one attack or another only after several years. Others have recurrent attacks which merge into each other.
- A single attack is rarely associated with any residual disability but recurrent attacks will lead to tophi, bone erosion and secondary arthritis.
- Some 10% of gout patients have an attack of renal colic and 5% of all stones are composed of uric acid[3].
- Progressive chronic renal failure accounts for 25% of deaths in patients with untreated tophaceous gout.
- Gout in men is associated with hypertension, ischaemic heart disease and hyperlipoproteinaemia but obesity is probably the linking factor.
- Tophi should resolve under treatment with allopurinol.
- There is no need for dietary restriction but obesity should be treated.

TREATMENT

Acute gout

1. Treatment with an adequate dose of an NSAID will relieve symptoms rapidly and can then be tailed off over a week. Any NSAID can be used but indomethacin 50 mg, 6-hourly is inexpensive and effective.

2. Colchicine 1 mg stat followed by 0.5 mg 2-hourly produces more rapid relief but there is a high incidence of nausea and diarrhoea.
3. Rest helps the joint to resolve rapidly and the patient can be given a small supply of the NSAID to take as soon as a recurrence happens. Allopurinol should not be given alone as it will exacerbate symptoms.

Chronic gout

1. Lifelong allopurinol is advised if acute attacks are recurrent; if there are tophi or joint damage; if there is renal disease or if patient is young with a family history of heart disease and serum urate > 0.75 mmol/l.
2. Allopurinol 200–300 mg daily (adjusted according to serum urate) should be accompanied by an NSAID for the first month of treatment.
3. Patients with renal disease should be referred for investigation.

FOLLOW-UP

Patients on allopurinol should have their serum uric acid checked every 2 or 3 years. Otherwise patients need only be seen when symptoms occur.

---

[1] Morbidity Statistics from General Practice (1986) London: HMSO.
[2] Healey LA, Hall AP (1970) The epidemiology of gout and hyperuricaemia. *Bull. Rheum. Dis.*, **20**, 600.
[3] Fessel WJ (1978) Renal outcomes of gout and hyperuricaemia. *Am. J. Med.*, **67**, 74–82.

Pseudogout

Pseudogout is due to the deposit of calcium pyrophosphate dihydrate crystals and produces symptoms similar to gout. There is an equal sex distribution and the condition occurs in older patients. Diagnosis is confirmed by examination of joint aspirate.

PROGNOSIS

- Acute attacks tend to be recurrent and to last several weeks.
- Chronic patients slowly progress to arthritic symptoms.

TREATMENT

1. Any NSAID in adequate dose will relieve the symptoms.
2. An acutely inflamed joint with an effusion should be rested. Intra-articular steroid injection will produce rapid relief.

FOLLOW-UP

This is unnecessary.

Ankylosing Spondylitis

Ankylosing spondylitis is an inflammatory arthritis of the spine and sacroiliac joints. It has ocular, cardiac and lung features as well. It occurs in young adults below the age of 30 and the male to female ratio is 8:1[1]. There is a strong genetic factor in the aetiology and patients have a high frequency of human leukocyte antigen B27 antigen, a genetic marker found on lymphocytes.

The incidence of new cases is about 1:10 000 people per year.

PROGNOSIS

- Ankylosing spondylitis without complications does not shorten life, although it may seriously affect quality of life.
- Proper treatment with physiotherapy and anti-inflammatory drugs can keep patients reasonably mobile.
- Severe ankylosis of the spine can occur in a few patients.
- Some 25% develop conjunctivitis or iritis, and 35% develop peripheral joint involvement.
- Only 3% develop cardiac involvement[2].

TREATMENT

1. Early referral for specialist advice is important.
2. NSAIDs, especially indomethacin 25–50 mg t.d.s. orally or 100 mg as a suppository at night, will relieve pain and maintain mobility.
3. Physiotherapy has an important role in maintaining mobility, muscle power and preventing deformity, especially of the spine.
4. Eye complications (conjunctivitis or uveitis) are best referred for specialist advice, but recurrences can be managed in practice.
5. Prompt treatment with steroid eye drops (betamethasone 0.1% 2-hourly) can prevent adhesions and secondary glaucoma.

FOLLOW-UP

Long-term follow-up at 6-monthly intervals to monitor progress should be adopted.

Social and employment considerations are particularly important. The National Ankylosing Spondylitis Society (4 Beaconsfield Rd, Bristol 8; telephone 0272-3629) may be of assistance.

---

[1] Lawrence JS (1958) *Br. J. Clin. Pract.*, **17,** 699.
[2] Moll JMH (1980) *Ankylosing Spondylitis.* London: Churchill Livingstone.

Polymyalgia Rheumatica and Giant Cell Arteritis

Polymyalgia is a disease of unknown origin which mainly affects the elderly but an association with viral infection is suspected. The true annual incidence is uncertain but is believed to be about 4/1000 in over 65-year-olds and is twice as common in females[1]. It is associated with malaise, fatigue, depression and muscle pains (usually bilateral) and in the shoulder or pelvic girdle. The erythrocyte sedimentation rate is usually markedly raised but this is not an invariable feature. Anaemia is often present and liver function may be depressed. There is an important overlap with the potentially more serious condition—giant cell arteritis. Headache and scalp hypersensitivity are common symptoms of temporal artery involvement.

PROGNOSIS

Polymyalgia

- The disease usually remits within 2 years but may recur and is occasionally prolonged.
- The height of the sedimentation rate is a useful guide to the degree of activity.
- There are no serious complications of the condition but unless treated, lack of mobility and depression can be troublesome.

Temporal arteritis

- This can occur separately from polymyalgia rheumatica but is associated with it in 40–50% of cases.
- Involvement of the temporal artery may lead to blindness in 10%[2] of patients unless adequately treated.
- Temporal arteritis can involve other arteries, producing cranial neuropathies, myocardial ischaemia, intermittent claudication and aortic arch syndrome.
- Treatment with adequate doses of steroids will suppress the condition, which will usually remit within 2 years. Relapse or chronic disease is possible, as with polymyalgia rheumatica.

TREATMENT

Polymyalgia

1. In very mild cases ibuprofen 400 mg t.d.s. may be sufficient.
2. In all other cases prednisolone is required. The response is usually dramatic. Indeed, if symp-toms have not resolved within 48 hours of commencing steroids there should be doubt about the diagnosis.
3. The dose of prednisolone is 20 mg daily for 14 days, thereafter reducing by 5 mg every 2 weeks until the lowest controlling dose is achieved. Dosage should be guided by symptomatic response rather than erythrocyte sedimentation rate.
4. Treatment is usually needed for about 12 months and has to be restarted if relapses occur.

Temporal arteritis

1. This condition should be sought for in every case of polymyalgia rheumatica.
2. Referral for confirmatory biopsy should be considered.
3. Prednisolone therapy should be given at a dose of 40 mg daily, reducing after 1 month to controlling levels guided by the sedimentation rate.

FOLLOW-UP

Follow-up can be carried out in general practice with regular monitoring of the sedimentation rate. The potential for side-effects from steroid therapy in the elderly should be carefully considered.

When in remission a 6-monthly follow-up is advisable for several years to identify recurrence. Patients should be advised to contact their general practitioner immediately if this is suspected.

[1] Hunder GG et al. (1978) Bull. Rheum. Dis., **29**, 280.
[2] Hunder GG et al. (1969) Mayo Clin. Proc., **44**, 84.

Systemic Lupus Erythematosus

Systemic lupus erythematosus is a connective tissue disease with widespread immunological abnormalities. Its aetiology is uncertain but genetic factors and virus infections have been suggested. The prevalence is about 1 in 2000. It has a ratio of 9:1 in women and this rises to 15:1 in women of childbearing age, when it is most common. In negro women prevalence may be as high as 1 in 250[1]. Arthralgia occurs in nearly 100% of patients and skin changes, including the classical 'butterfly' rash, in 80%. Renal, central nervous system, pulmonary and cardiac involvement is also frequent.

PROGNOSIS

- The mild form of disease may masquerade as other disease for many years. There is a mean 5-year survival rate of 90%[2].
- Renal disease carries the gravest prognosis, with a survival rate of 76% at 5 years and 57% at 10 years.
- Central nervous system involvement, producing manifestations ranging from depression to a stroke, probably affects up to 70% of patients.
- Systemic lupus erythematosus arthritis is rarely as disabling as rheumatoid disease, but muscle weakness can be pronounced.

TREATMENT

1. Referral for specialist supervision is advisable.
2. Systemic lupus erythematosus is a disease that waxes and wanes and it is not certain whether treatment during remission is of any value. It is therefore best avoided.
3. It is important that the patient should avoid excessive sun exposure; the use of high-factor sunscreens is advisable.
4. Sulphonamides and penicillin are precipitants so should be avoided. Some patients are sensitive to oral contraceptives.
5. In patients with drug-induced lupus, stopping the drug usually results in remission.
6. Mild disease producing arthralgia or chest pain may respond to NSAIDs such as ibuprofen or indomethacin, but aspirin should be avoided as it may be hepatotoxic.
7. More severe disease may be treated with steroids at high dose, antimalarials such as hydroxychloroquine, cytotoxic agents or plasmapheresis under specialist supervision.

FOLLOW-UP

Patients with mild disease may be supervised by their general practitioner at 6- or 12-monthly intervals but more severe disease or major organ involvement needs specialist follow-up.

[1] Hughes GRV (1979) *Connective Tissue Disease*, 2nd edn. Oxford: Blackwell Scientific Publications.
[2] Grigor RR *et al.* (1978) *Ann. Rheum. Dis.*, **37**, 121.
[3] Hughes GRV (1986) *Treatment and Prognosis in Medicine* (Hawkins RL ed). Oxford: Heinemann.

Paget's Disease

This is a disease in which there is disorganization of normal structure due to continuous absorption and replacement of the bone with associated fibrosis of the marrow. It may produce pain, fractures and arthritis, deafness, heart failure due to increased cardiac output and, rarely, osteosarcoma. It occurs in 3–4% of people over 40 years of age and is commonest in men[1].

PROGNOSIS

- Whilst being radiologically common, less than 5% of patients with the disease will have symptoms. These are usually bone pain and deformity[2].
- Some degree of deafness will occur in 4% of those patients who have symptoms[3]. This has many causes including nerve compression and is not usually amenable to treatment.
- Malignant changes occur in about 1% of those with symptoms[2]. The humerus is a high-risk site; rapidly worsening pain is the main symptom.

TREATMENT

1. No treatment is required for asymptomatic patients whose disease is usually discovered radiologically.
2. Mild bone pain will usually respond to an NSAID.
3. Patients whose pain fails to respond to NSAIDs should be referred for specialist assessment.

Their treatment will usually consist of mithramycin, an antimitotic drug (given intravenously in courses), diphosphonates given orally which reduce bone turnover, or calcitonins. Salmon calcitonin is usually given three times weekly by injection and may cause nausea and vomiting.

4. Fractures through pagetic bone should be treated normally, though union may be delayed.

FOLLOW-UP

Regular follow-up is only required for patients with symptoms.

[1] Barker DJP et al. (1977) Paget's disease of bone on 14 British towns. Br. Med. J., 1, 1181–3.
[2] Smith R (1987) Disorders of the skeleton. In Oxford Textbook of Medicine. (Weatherall DJ et al. ed.) Oxford: Oxford University Press.
[3] Morrison AW (1979) Diseases of the optic capsule. In Scott–Brown's Diseases of the Ear, Nose and Throat. (Ballantyne J, Groves J) London: Butterworth.

12

Orthopaedics

D. W. Wall

Fractures and Dislocations

Fractures

Fractures are common. Hodgkin[1] found suspected fractures in 21.4 per 1000 patients, and 14.3 probable fractures per year. In general practice fractures may be divided into two groups—classical and concealed fractures[2]. With classical fractures, the diagnosis is obvious; there is trauma followed by pain, swelling, immobility and deformity. With concealed fractures, the diagnosis may be overlooked. Such sites include the skull, vertebrae, scaphoid, neck of femur, fibula, malleoli, ribs, and all fractures in children. In children, ligaments are far stronger than the bones to which they are attached.

If there is swelling, pain and loss of function then a fracture is nearly always present[3]. Risk factors include trauma (sometimes trivial), being elderly, carcinomatosis, osteoporosis, confusion, alcohol and medication (especially antidepressants, hypnotics and tranquillizers).

Osteoporosis is a major risk factor[4] since bone mass is lost with age, more so in women than in men. Colles' fracture, neck of femur and vertebral fractures all correlate with increasing age (15% of the population have had one of these fractures by the age of 80 years). The frequency of osteoporotic fracture is increasing in the UK and USA as the population ages.

Complications of fractures include shock, fat embolism, deep vein thrombosis, damage to blood vessels and major nerves, pneumonia, non-union, poor functional result and even death.

PROGNOSIS

- Prognosis depends on age, the presence of complications and the type of fracture.
- Fracture of the scaphoid is prone to non-union and secondary osteoarthritis of the wrist[2].
- Greenstick fractures in children may heal in 14 days[1].
- Elderly patients with hip fractures may never recover[1]. There is a 60% mortality rate in patients over 95 years, often from pneumonia[5].

TREATMENT

Preventive treatment

1. Avoid overmedication of elderly patients.
2. Encourage your patients to avoid accidents in the home, at work, during sport and in icy conditions, if possible.
3. Osteoporosis may be diagnosed by X-ray and treatment can then be considered. Calcium in the diet, postmenopausal hormone replacement and physical activity may all help[4].

Surgery

1. Refer for X-rays and surgical treatment. The surgical treatment depends on the site and type of fracture.
2. Reduction of the fracture and immobilization are basic principles of treatment.

Post-hospital treatment

1. Refer for physiotherapy if indicated.
2. Check other medication.
3. Assess for aids in the home.
4. Check for full mobilization and recovery.
5. Analgesia is important, especially early after the fracture has occurred.

Dislocations

Hodgkin[1] gives an incidence of 0.5 per 1000 patients per year. The shoulder is the joint most commonly affected.

PROGNOSIS

- Dislocations, especially of the shoulder, often become recurrent: recurrence rates of 57% have been reported. Surgical treatment may then be needed[2]. Stiffness may be a problem.

TREATMENT

1. Referral for X-ray to make diagnosis and exclude a coexisting fracture.
2. Referral for reduction (often under general anaesthesia).
3. After reduction, arrange adequate analgesia and physiotherapy exercises to aid full recovery of function.

[1] Hodgkin K (1985) *Towards Earlier Diagnosis*, 5th edn, pp. 664–8. Edinburgh: Churchill Livingstone.
[2] Apley AG, Solomon L (1982) *Apley's System of Orthopaedics and Fractures*, 6th edn. London: Butterworths.
[3] Jones PG, Woodward AA (1986) *Clinical Paediatric Surgery: Diagnosis and Management*, 3rd edn. Carlton, Victoria: Blackwell Scientific Publications.
[4] Lindsay R (1985) *The osteoporoses. Med. Int.*, **2,** 609–14.
[5] Martin A (1981) *Problems in Geriatric Medicine*, pp. 153–66. Lancaster: MTP Press.

Osteochondritis

There are several types of osteochondritis, often named eponymously. They are classified together because of some common features and include: Perthes' disease of the hip; Osgood–Schlatter's disease of the anterior tibial tubercle; Scheuermann's disease of the vertebral epiphysis; Köhler's disease of the navicular; Kienböck's disease of the lunate; Sever's disease of the os calcis, and Freiberg's disease of the metatarsal head[1].

Osteochondritis affects growing bones. There is active disease in the epiphysis in children and adolescents, lasting several months and leading to bone deformity and spontaneous healing. X-ray changes show the typical deformity. A single bone—rarely more—is usually affected in any one individual. Early diagnosis is needed to avoid later problems. The osteochondritic conditions have a range of 0.2–1.2 occurrences per 1000 patients per year[2].

Trauma is implicated as a possible cause. The spine and lower limbs are affected most commonly. There is vascular impairment of the bone. Osteochondritis tends to occur more commonly in families.

Two forms are described here. Perthes' disease is a serious disorder, needing early diagnosis and assessment. Osgood–Schlatter's disease is the most common of the group.

Perthes' disease

Perthes' disease is osteochondritis of the femoral head, which may become deformed and lead to the development of osteoarthritis of the hip later in life. The bone of the epiphysis undergoes necrosis and may become softened and flattened, especially if weight-bearing continues. Eventually the bone is revascularized and hardens again—but if deformed, it may never regain its original shape. The whole process may take 2 years or more. The ratio of boys to girls is 4:1: 80% of cases occur in the 4–9-year age group. Bone age is delayed in such children, for up to 3 years in some cases. Stature is short. There is a higher incidence in lower social class, and in low-birthweight and breech presentation babies[3]. The patient presents with limb pain around the hip radiating to the knee, often for several weeks. On examination the hip movements are limited and painful. Diagnosis is made by X-ray.

PROGNOSIS

- Untreated, 57% recover well, 19% fairly well and 24% poorly. Limb shortening and early arthritis characterize the latter group[3].
- Several factors influence whether a patient falls into the 60% group who do well without treatment, or the 40% group who need treatment. Younger patients, boys, and early diagnosed cases do best.
- Prognosis depends on the X-ray changes in the hip[3]. Catterall[3] proposed a classification indicating the degree of involvement of the femoral head, and therefore the severity of the disease,

aimed at clarifying prognosis and the need for surgical treatment. X-rays allow grading into four groups; grade 1 represents the least change, and grade 4 the most—with complete collapse of the epiphysis. Grades 1 and 2 heal very well, whereas grades 3 and 4 will often need surgical treatment and have a worse long-term prognosis. In practice, this grading has been extremely useful.

- By age 65 years, 86% of patients who had Perthes' disease will have arthritis of the affected hip.

TREATMENT

1. Refer to an orthopaedic surgeon urgently once the diagnosis has been made or is suspected by the general practitioner.
2. Assessment needs specialized X-rays by an expert. Following assessment, 60% of patients need no further action.
3. The principle of treatment is to contain the hip in the acetabulum. A broomstock plaster with progressive adjustment may be used.
4. Surgery may be necessary in the severe forms—femoral osteotomy may be done[3].

FOLLOW-UP

Follow-up is usually done by the orthopaedic surgeon for several years.

Osgood–Schlatter's disease

Osgood–Schlatter's disease is the commonest of the osteochondritis group of disorders. It is a traction injury of the epiphysis of the tibial tubercle of the insertion of the patellar tendon. It affects children aged 10–16 years. The tibial tubercle becomes swollen and tender. It may be recurrent and bilateral and may cause pain for several years. Pain is aggravated by exercise and jumping[2]. The differential diagnosis includes osteomyelitis, sar-

coma of the tibia, bone cyst and infrapatellar bursitis. X-rays in severe cases show fragmentation of the bone of the epiphysis.

PROGNOSIS

1. Prognosis is excellent. Spontaneous recovery is the rule[4].
2. Osgood–Schlatter's disease may recur until the epiphysis is fully fused with the tibia at age 16–18 years.
3. Very rarely, the epiphysis is pulled upwards by the patellar tendon, causing early fusion, osteoarthritis and genu recurvation of the knee[1].

TREATMENT

1. Reassurance is the main treatment[5].
2. Reduce activity—restrict sport, especially cycling and soccer.
3. Refer if the patient (and parents) are anxious and cannot be reassured. Most orthopaedic surgeons adopt a policy of masterly inactivity.
4. In very severe cases, a few surgeons recommend a plaster of Paris case to immobilize the kneejoint, or even surgical opening of the tibial tubercle and curetting of the inflamed bone[2].

FOLLOW-UP

Follow-up is at 3 and 6 months—most knees have settled by then.

[1] Duthie RB, Bentley G (1983) *Mercer's Orthopaedic Surgery*, 8th edn, pp. 310–27. London: Edward Arnold.
[2] Hodgkin K (1985) *Towards Earlier Diagnosis: A Guide to Primary Care*, 5th edn, pp. 639–40. Edinburgh: Churchill Livingstone.
[3] Catterall A (1985) Perthes' disease. *Surgery*, **1**, 388–92.
[4] Apley AG, Solomon L (1982) *Apley's System of Orthopaedics and Fractures*, 6th edn, pp. 66–8. London: Butterworths.
[5] Modell M, Boyd R (1982) *Paediatric Problems in General Practice*, p. 203. Oxford: Oxford University Press.

Tenosynovitis

Tenosynovitis is a painful disorder caused by inflamed tendon sheaths and surrounding tissue, usually due to unaccustomed use and repetitive movement. Awkward working positions, badly designed tools, lack of job variation and inadequate breaks for rest are predisposing factors[1]. Hodgkin[2] found 11.9 cases per 1000 patients, with the most common sites as follows: hand and wrist, 47%; foot and ankle, 45%; Achilles tendon, 8%. Tenosynovitis is now the second most common 'prescribed industrial disease' in the UK.

PROGNOSIS

- The overall prognosis is excellent. Most settle within a few days, often spontaneously[1]. Some may need a little longer—1–4 weeks[2].
- A very few go on to need surgery, and a few of these may have a stiff wrist which is permanently incapacitated for repetitive work[1].

TREATMENT

1. Prevention, particularly in the industrial setting, should be actively promoted.
2. It is important to exclude infection as a cause of the patient's problems before making the diagnosis of tenosynovitis.
3. Rest for a few days is helpful but not always possible.
4. NSAIDs have a role[3]. Ibuprofen 400 mg t.d.s. daily, ketoprofen 50 mg b.d. daily and flurbiprofen 50 mg t.d.s. daily are suitable choices.
5. Local injection of corticosteroid into the sheath (1 ml hydrocortisone acetate or methylpred-nisolone acetate) has a dramatic effect, but care must be taken not to inject into the tendon.
6. Ultrasound may be helpful.
7. Surgical release of the tendon sheath may be necessary if all else fails, or if there is an associated carpal tunnel syndrome.

FOLLOW-UP

Watch for the development of chronic tenosynovitis which may need surgery; refer for an orthopaedic surgeon's opinion in such cases. Rheumatoid arthritis and gout may first present as tenosynovitis[4].

[1] Evans G (1987) Tenosynovitis in industry: menace or misnomer? *Br. Med. J.*, **294**, 1469–570.
[2] Hodgkin K (1985) *Towards Earlier Diagnosis. A Guide to Primary Care*, 5th edn, pp. 644–5. Edinburgh: Churchill Livingstone.
[3] Anonymous (1987) Which NSAID? *Drugs Ther. Bull.*, **25**, 81–4.
[4] Golding DN (1981) *Problems in Arthritis and Rheumatism*, pp. 81–82. Lancaster: MTP Press.

Ganglia

Ganglia occur mainly in the hand and foot, occasionally around the knee. They may be soft and fluctuant, or hard and tense. A ganglion contains a thick jelly-like colloid. It is now thought that it does not arise from a joint or tendon, but from small bursae or islands of mesoderm around the joint capsule or fibrous sheath[1].

Ganglia occur most commonly in the age group 20–50 years, more in women, and less commonly in older people. They are usually symptomless, but occasionally compress a nerve[2]. Ganglia account for two-thirds of all hand tumours[3].

PROGNOSIS

- Explanation and reassurance are all that is required in many cases. Some ganglia disappear spontaneously (less than 50%).
- The outcome of treatment depends on the particular treatment used. There is, however, a recurrence rate with all methods[4].
  1. Rupture by pressure: 66% cure rate at 8-year follow-up.
  2. Aspiration and injection; an initial 65% cure rate, but less effective when repeated.
  3. Surgery under local anaesthesia and tourniquet; 84% cure rate.
  4. Surgery under general anaesthesia and tourniquet; 94% cure rate.

TREATMENT

1. Direct pressure or a sudden blow are traditional methods of treatment. If the wall of the ganglion resists rupture, it may be pierced with a large needle or tenotomy knife first.
2. Aspiration and injection with corticosteroid is sometimes difficult because the contents of the ganglion may be very thick. After aspiration, inject 0.5 ml hydrocortisone acetate or methyl-prednisolone acetate.
3. Surgery: most general practitioners would refer to an orthopaedic surgeon for excision. A few enthusiasts would operate themselves. A careful dissection in a bloodless field is essential. Beware the ganglion near the pisiform bone of the wrist, since this is very near the ulnar nerve, and the ganglion may extend deeply around it—refer these cases.

FOLLOW-UP

There is a recurrence rate for all methods of treatment. Explain this to the patient beforehand.

[1] Apley AG, Solomon L (1986) *Apley's System of Orthopaedics and Fractures*, 6th edn, pp. 183–4. London: Butterworths.
[2] Duthie RB, Bentley G (1983) *Mercer's Orthopaedic Surgery*, 8th edn, pp. 932–4. London: Edward Arnold.
[3] Wenger RJJ (1984) Operations for ganglion. In *Rob and Smith's Operative Surgery*, 4th edn, pp. 466–8 (Dudley H, Carter D eds). London: Butterworths.
[4] Nelson CL *et al.* (1972) Ganglions of the wrist and hand. *Bone Joint Surg.*, **54a,** 1459–64.
[5] Brown JS (1986) *Minor Surgery. A Text and Atlas.* London: Chapman & Hall.

Neck Pain

Neck pain is a very common symptom. Hodgkin[1] found 5 cases per 1000 patients per year, but this may understate the true numbers. As many as 93% of cases are aged over 30 years, and women predominate over men in a ratio of 2:1. Risk factors include middle age, cervical rib, osteoarthrosis of the cervical spine and the carrying of heavy loads such as shopping bags.

Mechanisms of neck pain are poorly understood. However, in young adults Cyriax and Cyriax[2] felt that most neck pain is due to intervertebral disc displacements. In older people cervical spondylosis (disc degeneration) is the most common cause[3]. Other common presentations include torticollis, acute cervical disc protrusion, whiplash injury, cervical spondylosis (stiff neck) and fibrositis[3].

The condition is usually benign and transient. However, a small number of rare pathological causes must be excluded. These include meningitis and meningism, tumours (primary and secondary), thyroiditis, inflammatory arthropathies, polymyalgia rheumatica and dental causes.

PROGNOSIS

- Neck pain is a benign self-limiting condition in most cases, whatever treatment is given.
- Some 85% of patients are symptom-free in 1–4 weeks. Most of the other 15% have settled in 2–3 months[1]. Almost all cases have settled in 4 months[2].
- Relapses are, however, common (18% in 2 years). It is as well to tell the patients that the condition may come and go, but is not serious or crippling.
- For more serious pathological causes (see above) the prognosis is that of the underlying disorder.

TREATMENT

1. A soft cervical collar is a traditional treatment[3]. There is no objective evidence of benefit but many patients find them comfortable, although others are not helped. National Health Service general practitioners in England and Wales cannot prescribe cervical collars.
2. Care with posture whilst standing and sitting, and lying with one pillow may help.
3. Analgesia such as paracetamol, co-codamol and co-dydramol usually gives the patient some pain relief.
4. NSAIDs have a role[4]. A recent review[4] gives ibuprofen 400 mg daily, ketoprofen 50 mg b.d. daily and flurbiprofen 50 mg daily as the three best choices.
5. Muscle relaxants: diazepam 2–5 mg three times daily is very useful together with an anti-inflammatory drug for a short course of about a week. Warn the patient about driving and sedation.
6. Physiotherapy: several treatments may be used, including a collar, exercises, traction and manipulation. Physiotherapists trained in the methods of manipulation described by Cyriax and Cyriax[2] will produce excellent results in selected patients.
7. There is very little place for surgery in neck pain. Operation on lateral disc displacements is dangerous and difficult. However, a central disc displacement with cervical spinal cord compression does need to be recognized and referred for immediate neurosurgical admission.

FOLLOW-UP

Normally the condition settles quickly with simple treatment. It is as well to ensure it does. If not, further investigation may be necessary. X-rays are not usually much help. Where infection or malignancy is suspected, bone scan may give more information. Cervical spondylosis can occasionally cause spinal cord compression, with long tract signs in the legs and bladder problems. This needs immediate hospital referral.

[1] Hodgkin K (1985) *Towards Earlier Diagnosis. A Guide*

to *Primary Care*, 5th edn, pp. 297–9. Edinburgh: Churchill Livingstone.
[2] Cyriax JH, Cyriax PJ (1983) *Illustrated Manual of Orthopaedic Medicine*, pp. 145–66. London: Butterworth.
[3] Berry H, Jawad ASM (1985) *Rheumatology*, pp. 55–64. Lancaster: MTP Press.
[4] Anonymous (1987) Which NSAID? *Drugs Ther. Bull.*, **25**, 81–4.

Lower Back Pain

Lower back pain is a very common problem. A total of 64 million working days are lost per annum in the UK and 1.5 million new general practitioner consultations and 5 million total consultations occur for this reason each year[1]. A general practitioner will, on average, see 75 new cases of acute backache per year, and have 3 or 4 chronic back invalids on his or her list[2]. The range of presentation within general practice occurs as follows: acute backache only, 80%; acute backache with sciatica, 15%, and acute backache with nerve damage, 5%[2].

The cause of most cases of backache is uncertain. Most are presumed 'mechanical'. Rarer causes are spondylolisthesis, sacroileitis, osteomalacia, osteoporosis, Paget's disease, tuberculosis and primary and secondary malignant disease. In immigrants of Asian origin, osteomalacia and tuberculosis should be considered.

Investigations are not often needed. X-rays are often unhelpful and unnecessary. If malignancy is suspected, a bone scan is a better investigation.

PROGNOSIS

- Overall the prognosis for acute lower back pain is excellent[2]. 75% of patients recover with a minimum of treatment within 1 month and 98% of patients recover within 3 months.
- Only 5% of patients are referred to hospital, and half of these do not attend because their back has got better while waiting for an appointment. Of those actually treated, 20% are not relieved and have persistent symptoms.
- Of all backache patients seen by a general practitioner, only 1 in 1000 eventually has surgery and, of these, only 10% continue to have chronic backache.
- The general practitioner must identify those with underlying serious disease, and refer them appropriately. The prognosis then depends on the underlying disorder.

TREATMENT

Prevention

1. Advice on posture and the correct way to lift objects, and the use of back and postural exercises may help prevent recurrence of low back pain problems.

General

1. Rest in a firm bed with a pillow beneath the knee is useful in the acute stage.
2. Analgesia: paracetamol, aspirin, co-proxomol and co-dydramol are useful analgesics (guard against constipation by advising a simultaneous high-fibre diet).
3. Of NSAIDs, ibuprofen, ketoprofen and flurbiprofen are three suitable choices[3].
4. Muscle relaxants; diazepam is useful in cases of hyperacute lumbar backache and can be used in combination with NSAIDs.
5. Corsets are widely prescribed and acupuncture recommended by some, but there is little scientific evidence of their value.
6. Using the measures described in points 1–4 above most patients will settle within 1–2 weeks[2].
7. Physiotherapy: posture, exercises and manipulation in selected cases will all help.
8. If all the above measures fail, referral to an

orthopaedic surgeon will be necessary. Indications for referral include:

a. Persistence of severe pain despite full medical treatment.
b. Progressive neurological signs, such as foot drop.
c. Bladder and/or bowel paralysis; this needs **immediate hospital opinion**.

At this stage myelography and/or radiculography may be carried out. Other treatments may, in selected cases, include:

a. Epidural injection of local anaesthetic/cortocosteroid, which is an effective treatment in severe unremitting sciatica[4]. Cyriax and Cyriax[4] cited 94 patients treated and 69 restored to full painless movement[4].
b. Surgery: apart from urgent decompression of the spinal cord or cauda equina, surgery is the very last resort. Only 1 in 1000 backache patients have surgery. The results are not always good and over 10% may continue to have severe problems[2].

FOLLOW-UP

Advice on posture, correct lifting and exercises is of value. A physiotherapist may teach the patient the valuable McKenzie exercises[5] which will enable him or her to control the back and keep it free of pain.

[1] Berry H, Jawad ASM (1985) *Rheumatology*, pp. 47–53. Lancaster: MTP Press.
[2] Fry J *et al.* (1986) *Disease Data Book*, pp. 318–36. Lancaster: MTP Press.
[3] Anonymous (1987) Which NSAID? *Drugs Ther. Bull.*, **25**, 81–4.
[4] Cyriax JH, Cyriax PJ. (1983) *Illustrated Manual of Orthopaedic Medicine*. London: Butterworths.
[5] McKenzie RA (1981) *The Lumbar Spine: Mechanical Diagnosis and Therapy*. New Zealand: Spinal Publications.

Dupuytren's Contracture

Dupuytren's contracture is a thickening of the fibrofatty tissue of the palm of the hand, progressing with fibrosis and contracture to draw the affected finger into a fixed flexion deformity. The contracture usually affects the fourth (ring) finger. It is inherited as an autosomal dominant and is most common in Anglo-Saxon peoples. It is associated with epilepsy, diabetes mellitus, alcoholic cirrhosis and pulmonary tuberculosis[1]. Injury may play a part in the causation of this disorder. The condition is usually painless, although occasionally nodules may be tender[2].

PROGNOSIS

- Minor cases with normal hand function are probably best left alone.
- Surgical treatment presents problems, as recurrences after surgery are common, especially in patients under age 40 years, when up to 70% may recur.
- The little finger has the worst prognosis.
- Most recurrences occur within 2 or 3 years of operation. In 224 cases, 106 were cured, 56 showed extension and 63 recurrence of the contracture.

TREATMENT

1. In mild cases with no loss of movement or function, no treatment is needed. Check for underlying causes, as described above.
2. Surgical treatment is indicated when the hand cannot be placed flat on a tabletop; refer these cases.
3. Postoperative complications include haematoma, damage to nerves and arteries in the fingers, ischaemic skin necrosis, scar contracture and joint stiffness. The general practitioner should refer such patients very carefully only when necessary. An experienced hand or plastic surgeon must be chosen for these cases. Patients with minor thickening and normal hand function are probably best left alone. Surgery may worsen the problem.

Check for underlying causes and treat these if possible. The healing after surgery is slow. The surgeon should follow these patients for at least 6 months, and probably for several years.

[1] Duthie RB, Bentley G (1983) *Mercer's Orthopaedic Surgery*, 8th edn, pp. 928–31. London: Edward Arnold.
[2] Apley AG, Solomon L (1982) *Apley's System of Orthopaedics and Fractures*, 6th edn, pp. 188–90. London: Butterworths.
[3] Huelston JT (1984) Dupuytren's disease. In *Ron and Smith's Operative Surgery*, 4th edn (Dudley H, Carter D eds), pp. 444–60. London: Butterworths.
[4] Huelston JT (1963) Recurrent Dupuytren's contracture. *Plast. Reconstr. Surg.*, **31**, 66–9.

Carpal Tunnel Syndrome

Carpal tunnel syndrome is due to compression of the median nerve under the flexor retinaculum of the wrist. It is more common in the dominant hand, and is aggravated by strenuous physical activity. The incidence is about 1 per 1000 patients per year[1]. Women are affected 8 times more commonly than men, with a peak age of 40–50 years[2]. Carpal tunnel syndrome may be an isolated condition or may be secondary to rheumatoid arthritis, hypothyroidism, acromegaly, diabetes, pregnancy or Colles' fracture.

PROGNOSIS

- Prognosis depends on the cause. It is easy to miss rheumatoid arthritis and especially hypothyroidism. Always do blood investigations for these conditions.
- Some 60% of patients will get better with conservative treatment; 40% will require surgical treatment to divide the flexor retinaculum[3].
- The results of surgery show relief of symptoms in 85% of cases, but 10–15% may have persistent pain, muscle-wasting and incomplete recovery, especially when surgery is done more than 6 months after onset[4]. Recurrence can occur in up to 10%[4] (usually due to incomplete division of flexor retinaculum) and will need repeat surgery.

TREATMENT

1. Conservative treatment should usually be tried first, unless indications for surgery are present at the time of diagnosis (see below)[3].
   a. Splinting with a resting wrist splint at night will give temporary relief to 70% of patients.
   b. A diuretic such as bendrofluazide 5 mg can be tried for 1–2 months.
   c. Corticosteroid injection: 1 ml hydrocortisone acetate or methylprednisolone acetate can be injected under the flexor retinaculum.
2. About 40% of cases require surgery eventually. The indications for surgery are:
   a. In acute carpal tunnel syndrome:
      i. Progressive impairment of nerve function.
   b. In chronic carpal tunnel syndrome:
      i. failure of conservative treatment.
      ii. signs of sensory loss, thenar muscle-wasting or weakness.
      iii. a space-occupying lesion in the carpal canal, especially a fracture or a bony tumour.
      Surgical treatment involves division of the flexor retinaculum at the wrist. Most general practitioners would refer the patient to an orthopaedic surgeon, although a few enthusiasts operate themselves[5].

FOLLOW-UP

Watch for recurrence of carpal tunnel syndrome after surgery. Watch for hypothyroidism which may only manifest itself clinically and biochemically after the carpal tunnel syndrome has been treated.

[1] Hodgkin K (1985) *Towards Earlier Diagnosis. A Guide to Primary Care*, pp. 299–300. Edinburgh: Churchill Livingstone.
[2] Apley AG, Solomon L (1986) *Apley's System of Orthopaedics and Fractures*, 6th edn. London: Butterworths.
[3] Berry H, Jawad ASM (1985) *Rheumatology*, p. 76. Lancaster: MTP Press.
[4] Conolly WB (1984) *A Colour Atlas of Treatment of Carpal Tunnel Syndrome*. Weert, Netherlands: Wolfe Medical.
[5] Brown JS (1986) *Minor Surgery. A Text and Atlas*, pp. 182–7. London: Chapman & Hall.

Congenital Dislocation of the Hip

The term 'congenital dislocation of the hip' is a misnomer. Most hips so described are unstable (dysplastic) at birth and have the potential for complete dislocation if not treated. In all, 15–20 children per 1000 livebirths have unstable hips. Perhaps 2–4 will go on, if untreated, to full dislocation[1]. Other studies show a prevalence of 1 in 1000 in white races, higher in American Indians and Laplanders, and very rare in Chinese and African races[2]. The condition is more common in first-born children, increases by 10 times in siblings of affected children, and is more common in breech-presentation babies[2].

There are two main features: dysplasia of the acetabulum and laxity of the ligaments of the hip joint. All newborn infants should be examined by a competent and experienced person, using Barlow's test. The examination should be repeated at 6 weeks, 3 months and 6 months.

PROGNOSIS

- The best results are obtained in children in whom the diagnosis is made early, hence screening programmes for early diagnosis are very important[1,3].
- If the dysplastic hip is recognized and treated early and stabilized in the acetabulum, the hip is likely to develop normally.
- If the condition is unrecognized and untreated in the first few months of life, dysplasia in the acetabulum worsens. The head of the femur comes to lie on the outer surface of the ilium where it forms a false joint. The deformed hip joint is prone to severe distortion and degenerative osteoarthritis in early adult life. Studies show 71.5% of hips are normal on X-ray criteria when treated in the first year of life, falling to only 11.9% with a normal hip when treated in the ninth year.
- The later the diagnosis is made, the less successful the outcome and the longer and more complex the course of treatment is likely to be. The risk of complications is greater in babies treated late—the risk of necrosis of the epiphysis of the head of the femur is especially high. Such necrosis results in permanent deformity.

TREATMENT

1. The general practitioner should ensure every baby has had screening examinations and that suspected cases are referred for an orthopaedic opinion. Subsequent management will depend on the individual presentation.

2. *Conservative treatment*
   a. Follow-up examination may be all that is needed for a minor neonatal instability that disappears at 1–2 weeks of age.
   b. The hips can be splinted in abduction— often for 3 months—with check X-rays
   c. Traction for the totally dislocated hip at birth, or the baby when the diagnosis is made late (after 4 months of age). Traction continues until 20–30° of abduction and 15–20° of internal rotation of the femoral head leads to a perfect position of the femur in the hip joint. This may take some weeks. Traction is followed by immobilization in plaster for 3–6 months, with a plaster change after 3 months.

3. Operative treatment is reserved for more severe cases, and those where conservative treatment falls. There may be a rim of joint capsule folded inwards to form a limbus, pre-

venting full reduction. After surgery, the hip will need immobilization for at least 3 months in a hip plaster. In addition, a derotation osteotomy of the femur or surgery on the pelvic bones to make a deeper acetabulum may be necessary.

4. All complications occur more frequently the later treatment begins.
   a. Avascular necrosis of the femoral head epiphysis may occur, producing a permanent deformity.
   b. Cartilage necrosis may occur, producing a stiff painful joint.
   c. Osteoarthritis may set in by early adult life, and may need a total hip replacement operation at that time.

FOLLOW-UP

Barlow's test should be repeated at 6 weeks, 3 months and 6 months of age. X-rays may be a valuable aid to diagnosis, but are less useful in neonates. In these babies ultrasound is the best investigation[4]. The general practitioner should re-check all babies at 6 weeks of age.

[1] MacFarlane A (1987) Screening for congenital dislocation of the hip. *Br. Med. J.*, **294,** 1047.
[2] Duckworth T (1983) Congenital dislocation of the hip. *Surgery,* **1,** 7–12.
[3] Standing Medical Advisory Committee and Standing Nursing and Midwifery Advisory Committee for the Secretaries of State for Social Services and Wales (1986) *Screening for the Detection of Congenital Dislocation of the Hip.* London: DHSS.
[4] Clark NMP (1987) Screening for congenital dislocation of the hip. *Br. Med. J.*, **294,** 1417.

Bow Legs

In the first 2 years of life the tibia is normally bowed, with an outward curve. This is usually unnoticed until the child stands, and then appears bow-legged. The bowing appears most pronounced in very sturdy children. It increases in the first 6 months after walking begins. Later, improvement occurs spontaneously and the legs become normal by the age of 2–3 years[1,2].

To measure the bowing, lay the child down with the legs extended. With the malleoli together, measure the distance between the condyles of the knees. Up to 5 cm distance may be normal.

PROGNOSIS

- Physiological bowing is bilateral and symmetrical and corrects itself by the age of 3 years.
- Pathological bowing is due to rickets, trauma, infection causing epiphyseal damage, and the rare Blount's disease of the upper tibial epiphysis in West Indian children. The child will need referral for osteotomy which may need to be repeated throughout childhood. Despite surgery, some results are poor[1]. It may be impossible to achieve a straight leg and equal leg length for both legs, especially when the growing epiphysis has been damaged.

TREATMENT

1. When there is bilateral bowing in young children, with separation of 5 cm or less at the knees, explanation is all that is necessary in most cases.
2. Pathological bowing (unilateral cases or those with more than 5 cm of separation): the child should be referred to an orthopaedic surgeon. Surgical treatment, such as repeated osteotomy or epiphyseal stapling, may be needed throughout childhood.

FOLLOW-UP

In young babies, a 6-month follow-up in the well baby clinic, with serial measurements of the bowing, up to the age of 3 years is often all that is needed. Most children will settle spontaneously. For those children with pathological bowing the orthopaedic surgeon will follow up.

[1] Jones PG, Woodward AA (1986) *Clinical Paediatric Surgery. Diagnosis and Management*, 3rd edn. Carlton, Victoria: Blackwell Scientific Publications.
[2] Duthie RB, Bentley G (1983) *Mercer's Orthopaedic Surgery*, 8th edn. London: Edward Arnold.

Knock Knees

Soon after the age of 2 years, the child's knees develop a knock-knee posture (genu valgum). This increases to a maximum at age $3\frac{1}{2}$ years, and then gradually improves, until the legs of most children are 'straight' at age 6–7 years[1]. Knock knees are due to unequal growth of the femoral condyles (*not* laxity of the knee ligaments).

Between the age of 3 and $3\frac{1}{2}$, 22% of children have knock knees of 5 cm or more[2]. Measure the distance between both medical malleoli of the ankle joints with the child lying on a couch, with the extended knees just touching each other.

In adults, knock knees may be due to Paget's disease, osteoarthritis of the knee and previous fracture of the lateral tibial condyle.

PROGNOSIS

- In children the prognosis is excellent. The vast majority correct themselves by the age of 6–7 years with no treatment.
- Severe genu valgum at age 10 and onwards often need surgery.
- In adults the prognosis is that of the underlying disease. Paget's disease may be difficult to treat. Osteoarthritis may be helped by surgery (osteotomy or knee joint replacement).

TREATMENT

1. Explanation and reassurance are usually all that is required in most young children. Six-monthly follow-up measurements are made.
2. Referral to an orthopaedic surgeon will be required for severe knock knees (10 cm or more) by age 10 years and unilateral knock knees. In children supracondylar osteotomy of the femur, or tibial osteotomy is carried out. The decision rests on the site of maximum deformity.
3. Surgery may be required for unilateral knock knee. Also, in adults, osteotomy and/or knee joint replacement may correct deformity or osteoarthritis.

FOLLOW-UP

The general practitioner is ideally placed to follow up young children with knock knees in the well baby clinic. Serial measurements of the intermalleolar distance are reassuring to doctor and parents.

[1] Jones PG, Woodward AA (1986) *Clinical Paediatric Surgery. Diagnosis and Management*, 3rd edn. Carlton, Victoria: Blackwell Scientific Publications.
[2] Duthie RB, Bentley G (1983) *Mercer's Orthopaedic Surgery*, 8th edn, pp. 1006–8. London: Edward Arnold.

Flat Feet

Flat feet are common. An incidence of 1.9 per 1000 patients is probably an underestimate, as many cases are never reported[1]. The feet of all babies are flat because a pad of fat fills the longitudinal arch of the feet. When the child stands, the foot rolls into valgus because of incomplete muscle control. The foot gradually approaches the adult form over the first 3 years of life[2]. In older children with flat feet there may be an outward twisting of the foot (valgus), prominence of the navicular tuberosity, and excessive heel wear on the shoe's inner edges[3]. A tiptoe test is useful. If the arch appears on standing on tiptoe and the foot is flexible, then the flat foot is of no significance and requires no treatment other than explanation.

PROGNOSIS

- In most cases under the age of 16 years the prognosis is excellent and no treatment is needed. The tiptoe test indicates a flexible foot[1].
- Over the age of 16 years, arthritis may occur and surgery may be needed. The foot may remain stiff and painful.

TREATMENT

1. Explanation and reassurance is the main treatment. Referral to an orthopaedic surgeon may be necessary to reinforce this to patients.
2. In babies, flat feet are normal[2].
3. In children, explanation is the best treatment. In very few cases is any treatment necessary[3]. If so, the following may be used.
   a. Exercises by the physiotherapist to strengthen muscles.
   b. Supports in the shoes to support a sagging arch.
   c. Heel wedges may lessen excessive wear on the shoes.
   d. Diet to control obesity.
   Referral to an orthopaedic surgeon may be necessary to gain access to an orthoptist for shoe supports and heel wedges.
4. In teenagers spasmodic flat foot may occur[4]. This is an acute condition of pain, spasm and tightness of the peroneal muscles, often after starting a new job with prolonged standing. The prognosis is excellent, without recourse to surgery. Treatment includes rest, analgesics and anti-inflammatory drugs. Occasionally a manipulation under anaesthesia and 6 weeks in plaster will be necessary to produce a neutral position for the foot.
5. In adults no treatment is necessary unless there are symptoms—usually pain and stiffness. Measures listed as above (point 3a–d) should be tried first. Rarely, in severe cases of rigid flat foot there is arthritis of the talonavicular joint. Operative fusion may be advised by the orthopaedic surgeon.

FOLLOW-UP

In small children a yearly follow-up may be needed to reassure the parent. Very occasionally flat foot may be the first sign of a muscular dystrophy or a neurological disorder.

[1] Hodgkin K (1985) *Towards Earlier Diagnosis. A Guide to Primary Care*, 5th edn, p. 651. Edinburgh: Churchill Livingstone.
[2] Jones PG, Woodward AA (1986) *Clinical Paediatric Surgery. Diagnosis and Management*, 3rd edn. Carlton, Victoria: Blackwell Scientific Publications.
[3] Apley AG, Solomon L (1986) *Apley's System of Orthopaedics and Fractures*, 6th edn. London: Butterworths.
[4] Duthie RB, Bentley G (1983) *Mercer's Orthopaedic Surgery*, 8th edn. London: Edward Arnold.

Hallux Valgus and Bunions

Hodgkin[1] gave 2 per 1000 incidence of patients with bunions, and a 10:1 female predominance. Hallux valgus is the most common of the foot deformities[2]. Often there is a congenital familial problem, with the first metatarsal rotated like a thumb. In acquired cases, increasing weight and tight shoes will add to the deformity. It is most common in women in the sixth decade, and is usually bilateral[2].

PROGNOSIS

- All cases can be made comfortable by careful attention to footwear[2].
- Results of surgical treatment are good where the deformity is not too severe. Results are poor in severely deformed and clawed feet—surgical shoes are better treatment[2].
- In a 6-year follow-up of metatarsal osteotomy in the treatment of hallux valgus, for 130 operations on 77 patients results were good in 45%, fair in 21% and poor in 34%[3].
- Of the many complications of bunion surgery, circulatory problems are the commonest, including gangrene, dead tissue and local skin necrosis[4]. Others include metatarsalgia (especially when the first metatarsal is shortened), recurrence of the bunion, floppy toe, foreign body reaction to silastic implants, and recurrent hammer toe. Also, the first toe may turn outwards again, rotate inwards or become fixed in an extended position.

TREATMENT

1. *Preventive treatment*: patients at risk should be advised to avoid ill-fitting shoes with pointed toes; not to wear very high-heeled shoes and to keep their weight down.
2. *Conservative treatment*
   a. Acute exacerbations of pain and cellulitis may require analgesics, antibiotics and NSAIDs.
   b. Refer the patient to an orthopaedic surgeon to obtain surgical footwear (wide shoes with very soft uppers).
   c. Refer the patient to a chiropodist to obtain foot padding.
3. *Surgery*: refer to an orthopaedic surgeon. Several procedures may be done, usually involving trimming of the bony exostosis and osteotomy of the first metatarsal. Indications include pain unresponsive to the above conservative treatments and the presence of osteoarthritis in the metatarsophalangeal joint.

FOLLOW-UP

Remember gout as a possible cause of symptoms. Refer the patient early if you think surgery is indicated.

[1] Hodgkin K (1985) *Towards Earlier Diagnosis. A Guide to Primary Care*, 5th edn, pp. 633–44. Edinburgh: Churchill Livingstone.
[2] Apley AG, Solomon L (1986) *Apley's System of Orthopaedics and Fractures*, 6th edn, pp. 215–318. London: Butterworths.
[3] Hart JAL, Bentley G (1976) Metatarsal osteotomy in the treatment of hallux valgus. *J. Bone Joint Surg.*, **58B,** 261.
[4] Epps CH Jr (1986) *Complications in Orthopaedic Surgery*, vol 2, 2nd edn, pp. 1268–87. Philadelphia: JB Lippincott Company.

13

Ophthalmology

V. W. M. Drury

Conjunctivitis

Inflammation of the conjunctiva is the commonest eye problem seen by the general practitioner and accounts for 30% of eye consultations. It may be caused by bacterial or viral infection, by chemical reactions or eyelid abnormalities or may be due to allergy. Except in cases of bilateral conjunctivitis in children, the cornea should be stained with fluorescein to ascertain that the epithelium is intact.

Bacterial Infection

This is usually caused by *Haemophilus influenzae*, streptococcus, staphylococcus or *Moraxella lacumata*. The discharge is mucopurulent and there is crusting on the lashes. Chlamydial infection is acquired by genital contact. It is seen in sexually active adults and the conjunctivitis affects particularly the lower fornix with follicle formation.

Conjunctivitis in the newborn is notifiable. A swab should always be taken. The same organisms that affect adults are found, with the addition of *Neisseria gonorrhoea*.

PROGNOSIS

● Treatment will normally cure the condition in a few days. Conjunctivitis is contagious and separate towels and flannels should be used in a family.
● Some cases of chronic conjunctivitis are difficult to treat.

TREATMENT

1. Swabs should be taken from all newborn babies with conjunctivitis and from adults where possible. Special transport medium is required for *Chlamydia* culture.
2. Chloramphenicol eyedrops or ointment used 3–4 times daily for 5 days is appropriate.
3. Chlamydial infection is usually diagnosed by failure to respond to this treatment. Swabs should then be taken and in adults tetracycline ointment used three times daily; erythromycin orally 500 mg 4 times daily for 3 weeks should eradicate the eye and genital infection. Treatment of sexual partners is advisable.
4. Conjunctivitis in the newborn normally responds to chloramphenicol eye ointment 6 times daily.

5. Chlamydial infection (trachoma) is a common cause of blindness in some countries.

FOLLOW-UP

Failure to respond to treatment within 48 hours needs review to check the diagnosis.

Viral Infection

The commonest cause is the adenovirus and it is most frequently seen in epidemics in schools and families[1]. Rapid onset is common, the preauricular glands are often enlarged and there is no purulent discharge. Tiny corneal ulcers may be present. Viral infection is potentially serious. Viral swabs should be taken.

PROGNOSIS

● Most patients present trivial and transient symptoms and the condition resolves in 10–14 days.
● Keratitis and uveitis produce blurring of the vision, photophobia and pain and may give rise to conjunctival scarring.
● In a few patients the symptoms may persist for months or years. It is not known how frequently the complications occur.
● Herpes simplex infections are usually short-lived (see p. 227).

TREATMENT

1. The most important step is strict personal hygiene to prevent spread of infection.
2. No specific treatment is available except the use of vasoconstrictors to relieve pain (1% adrenaline eyedrops).

3. Viral swabs should be taken whenever possible.
4. Referral is indicated in all patients in whom ulceration, keratitis or uveitis is suspected.

Allergic Conjunctivitis

Allergic conjunctivitis may occur acutely with gross conjunctival oedema which settles equally quickly, or may present as a mild inflammation, usually at hayfever time and associated with much itching.

Atopic individuals can develop vernal conjunctivitis ('spring catarrh') with characteristic 'cobblestones' on the tarsal conjunctiva.

PROGNOSIS

● Allergic conjunctivitis, like hayfever, is a disease of children and young adults and normally resolves in middle age.

TREATMENT

1. Acute conjunctival oedema will resolve quickly with Otrivine-Antistin drops instilled hourly. An oral antihistamine can be administered at the start. The conjunctivitis of hayfever may be prevented by regular use of sodium cromoglycate (Opticrom) drops supplemented by Otrivine-Antistin as required.

FOLLOW-UP

None is necessary.

---

[1] Gigliotti F et al. (1981) Etiology of acute conjunctivitis in children. J. Pediat., **98,** 531–6.

Diseases of the Eyelids

Styes and meibomian infections

Styes are infections of eyelash follicles. Meibomian glands lie inside the lids and may become infected and form cysts. Both styes and meibomian infections present as painful swellings of the lid often with a yellow, pointing area. They are reported in 5–20/1000 patients per year but many mild cases are never reported[1].

PROGNOSIS

● Once styes have drained resolution is complete. If styes are recurrent then the urine should be checked for sugar. Patients who develop one meibomian cyst may develop others.

TREATMENT

1. Styes are treated with hot bathing and removal of the offending lash once pus is seen.
2. Meibomian infection is treated with local heat. Topical antibiotics may help to prevent recurrence.
3. Antibiotics (flucloxacillin 250 mg 6-hourly or phenoxymethylpenicillin 250 mg 6-hourly) are required if cellulitis occurs.
4. A residual cyst is treated with incision and curetting under local anaesthetic, followed by an antibiotic ointment for several days.

FOLLOW-UP

No follow-up is required after resolution has occurred.

Blepharitis

This is a chronic inflammation of the margin of the eyelid. It is usually caused by the staphylococcus. In its more severe forms it can destroy the follicles and distort the lids. It is often associated with seborrhoea.

PROGNOSIS

● Blepharitis tends to recur unless the patient can be persuaded to avoid touching and rubbing the eye.

TREATMENT

1. Blepharitis requires regular and meticulous treatment. Careful explanation should be given to the patient, who should be exhorted to avoid touching or rubbing the eyes.
2. The lid margin should be swabbed daily with warm bicarbonate solution to remove scales and crusts
3. A local antibiotic cream (chloramphenicol or framycetin) should be applied twice daily.
4. An antibiotic and steroid cream may be more effective but care must be taken when putting steroids into the eye, and prolonged treatment must be avoided.

5. Seborrhoea of the scalp should be treated if present with salicylic and sulphur cream or a selenium sulphide preparation.

FOLLOW-UP

The patient will need to be seen regularly until cured and then told to return promptly if the condition recurs.

[1] Hodgkin K (1978) *Towards Earlier Diagnosis*. Edinburgh: Churchill Livingstone.

The Watering Eye

The watering eye may occur at any age, and usually is due to an obstruction of the tear drainage mechanism.

PROGNOSIS

- In infants the watering eye is always curable.
- In adults a block in the lacrimal sac or beyond can be cured in 90% of cases. Stenosis proximal to the sac may require radical reconstructive surgery and the cure rate is less than 50%[1].

TREATMENT

Infants

1. The mother is shown how to press gently with her index finger over the medial palpebral ligament to squeeze out infected material. The aim is to express the sac contents into the nose and this is frequently curative. This is done twice a day and chloramphenicol eyedrops are instilled four times a day.

2. If the problem is not resolved by 6 months the infant should be referred for surgical probing under general anaesthetic.

Adults

1. If there is a block in an otherwise normal drainage system the duct can be syringed under local anaesthetic but this rarely gives lasting benefit. If this is unsuccessful the patient has to choose between accepting the condition and surgery. Dacrocystorhinostomy is successful in more than 90% of patients[2].

[1] Glasspole M (1982) *Problems in Ophthalmology*. Lancaster–MTP Press.
[2] Roper Hall MJ (1980) *Stallards Eye Surgery*, 6th edn. Bristol: John Wright.

The Dry Eye

The dry eye due to deficiency of tears (Sjögren's syndrome), deficiency of mucus (Stevens–Johnson's syndrome etc.) or to problems with the corneal surface. The symptoms can be mimicked by low-grade inflammation, such as that due to low-grade allergy, and this must be excluded.

PROGNOSIS

- The condition is incurable.

TREATMENT

1. Artificial teardrops—hypromellose or poly- vinyl alcohol—can be applied hourly or even more frequently.
2. Closure of lacrimal puncta to prevent tear drainage can be very effective, and enhances the effects of tear supplements.
3. Hydrogel contact lenses have proved valuable in protecting the cornea.

Dacrocystitis

Infection of the lacrimal sac can present as a watering eye and is diagnosed by feeling a tender sac. Chronic infection is usually associated with recurrent conjunctivitis. Dacryocystitis can occur in infants but is most common in middle-aged females.

PROGNOSIS

- Normally dacryocystitis resolves following treatment without leading to any permanent block of the duct. Incision, if necessary, will heal without leaving a scar, though in a few cases recurrence occurs.

TREATMENT

1. In the early stages a systemic antibiotic and warm compresses will produce resolution.
2. If an abscess has formed this should be incised under general anaesthetic.

Iritis

The iris, the ciliary body and the choroid form the uveal tract and are anatomically so close together that disease usually involves all three parts. The cause of inflammation is often difficult to identify. Infection and allergy are the usual factors but a specific cause is found in less than half the cases seen. There is an association between anterior uveitis and ankylosing spondylitis, Reiter's disease, and some other diseases, in that about 90% of patients suffering from these conditions carry the tissue type HLA-27, compared to between 4 and 8% of the normal population. Anterior uveitis occurs in 20% of patients with ankylosing spondylitis and 10% of patients with Reiter's disease[1].

PROGNOSIS

- Early and appropriate medical treatment will usually render the eye quiet in 3 or 4 weeks but more severe cases may take several months to resolve. Uveitis may take a relapsing chronic course over many years, especially when associated with some other condition such as ankylosing spondylitis.
- Residual damage may lead to secondary glaucoma and cataract formation in 1–2% of patients.

TREATMENT

1. Early referral of new cases for specialist advice is indicated.
2. Occasionally chronic relapsing cases can have a recurrence dealt with without referral.
3. Dilatation of the pupil with 1% atropine eye-drops 4-hourly rests the pupil and prevents synechiae (adhesions). Treatment should be continued until the eye has been quiet for 2 weeks.
4. Hot applications and aspirin will relieve pain.
5. Prednisolone 0.5% eyedrops used 2-hourly are essential to suppress inflammation.

FOLLOW-UP

The patient should be seen regularly until the eye is quiet. Instructions should be given to return if there is any recurrence.

---

[1] Hughes GRV (1979) *Connective Tissue Diseases*, 2nd edn. Oxford: Blackwell Scientific Publications.

Corneal Ulcer

The cornea is highly susceptible to damage and whenever a breach of the corneal epithelium is suspected 2% fluorescein drops should be instilled to confirm the diagnosis. Commonest causes include traumatic abrasions which, if infected, may proceed to ulceration, herpes simplex infections and herpes zoster ophthalmicus.

PROGNOSIS

- An abrasion will normally heal within 12–24 hours unless secondary infection occurs.
- With any ulcer anterior uveitis may occur leading to secondary glaucoma.
- Herpes simplex infections should heal with treatment with topical acyclovir in 6–10 days but occasionally longer treatment is required. Recurrence is unusual (5%) if treatment is prompt, i.e. before the virus reaches the corneal stroma[1]. Recurrence is unlikely in epithelial herpes but common in stromal herpes.
- Visual acuity may be decreased in up to 6% of patients—usually those with geographic ulcers[2].
- Visual acuity will be affected if the central cornea is affected, but unlikely if the ulcer is peripheral.

TREATMENT

Corneal abrasion or traumatic ulcer

1. 1% cyclopentolate is applied 3-hourly to rest the eye by preventing ciliary spasm, followed by chloramphenicol eye ointment 3 times daily to prevent secondary infection. The lid margins are closed with micropore and a pad and bandage are applied.
2. The eye is inspected daily until healing has occurred.

Herpes simplex ulcer

1. Dendritic ulcers, diagnostic of herpes simplex, should always be considered in patients with a red or sore eye.
2. A 1 cm ribbon of acyclovir ointment is instilled into the lower conjunctival sac 5 times daily and continued for 3 days after healing has taken place.
3. Referral to an eye specialist is usually required because of the potential threat to vision.

Herpes zoster ophthalmicus

1. Acyclovir ointment is used as described above. Mydriatics, such as 1% atropine drops, will relieve pain. Early referral to an eye specialist is indicated.

FOLLOW-UP

All patients with corneal ulceration must be seen regularly until healing has occurred. Referral to an eye-specialist is indicated in all but minor abrasions.

---

[1] McGill J et al. (1983) Trans. Ophthal. Soc. U.K., **103**, 111–14.
[2] Wilhelmus K et al. (1981) Arch. Ophthal., **99**, 1578–82.

Retinal Detachment

Retinal detachment occurs as a result of fluid (or rarely a solid tumour) accumulating between the two layers of the retina. The vast majority of cases are due to a hole in the retina. Common predisposing conditions are myopia associated with vitreous degeneration which pulls the retina away, aphakia, advancing age and, occasionally, trauma. The classical symptoms are a sudden flash of light followed by black 'floaters' and then a 'shadow' or 'curtain' over the vision. Examination may reveal field loss and/or funduscopic change. The general practitioner might see a case every 2–3 years.

PROGNOSIS

- The success rate for early surgery is around 90%.
- If the subretinal fluid involves the macular area visual acuity can rarely be improved beyond 6/10[1].
- Even when the detachment has been present for 2–3 years some useful vision can be regained by surgery.

TREATMENT

1. Treatment consists of immediate referral to an ophthalmologist for surgery. The aim is to seal the retinal hole. Occasionally surgery has to be repeated several times.

FOLLOW-UP

This is carried out by a specialist department but, once the patient has been cured, long-term follow-up is unnecessary. In about one-fifth of cases the other eye becomes affected at a later date[2].

[1] Crick R, Trimble R (1986) *Textbook of Clinical Ophthalmology*. London: Hodder & Stoughton.
[2] Galloway NR (1985) *Common Eye Diseases and their Management*. Berlin: Springer-Verlag.

Squint

Squint (strabismus) is present when the visual axes of the eyes fail to meet at the point of regard. During the first few weeks of life the eyes seem to be wandering about and intermittent squint is common and can be ignored. However, a fixed squint at any age must be taken seriously as it may indicate other pathology such as cataract or retinoblastoma and so must be referred. By 6 months of age squinting is significant if present and action must be taken if it is to be effectively treated. It is described as convergent (esotropic) if one eye turns inwards and divergent (exotropic) if one eye turns outward. In children, squint is usually non-paralytic (concomitant) and is constant in every direction. A paralytic squint (incomitant), most common in adults, increases or occurs at a particular position of gaze at all ages, and indicates serious underlying disease. A non-paralytic squint that develops in a child aged 2–3 is usually associated with hypermetropia. False squint, due to prominent epicanthic folds, can be excluded by the cover test. Each eye is covered in turn to ensure that there is no movement of either eye during the test. The alternate cover test, consisting of rapidly and repeatedly occluding one eye after the other will reveal a latent squint by demonstrating slow recovery of vision.

Squint in childhood

Squint in childhood occurs in 5–6% of children and is more common among handicapped children[1]. There is a familial tendency. Twenty per cent of squints are exotropes, the remaining 80% are esotropes. Squints should be screened for between 6–9 months by the GP and if a squint is obvious before then referral should not be delayed.

PROGNOSIS

- If not treated amblyopia (lazy eye) will become fixed in the squinting eye by the age of 6 years[2]. It usually responds rapidly to treatment before that age, but poorly in older children.
- Cosmetic improvement can be affected at any age. The absence of binocular vision is less important. If there is any delay in controlling early onset squint, the prognosis for binocular vision is poor. In later onset squint, 4 years and upwards, the prognosis for restoring binocular vision is good.

TREATMENT

1. Suspected squint must always be referred to an ophthalmologist. If squint is due to an abnormality such as cataract or retinoblastoma even 6 months could be too late.
2. Amblyopia is treated by forcing the child to use the squinting eye. The normal eye must be covered completely with a patch for a period, depending on severity, varying from a few weeks to more than a year. If a patch is not tolerated blurring the vision in the good eye with 1% atropine drops may help. Older children also receive orthoptic treatment.
3. Exotropes normally require surgery.
4. Only 70% of esotropes require surgery.
5. Cosmetic success should be regularly obtainable.
6. Attaining binocular vision depends on age of onset and prompt treatment.

Squint in adults

This is usually extremely disabling and is usually due to ocular muscle palsy caused by conditions such as multiple sclerosis or cerebrovascular disease[3].

PROGNOSIS

- If the continuing cause can be treated, recovery may occur within 6 months.
- Many cases recover spontaneously within a period of 6–9 months[4].

TREATMENT

1. Occlusion of the other eye helps and prisms

may help in less severe cases. If there is no continuing pathology, surgery to restore binocular vision is indicated after 9 months[5].

FOLLOW-UP

No special follow-up is required by the GP, but the GP should always reinforce the advice given to parents about occluding the non-squinting eye as directed and making the child use the non-occluded eye at such times by playing appropriate games with them.

[1] Graham PA (1974) Epidemiology of strabismus. *Br. J. Ophthalmol.*, **58**, 224–31.
[2] Fletcher MC, Silvermans J (1966) Strabismus: a study of 1110 cases. *Am. J. Ophthal.*, **61**, 86–9.
[3] Douglas A (1963) Visual disorder and cerebral palsy. *Little Club Clin. Dev. Med.*, **9**, 9–21.
[4] Glasspole M (1982) *Problems in Ophthalmology*. Lancaster, MTP.
[5] Miller D (1979) *Ophthalmology: The Essentials*. New York: Houghton Mifflin.

Glaucoma

The normal intraocular pressure is between 16 and 22 mmHg. Ideally it should be measured routinely in eye-testing of persons over 40 years of age. Glaucoma is present when the eye has an abnormally high internal pressure, but the extent of this is variable in different persons and may be variable and intermittent in individuals. Prevention or early diagnosis is particularly important. Glaucoma is manifested as acute (closed angle) glaucoma, chronic (open angle) glaucoma, secondary glaucoma or, very rarely, congenital and juvenile glaucoma. Chronic glaucoma has an insidious onset.

Acute glaucoma

This is associated mainly with middle-age, long-sighted people and occurs in women more often than men. It was an hereditary incidence and occurs in 5% of first-degree relatives. Acute glaucoma may present with attacks of coloured rings around lights occurring in the evening or, more acutely, with sudden headache, visual disturbance and vomiting associated with a painful red eye.

Chronic glaucoma

Chronic glaucoma occurs in 1% of the population over 50 years of age and accounts for 95% of cases of glaucoma. Some 5% of cases present as acute glaucoma[1].

Chronic glaucoma is three times more common in diabetics and has a 5% hereditary incidence in first-degree relatives.

PROGNOSIS

● Untreated glaucoma leads to blindness; 5% of visual disability is due to the condition[2].

● In acute glaucoma, treatment applied in the prodromal phase (transient blurring of vision, headache or—especially significant—haloes around lights) results in cure in almost 100% of patients. In the acute phase delay of more than a few hours will cause blindness.

● In chronic glaucoma prognosis is good only if treatment is started early, continued regularly, and control is adequate. Otherwise vision may continue to deteriorate. Therefore if in doubt about the diagnosis, always refer for specialist opinion.

● More than 90% of patients with chronic glaucoma can be treated medically; the remainder require surgical treatment[3].

● Compliance is often suspect—reinforcement is needed from the general practioner, especially in the early months after diagnosis.

TREATMENT

Acute glaucoma

1. Pilocarpine 4% drops in the affected eye every

5 minutes should be given during urgent transfer to specialist care.
2. Pilocarpine 2% drops should be administered prophylactically in the other eye 3-hourly.
3. Acetazolamide (Diamox) 500 mg can be injected intramuscularly.
4. Further treatment is normally surgical, laser or surgical iridectomy and is usually curative.

Chronic glaucoma

1. Pilocarpine 0.5–4% drops can be applied 3–4 times daily. This causes blurring and dimness of vision because of pupil constriction, and careful explanation to the patient is thus required.
2. A topical beta-blocker 0.25–0.5% 1–2 times daily is now a common alternative to pilocarpine. It suppresses secretion of aqueous humour but its absorption may cause common beta-blocker side-effects.
3. Acetazolamide (Diamox) tablets 500 mg daily reduces the volume of fluid secreted into the eye.

4. Surgery is required when medical control is unsatisfactory in less than 5% of cases.

Secondary glaucoma

1. This occurs in 5% of patients with iridocyclitis. It may be induced by the use of steroids in the eye for more than 3 weeks. Early referral for specialist care is mandatory.

FOLLOW-UP

In general, patients with glaucoma will be followed up in a specialist department. The general practitioner's main role will be explanation and encouraging patients to comply with advice.

[1] Galloway NR (1985) *Common Eye Diseases and their Management*. Berlin: Springer-Verlag.
[2] Cullinan TR (1977) *The Epidemiology of Visual Disability—Studies of visually Disabled People in the Community*. HSRU report no. 28. Canterbury: University of Kent.
[3] Miller S (ed) (1984) Parsons' Diseases of the Eye, 17th edn. Edinburgh: Churchill Livingstone.

Cataracts

A cataract is an opacity within the lens or its capsule. It may be developmental or acquired.

Developmental cataract

Some degree of developmental cataract is very common and most people have minute areas of opacity. The incidence of such cataracts requiring treatment is unknown but they are uncommon. There is a great variety and their type depends upon the fetal age when the development was disturbed and the nature of the disturbance. Some 10% are hereditary. Other causes presenting at birth include maternal malnutrition, virus infection (especially rubella) and oxygen deprivation from placental haemorrhage. There is no known cause in 30% of cases[1].

Acquired cataract

The commonest cause of acquired cataract is age but it can be caused by trauma and is sometimes associated with conditions such as diabetes, Down's syndrome and hypoparathyroidism.

PROGNOSIS

- In congenital cataract, despite 'ideal' treatment to patients with otherwise normal eyes, only half the children achieve acuities that allow unimpeded schooling[3].
- Good control of diabetes may result in the

resolution of very early lens changes but apart from this, once established, cataracts are only amenable to surgical removal.

- In acquired cataract progress is inevitable but some cataracts may remain almost static for a period of years.
- The results of surgery are very satisfactory. For example, posterior lens implantation will give postoperative vision of 6/9 or better in more than 95% of patients without pre-existing eye disease. Retinal detachment occurs postoperatively in 1–2% of patients as a late complication[3].

TREATMENT

1. No medical treatment avails once opacities are present and lens protein has coagulated.
2. In incipient cataract the patient may be helped if dark glasses are worn outdoors and if reading and close work are done under bright light.
3. When the cataract is bilateral and visual acuity has been reduced to the extent that patients are unable to read, to make their way about independently or to follow their occupation, the operation is justifiable. It will obviously produce earlier handicap in a professional person than in an unskilled labourer.
4. Removal of the lens without an intraocular lens replacement results in a loss of accommodation, loss of refracting power, enlarged image sizes and alteration in colour vision. The disabilities of aphakia are treated with spectacles, contact lenses or secondary anterior or posterior chamber lens implantation. Spectacles need very thick lenses and can cause distortion of vision. Contact lenses are difficult to manage for some, such as elderly people or those with arthritis of the fingers, so intraocular lenses are now the most popular choice.
5. Rehabilitation with intraocular lenses is much easier than with other methods. Postoperative vision is similar to the patient's previous experience and there may be an improved depth of focus. Some 30% of patients can achieve 6/9 or better and more than half achieve[4] 6/18. Problems occur due to degradation of supports but in good hands the operation should give at least as good results as other forms of cataract removal.

FOLLOW-UP

This is normally carried out by the ophthalmologist but if a patient is otherwise handicapped, supervision may be required on discharge from hospital and if a complication occurs immediate referral should be made.

[1] Merin S, Crawford JS (197) The aetiology of congenital cataracts. *Can. J. Ophthalmol.*, **6,** 178.
[2] Taylor D (1982) Risks and difficulties of treatment of aphakia in infancy. *Trans. Ophthal. Soc. U.K.*, **102,** 403.
[3] Roper-Hall MJ (1980) *Stallard's Eye Surgery*, 6th edn. Bristol: John Wright.
[4] Rich W (1982) Advantages and disadvantages of different methods of senile cataract surgery. *Trans. Ophthal. Soc. U.K.*, **102,** 407–9.

14

Endocrinology

M. D. Jewell

Diabetes Mellitus

Diabetes mellitus is a condition characterized by raised blood glucose, with a prevalence of approximately 1%. The majority of those with diabetes have non-insulin-dependent diabetes mellitus (NIDDM) which begins later in life and reaches a peak prevalence in the 60s, and is associated with obesity in 60–90% of cases. The remainder have insulin-dependent diabetes mellitus (IDDM), which starts in younger age groups. It will usually present with classical symptoms of hyperglycaemia: thirst, polyuria, tiredness and loss of weight. The symptoms in NIDDM are less marked: mild thirst, pruritus vulvae in women, and sometimes nocturia. Because of the mild symptoms, NIDDM often presents with one of the complications such as cataract.

Diagnosis is made by single venous blood sugar measurements > 10.0 mmol/L (random) or > 6.7 mmol/L (fasting). Only if fasting blood sugar is between 4.4 and 6.7 mmol/L, or random blood sugar is between 6.6 and 10.0 mmol/L is a glucose tolerance test required. Susceptibility to IDDM is inherited with some HLAs; NIDDM tends to run in families and is probably polygenic.

PROGNOSIS

- In IDDM use of insulin protects against the immediate metabolic consequences of the disease but life expectancy is still reduced by the complications of the disease.
- Life expectancy is considerably impaired in diabetes. Mortality from ischaemic heart disease and other cardiovascular disease is double that of non-diabetic patients[1].
- For an unselected group of diabetics diagnosed before the age of 31 and followed up from 1931 to 1973, 16% became blind, 20% had objective signs of myocardial infarction, 10% had had a stroke, 12% had had gangrene or an amputation and 22% had had uraemia[2].
- Diabetes is the commonest cause of blindness in those under the age of 65. The prevalence of retinopathy increases with increasing duration of diabetes, and is associated with high glycosylated haemoglobin (HbA1) levels, the presence of proteinuria and high diastolic blood pressure. The prevalence of background retinopathy in those aged less than 30 at diagnosis rises from 17% after 5 years to 97.5% after 15 years[3]. In the same group proliferative retinopathy rose from 1.2% in patients with diabetes lasting less than 10 years to 67% after 35 years. In older age groups diabetes causes blindness through maculopathy and increases the incidence of cataract[3]. Overall diabetes is responsible for 13% of blindness in men and 18% in women[4], although these figures largely predate

photocoagulation treatment; it remains to be seen whether these levels will be reduced in the future.

- In IDDM good prognosis is associated with good quality of metabolic control, low insulin dose, mean body weight 10% below the ideal, a mean blood pressure less than 100 mmHg and absence of proteinuria[2].
- Over a 40-year period, excess mortality among patients with proteinuria was 3–4 times that of patients without proteinuria[2].
- There is increasing evidence that good diabetic control delays the appearance or slows the development of microangiopathic complications[5]. Regular review of fundal changes with early referral for ophthalmological opinion and laser photocoagulation treatment, if required, will preserve vision in many patients[6]. Whether good control slows the progression of already established complications remains unclear.

TREATMENT

1. *Education*: An essential prerequisite for self-care in diabetes is that patients should understand their conditions. However there is no direct link between knowledge and behaviour, and merely giving the information will not automatically ensure compliance with medical advice. Effective counselling of diabetics, as for all other groups, is likely to start from the patients' own concerns and beliefs. The British

Diabetic Association (10 Queen Anne St, London W1M 0BD; telephone 01-323-1531) fulfils an important educational role for diabetic patients, through literature and meetings.

2. *Diet*: Current principles for diet in diabetics are similar to those being advised for the British diet nationwide. Energy intake from fat should be reduced from an average of 42% to approximately 30–35% of the total. The balance should be made up from carbohydrate, with preference given to complex carbohydrate found in bread, potatoes, pasta and pulses. Sugar should be avoided as far as possible; it should be noted that many foods sold as 'suitable for diabetics' contain sweetening substances other then sucrose which have a similar calorific value. Patients may need help to identify foods with a high fat content. For patients with IDDM the carbohydrate component of their diet is conveniently divided into exchanges. The eventual aim is to maintain a normal body weight as well as to allow unrestricted activity.

3. *Medication*

   a. *IDDM*: Insulin is usually given twice daily 20–30 minutes before breakfast and evening meals in a combination of soluble insulin to coincide with meals and longer-acting insulin to maintain control between meals and overnight. This can either be managed by mixing soluble and isophane insulins or by a fixed-dose combination such as Mixtard to avoid mistakes in drawing up the correct dose. Alternatively a single daily dose of longer-acting insulin such as ultralente can be supplemented by injections of soluble insulin before each meal.

   The physiological pattern of insulin secretion is not reproduced by two- or even three-times daily insulin injections, but is more closely approached by more frequent injections of short-acting preparations. This is simpler to achieve with the pen-syringe (Novo Labs), recently developed which can be carried around and used to inject small amounts of soluble insulin.

   Patients with IDDM must understand the importance of continuing with insulin injections (and possibly increasing the dose) when they are ill, even when the illness leads them to reduce their food intake. The dose may need to be reduced before vigorous exercise, or when meals are missed.

   b. *NIDDM*: Some patients will achieve control of blood sugar levels by dietary control alone, but many will also require oral hypoglycaemic agents.

   Sulphonylureas, such as tolbutamide, can be administered in doses up to 1 g twice daily, or glibenclamide up to 15 mg daily. Sulphonylureas have the troublesome side-effect of increasing appetite in patients who may already be overweight.

   Biguanides, such as metformin up to 1 g twice daily, may be given alone or in combination with a sulphonylurea and do not have the same effect on appetite.

   Hypoglycaemia is uncommon with oral hypoglycaemic drugs, but can be severe and difficult to treat if it does occur. Longer-acting sulphonylureas can cause nocturnal hypoglycaemia. Caution is required in patients with renal failure, as this increases the risk of hypoglycaemia with sulphonylureas, or lactic acidosis with metformin.

   Inadequate control of NIDDM with diet and drugs is an indication for treatment with insulin, but this decision may be difficult for doctors to negotiate, particularly where older patients are concerned, when arguments for prolonging life based on studies of younger groups carry less scientific and emotional weight.

4. *Pregnancy*: The problems for pregnant diabetic women of large babies, late intrauterine death and obstetric complications can be largely avoided if tight control is maintained throughout the pregnancy. Pregnant diabetic women will normally need to be supervised by specialist obstetricians and diabetologists working together, and may need short hospital admissions during the pregnancy.

5. *Monitoring*: Patients with IDDM are taught to use blood glucose testing strips for regular monitoring of their control. They should be encouraged to take measurements regularly at different times of the day. A series of several readings in a single day will also help to give a complete picture. For those with NIDDM, control can be effectively monitored by occasional measurement of a single fasting blood

sugar. For both groups additional information is given by glycosylated haemoglobin, which measures average control over the preceding 6–10 weeks. Blood fructosamine is a cheaper measure used in some laboratories as an indication of average control over the preceding 2–4 weeks.

6. *General measures*: As stated above, a large part of the morbidity and mortality associated with diabetes arises from its effect on atherosclerosis. It is important to reduce the risk of these complications as far as possible by attention to other risk factors, such as smoking, hyperlipidaemia and hypertension. Diabetes is one of the conditions that entitles patients to exemption from all prescription charges.

FOLLOW-UP

Regular review of diabetic patients enables early signs of complications, particularly retinopathy, neuropathy and ischaemia of the feet, to be appropriately treated. It is generally accepted that all diabetic patients should be seen at least once a year for assessment of overall control, fundoscopy through dilated pupils, visual acuities and foot examination.

Traditionally this work has been seen as the preserve of hospital diabetic clinics, but the cover is less than complete[7], and the increase in staffing levels required to achieve this would be considerable. Regular review is becoming accepted as appropriate activity for general practitioners. For general practitioners to provide high-quality care it may be necessary for the general practitioners or

the nurses working with them to acquire additional skills, for instance in dietary advice of foot care. However, above all a structured approach with clear targets and a system for regular recall and identifying defaulters are vital. Reviewing the evidence, it is clear that resources are not available in hospitals to provide the full service for all diabetic patients, but that the ability of general practitioners to offer an effective alternative on a large scale is not yet established[8–10].

[1] Jarrett RJ, Shipley MJ (1985) Mortality and associated risk factors in diabetes. *Acta Endocrinol.*, **110**, (suppl 272), 21–6.

[2] Deckert T *et al.* (1978) Prognosis of diabetics with diabetes onset before the age of 31. *Diabetologia*, **14**, 371–7.

[3] Klein R *et al.* (1984) The Wisconsin epidemiologic study of diabetic retinopathy. *Arch. Ophthalmol.*, **102**, 520–32.

[4] Jarrett RJ (1986) *Diabetes mellitus*. London: Croom Helm.

[5] Tchobroutsky G (1978) Relation of diabetic control to development of microvascular complications. *Diabetologia*, **15**, 143–52.

[6] Kohner EM, Barry PJ (1984) Prevention of blindness in diabetic retinopathy. *Diabetologia*, **26**, 173–9.

[7] Burrows PJ *et al.* (1987) Who cares for the patients with diabetes? Presentation and follow-up in seven Southampton practices. *J. R. Coll. Gen. Pract.* **37**, 65–9.

[8] Singh BM *et al.* (1984) Metabolic control of diabetes in general practice clinics: comparison with a hospital clinic. *Br. Med. J.*, **289**, 726–8.

[9] Hayes TM, Harries J (1984) Randomised controlled trial of routine hospital clinic care versus routine general practice care for type II diabetics. *Br. Med. J.*, **289**, 728–30.

[10] Day JL *et al.* (1987) Problems of shared diabetes care. *Br. Med. J.*, **294**, 1590–2.

Hypothyroidism

In the UK the prevalence of hypothyroidism, including treated and untreated cases, is 1%, with a preponderance of cases among women[1]. In all 95% of cases are the result of autoimmune disease, with other causes including drugs (lithium, amiodarone), surgical or radioactive iodine treatment of hyperthyroidism, and pituitary failure. Congenital hypothyroidism occurs in up to 1 in 3000 births and is detected in screening programmes for raised thyroid-stimulating hormone levels soon after birth. Clinical features include fatigue, cold intolerance, constipation, hoarse voice, dry skin and hair, bradycardia, slow tendon reflexes and ataxia.

PROGNOSIS

- With appropriate thyroxine replacement patients lead a normal life with normal life expectancy.
- Myxoedema coma, of which the effects include hypothermia, is a rare complication with a high mortality rate.

TREATMENT

1. L-Thyroxine is given in a single daily dose, starting at 50 µg daily and increasing at 3–4-weekly intervals. The standard replacement dose is 200 µg daily. Some patients will be adequately maintained on less while a small number will require more.
2. In older patients the starting dose and increments may be half the above to avoid precipitating or exacerbating angina. In those with established ischaemic heart disease tri-iodothyronine can be used initially; its shorter duration of action allows more rapid withdrawal if angina develops.

FOLLOW-UP

Treatment is assessed by monitoring the patient's clinical condition and tetraiodothyronine or thyroid-stimulating hormone levels in the blood. Once the appropriate replacement dose has been established there is no need to review patients more often than once a year. Doctors should remember the possibility of patients with hypothyroidism developing associated conditions such as pernicious anaemia and diabetes.

Hypothyroidism is one of the conditions that entitles the sufferer to exemption from all prescription charges.

---

[1] Tunbridge WMG et al. (1977) The spectrum of thyroid disease in the community: the Wickham survey. Clin. Endocrinol., 7, 481–93.

Hyperthydroidism

The prevalence of hyperthyroidism, taking into account treated and untreated cases, is 1.9%, with a female : male ratio of 6 : 1 or higher[1]. Graves' disease is the cause in 70–85% of cases: together with toxic adenoma (hot nodule) and toxic multinodular goitre it accounts for approximately 90% of cases[2]. Thyrotoxicosis may occur transiently in the early stages of thyroiditis. Clinical features include weight loss with normal or increased appetite, heat intolerance with warm skin and excessive sweating and tachycardia.

PROGNOSIS

- *Graves' disease*: in most patients it has a relapsing and remitting course. Some patients will have a complete, spontaneous remission; this is more likely with mild disease and small goitres[3]. If untreated, the mortality is 11% with death caused by pulmonary embolism or heart failure.

  Up to 50% of patients have eye signs; the commonest are proptosis and lid retraction. The signs may appear for the first time coincidentally as treatment for thyrotoxicosis is started.
- Atrial fibrillation occurs in 10–19% of thyrotoxic patients. It is uncommon before the age of 40, but may be the only clinical feature of the disease in older patients.

TREATMENT

Graves' disease

1. Carbimazole can be given at a starting dose of 15 mg 3 times daily; it may take up to 8 weeks for the patient to become euthyroid. The dose is then reduced with the patient kept euthyroid, and then continued for at least a year before stopping treatment. The condition recurs in 50% of patients after medication is stopped[4]: in such patients it is reasonable to try a second course of carbimazole or refer to a specialist for more definitive treatment. Some patients may prefer to continue taking pills indefinitely rather than have any of the treatments suggested below. Carbimazole can cause rashes – in which case propylthiouracil can be used – or, rarely, agranulocytosis. Patients should be warned about this side-effect and asked to report sore throats without delay.
2. Radioiodine: I^{131} is conveniently given as a drink or tablets and two-thirds of patients will respond successfully to a single dose. The important complication of radioiodine treatment is subsequent hypothyroidism – approximately 15% in the first year and 3% annually thereafter, eventually rising to 100%. In the UK radioiodine is rarely used in women of childbearing age, although recommendations are more liberal in the USA and continental Europe. There is no evidence that radioiodine is carcinogenic.
3. Subtotal thyroidectomy: patients require preoperative treatment with carbimazole to make them euthyroid, and shortly before operation iodine to reduce vascularity.
4. Eye signs can be treated symptomatically with methylcellulose drops, and/or a mild diuretic. In more severe cases steroids (for instance, prednisolone 60 mg daily) are given, and at worst patients may need to be referred for surgical decompression or irradiation.

Multinodular goitre and toxic nodule

1. Treatment with thioureas may be tried according to the doctor's and patient's preference, but thioureas are less likely to be effective for nodular goitre than for Graves' disease, and spontaneous remission is less probable[3]. Otherwise patients will be referred for either surgery or radioiodine treatment.
2. Beta-blockers can help to control symptoms while treatment with carbimazole is taking effect, or if surgery is awaited.

Thyroid crisis

1. This is an attack of uncontrolled thyrotoxicosis, requiring immediate referral to hospital. Treatment consists of a combination of antithyroid drugs, iodine, cooling and beta-blockers.

FOLLOW-UP

Whichever treatment is chosen – radioactive

iodine or surgery – a system for dealing with the known risk of late hypothyroidism is indicated. Doctors should choose either to review the patient regularly to detect its development with thyroid function tests, or give L-thyroxine to prevent late hypothyroidism developing.

[1] Tunbridge WMG et al. (1977) The spectrum of thyroid disease in the community: the Wickham survey. Clin. Endocrinol., 7, 481–93.
[2] Spaulding SW, Lippes H (1985) Hyperthyroidism. Causes, clinical features and diagnosis. Med. Clin. North Am., 69, 937–51.
[3] Cooper DS, Ridgway EC (1985) Clinical management of patients with hyperthyroidism. Med Clin. North Am., 69, 953–71.
[4] Hennemann G et al. (1986) Place of radioactive iodine in the treatment of thyrotoxicosis. Lancet, i, 1369–72.

Thyroiditis

Thyroiditis most commonly follows a virus infection with viruses such as mumps, adenoviruses and measles (de Quervain's thyroiditis). Other forms are autoimmune (Hashimoto's) thyroiditis, or the rare fibrous infiltration of the thyroid (Riedel's thyroiditis). Apart from the results of functional thyroid disturbance, the only clinical features are an enlarged thyroid gland and usually mild pain.

PROGNOSIS

De Quervain's thyroiditis
- Spontaneous remission is the rule. There may be hyperthyroidism initially in 50%, and transient hypothyroidism can persist for some months. Permanent hypothyroidism is rare[1]. Pain, if present, may last 2–5 months, and complete recovery may take up to 10 months[2].

Hashimoto's thyroiditis
- Hyperthyroidism is seen in up to 10% of patients at presentation. Progression to hypothyroidism occurs in up to 20% over several years.

TREATMENT

1. Hypothyroidism is treated appropriately. Hyperthyroidism is usually mild and can be controlled symptomatically by beta-blockers.
2. In de Quervain's thyroiditis pain can be treated with simple analgesics or NSAIDs.

FOLLOW-UP

Regular follow-up is required to detect developing hypothyroidism.

[1] Hay ID (1985) Thyroiditis: a clinical update. Mayo Clin. Proc., 60, 836–43.
[2] Woolf PD (1985) Thyroiditis. Med. Clin. North Am., 69, 1035–48.

Thyroid Enlargement

Non-toxic thyroid enlargement (other than due to thyroiditis; see p. 297) can be simple goitre or nodular enlargement. Simple goitre (rare in the UK) is classically the result of inadequate iodine intake in particular areas, causing low levels of circulating tetraiodothyronine and high levels of thyroid-stimulating hormone. Nodular enlargement is presumed to result from fluctuating levels of thyroid-stimulating hormone. Clinically single nodules will frequently be shown by investigation or exploration to be multinodular goitres.

PROGNOSIS

- Thyroid nodules tend to increase slowly in size and may become toxic. The increase in size is variable. Multinodular enlargement can eventually cause obstruction to trachea, oesophagus or great veins.
- Some 10–20% of solitary nodules are malignant; this proportion rises to 30–50% in those cases where there is a history of exposure to radiation[1].
- The prognosis of malignant swellings varies with the histology. Five-year survival rates are 70% or more for follicular and papillary carcinomas, compared with less than 5% for anaplastic carcinoma[2].

TREATMENT

1. Any iodine deficiency should be corrected.
2. Thyroxine has been given to stop further growth in a multinodular goitre with varied success.
3. When a confident diagnosis of multinodular enlargement can be made clinically or from a scan, there is no immediate need for treatment. Surgery may become necessary either to relieve pressure symptoms or for cosmetic reasons.
4. For single nodules a tissue diagnosis must be made either by needle[3] or open biopsy. 'Cold' nodules on radioactive scan are slightly more likely to be malignant than 'hot' nodules, but the difference is not enough to use this test for differentiation. Needle biopsy has doubled the proportion of nodules found at operation to be malignant by reducing the numbers requiring removal[1]. In either case the patient will be referred to a surgeon. Benign nodules are not amenable to medical treatment but surgery may be advised to confirm the diagnosis or for cosmetic reasons. Surgical treatment of carcinomas depends on the histological type.

FOLLOW-UP

Hospital specialists will often take responsibility for review of patients treated for cancer. It is important to remember that recurrences of follicular or papillary carcinoma may be treatable. For patients with multinodular goitre, the responsibility can be left with them to return if symptoms worsen or they want to consider surgery for cosmetic reasons.

[1] Rojeski MT, Gharib H (1985) Nodular thyroid disease. Evaluation and management. *N. Eng. J. Med.*, **313**, 428–36.
[2] Beahrs OH (1984) Surgical treatment for thyroid cancer. *Br. J. Surg.*, **71**, 976–9.
[3] Franklyn JA, Sheppard MC (1987) Aspiration cytology of the thyroid. *Br. Med. J.*, **295**, 510–1.

Osteoporosis

The term 'osteoporosis' describes loss of bony tissue. The bone mass reaches a maximum at about the age of 30, and decreases thereafter. In women the loss of bone tissue is greatest immediately after the menopause. Other risk factors include family history, short stature, early menopause, immobilization and weightlessness, steroids (either drugs or in Cushing's syndrome), hypogonadism and thyrotoxicosis, cigarette smoking and heavy drinking[1,2]. The clinical features are those of the disease's secondary effects, such as fractures of the vertebrae and femoral neck.

PROGNOSIS

- Osteoporosis contributes to the increasing frequency of fractures with increasing age. The cumulative prevalence of fractures of wrist, spine and femur in women is 5, 2.5 and 0.6% respectively by the age of 60, compared with 15, 7.5 and 6% respectively by the age of 80.
- Fractures of the hip are associated with an excess mortality of 5–20% in the year immediately following the injury, as well as causing lasting disability in survivors.

TREATMENT[2,3]

1. At present no treatment is widely available to treat the established disease effectively, i.e. to increase bone mass. The aim must therefore be to prevent the disease developing.
2. Long-term prevention of osteoporosis may be achieved by encouraging the maximum possible peak bone mass. Dietary intake of calcium during childhood and adolescence may be a determinant of peak bone mass, although it is not known whether increasing calcium intake will improve bone mass. If this became established, future children and adolescents might be advised to increase their calcium intake by drinking more (skimmed) milk. At present there is no strong argument for such advice, but equally no reason to discourage such cheap and harmless behaviour.
3. Attention to risk factors: osteoporosis is another reason why general practitioners should ascertain patients' smoking and drinking habits and give appropriate advice. Exercise in the elderly may decrease bone loss, and may also help to preserve neurological functioning and so reduce the risk of falling. The risk of falls can also be reduced by minimizing hazards in the domestic environment, for instance by ensuring adequate lighting, secure fastening of carpets, and putting up handrails where appropriate.
4. Oestrogen therapy given after the menopause is the only effective treatment to slow bone loss. It is most effective if started immediately after the menopause. Unopposed oestrogens have potentially serious side-effects, particularly endometrial hyperplasia and cancer. They should therefore be given with cyclical progestogens to reduce this risk, although this causes a return of menstrual bleeding. In women who have had hysterectomies, oestrogens can be given continuously and alone. The major problem is deciding who should take oestrogens, and for how long. The risk factors have been described above, but it is not known how or to what extent they can be used to identify a high-risk group. The current consensus is to continue treatment for 10 years on the grounds that this will postpone the progression of the disease and therefore the onset of complicating fractures for that length of time. The recommended daily dosages are 0.625 mg conjugated oestrogen, 2 mg 17 beta-oestradiol, or 25 μg ethinyloestradiol.
5. As stated above, calcium may have an effect on the growing skeleton. There is little evidence that a high calcium intake reduces bone loss in adult life. Nevertheless, in the absence of evidence that it does positive harm, it is reasonable to recommend a daily calcium intake of at least 1500 mg, if necessary given in the form of tablets.
6. Fluoride is the only drug known to have a beneficial effect on established osteoporosis: it increases the trabecular bone mass and reduces the rate of vertebral fractures. However there

are concerns about its use, not least the possibility that it decreases cortical bone mass, and not all patients respond to it. It is recommended that fluoride should be used only in patients with severe vertebral osteoporosis under supervision by specialist centres.

7. Other drugs: calcitonin may reduce bone loss but its effectiveness and usefulness are not yet fully established. Vitamin D has no effect on bone loss. Anabolic steroids can increase bone mass in established osteoporosis but cause side-effects, including virilizing and atherogenic effects, which preclude their long-term use. Androgens may be used in the treatment of osteoporosis caused by hypogonadism in males.

8. Treatment of complications: fractures of the wrist and hip will require orthopaedic referral. Vertebral fractures can be treated with analgesics and bedrest if necessary. Physiotherapy may help to improve posture following vertebral fractures.

FOLLOW-UP

Follow-up will usually be required for patients taking oestrogens. For those known to have osteoporosis but who are not having any specific treatment, the only reason for review would be to encourage exercise and look for deteriorating balance and posture.

[1] Nordin BEC, et al. (1984) Osteoporosis. In: *Metabolic Bone and Stone Disease* (Nordin BEC ed). Edinburgh: Churchill Livingstone.
[2] Smith R (1987) Osteoporosis: cause and management. *Br. Med. J.*, **294**, 329–32.
[3] Anonymous editorial (1987) Consensus development conference: prophylaxis and treatment of osteoporosis. *Br. Med. J.*, **295**, 914–15.

Osteomalacia

Osteomalacia is the delayed mineralization of bone caused by lack of vitamin D. The clinical features include proximal myopathy and bone pain. Nutritional lack of vitamin D is rare, but may occur in malabsorption syndrome. More commonly in the UK, it now occurs as a combination of relative dietary lack and underexposure to sunlight in elderly and Asian immigrants. It also occurs secondary to renal disease. In the UK most vitamin D is derived from the skin rather than the diet, and therefore should be regarded more as a hormone than a vitamin.

PROGNOSIS

● Provided there are no skeletal deformities at the time of diagnosis, treatment restores the skeleton to normal[1].

TREATMENT

1. Treatment is given in the form of calcium with vitamin D tablets twice daily, thus providing 1000 units of vitamin D daily. Myopathy usually resolves within 2–3 weeks of starting treatment, while bone healing takes several months. An alternative is a single injection of 600 000 units of vitamin D which lasts for 6 months; this avoids the need for regular pills and may therefore suit older patients.

2. Pharmacological doses may be required when osteomalacia is secondary to malabsorption, usually with 1-alpha hydroxycholecalciferol, or in renal disease. In both cases patients will normally need specialist supervision, as over-treatment can lead to a decrease in renal function. Patients on such doses of vitamin D need to have their blood calcium concentrations measured intermittently.

FOLLOW-UP

Patients at risk, or with a previous history of osteomalacia, should have biochemical monitoring at intervals.

[1] Peacock M (1984) Osteomalacia and rickets. In: *Metabolic Bone and Stone Disease* (Nordin BEC ed). Edinburgh: Churchill Livingstone.

Hyperprolactinaemia

Elevation of serum prolactin levels can occur transiently through stress, surgery and eating. It can also be secondary to pregnancy and lactation, diseases of the hypothalamus, and some drugs including chlorpromazine, pimozide, haloperidol and sulpiride (all acting as dopamine receptor antagonists), oestrogens and methyldopa. Persistently elevated levels in the absence of any other cause are assumed to be a result of a prolactinoma. In women hyperprolactinaemia causes amenorrhoea or oligomenorrhoea and galactorrhoea, and loss of libido. In men hyperprolactinaemia is rarer and causes impotence.

PROGNOSIS

- Untreated, most prolactinomas remain static; some will enlarge gradually while a few regress spontaneously[1].
- Prolactinomas tend to present later in men and have a worse prognosis.
- The risk of tumour enlargement during pregnancy is less than 5% in women with microadenomas (tumours which are less than 1 cm across), but higher for those with less common macroadenomas (tumours greater than 1 cm across).
- Untreated, hyperprolactinaemia is associated with osteoporosis in the longterm[2].

TREATMENT

1. Bromocriptine is the most commonly used drug. It is started at a dose of 1.25 mg daily and gradually increased to a dose sufficient to reduce the prolactin levels to normal, usually 2.5 mg 2 or 3 times daily. Most patients respond symptomatically to this regime. Tumours decrease in size, so that pressure effects may resolve rapidly. Side-effects of bromocriptine include nausea, vomiting and dizziness, and are minimized by the slow increase in doses noted. Patients who are unresponsive to bromocriptine or who have persistent troublesome side-effects may respond to one of the related drugs such as lisuride and pergolide, but these are not yet generally available. When bromocriptine is stopped, there is a tendency for prolactin levels to rise again so treatment may need to be continued indefinitely.
2. Radiotherapy or surgery (trans-sphenoidal adenomectomy) is indicated when patients have either a partial or complete lack of response to bromocriptine. The success of surgery is inversely related to the preoperative level of prolactin levels; in one series high recurrence rates were reported after surgery, but this finding is not universal[3,4]. Radiotherapy may cause pituitary destruction, with deficiencies of growth hormone and gonadotrophin developing gradually.
3. Although bromocriptine has not been found to be teratogenic, women trying to conceive are advised to stop taking bromocriptine as soon as they know they are pregnant, and these women are monitored throughout pregnancy for evidence of tumour enlargement. In the case of macroprolactinomas, the risk of enlargement during pregnancy is greater so definitive treatment with surgery or radiotherapy is recommended before conception.

FOLLOW-UP

The tendency to recurrence of this condition dictates the need for longterm follow-up of all patients, whichever treatment has been used.

[1] Grossman A, Besser GM (1985) Prolactinomas. *Br. Med. J.*, **290,** 182–4.
[2] Klibanski A *et al.* (1980) Decreased bone density in hyperprolactinaemic women. *N. Engl. J. Med.*, **303,** 1511–3.
[3] Serri O *et al.* (1983) Recurrence of hyperprolactinaemia after selective transsphenoidal adenoidectomy in women with prolactinoma. *N. Engl. J. Med.*, **309,** 280–3.
[4] Scanlon MF *et al.* (1985) Management of selected patients with hyperprolactinaemia by partial hypophysectomy. *Br. Med. J.*, **291,** 1547–50.

15

Haematology

V. W. M. Drury

Megaloblastic Anaemia

Megaloblastic anaemia is caused by vitamin B_{12} deficiency, folate deficiency or certain rare conditions interfering in DNA synthesis, such as orotic aciduria or erythroleukaemia.

Vitamin B_{12} deficiency

Pernicious anaemia is the most common cause. The anaemia develops due to lack of intrinsic factor and severe atrophic gastritis. Strict vegetarianism is also a cause and may be associated with folate deficiency. Chronic alcoholism, gastrectomy, enteropathy and intestinal parasites are other causes.

PROGNOSIS

- Pernicious anaemia is inevitably fatal unless treatment is introduced.
- Treatment has to be lifelong. With B_{12} treatment the patient usually feels better in 1–2 days and bone marrow becomes normal as quickly[1].
- Macrocytosis usually disappears in 5–10 weeks but iron deficiency anaemia may supervene in the recovery phase.
- Anaemia due to chronic alcoholism disappears by 3 months after drinking has stopped.

Folate deficiency

The commonest cause is a diet deficient in meat and/or green vegetables. Other causes are enteropathy, and increased requirements occur during pregnancy and lactation. Anticonvulsants may cause folate deficiency.

PROGNOSIS

- If the cause cannot be removed folic acid will have to be given indefinitely.
- It takes 4 months to restore depleted stores.

TREATMENT

1. Treatment must be preceded by investigation and diagnosis. Referral to a haematologist is sometimes necessary.
2. Vitamin B_{12} deficiency is treated with i.m. injections of hydroxocobalamin 1 mg every 3 days × 5, followed by 1 mg 3-monthly for life unless the cause, e.g. dietary deficiency or alcohol, can be removed.
3. Folate deficiency can be corrected by 15 mg folic acid daily, orally. This can be reduced to 5 mg at weekly intervals. This needs lifetime treatment unless the cause can be removed.
4. Prophylaxis of folate deficiency in pregnancy requires 300–500 µg daily.

FOLLOW-UP

An annual full blood count is needed.

---

[1] Chanarin I (1979) *The Megaloblastic Anaemias*, 2nd edn. Oxford: Blackwell Scientific Publications.

Anaemia Associated with Chronic Disorders

This type of anaemia is caused mainly by a failure of red cell production. It is associated most commonly with chronic rheumatism, renal disease, neoplasia and burns and trauma.

PROGNOSIS

- The severity of the anaemia reflects the activity of the underlying disease. It is a cause of morbidity but not of mortality. Patients tolerate mild anaemia quite well.

TREATMENT

1. There may be several factors in the cause, including blood loss, and these should be dealt with.
2. Suppression of disease activity, such as the use of steroids in rheumatoid arthritis, will bring about some improvement in the anaemia.
3. The anaemia may respond to oral iron therapy (ferrous sulphate 200 mg t.d.s.) but this is slow; if there is a response treatment must be prolonged and continue until the disease process remits.

FOLLOW-UP

This is usually dictated by the underlying disorder but should include a blood count at 6-monthly intervals.

Hodgkin's Disease

Hodgkin's disease is a form of lymph node malignancy which, untreated, may metastasize or spread directly. It usually starts in cervical glands but may begin at other sites. It may occur at any time of life but is most common in the third and fourth decades. It is more common in men than women.

PROGNOSIS

- More than 75% of patients presenting live up to 15 years after treatment and can be considered cured. Rates are dependent on the clinical stage[1].

Stage I 5-year survival 94%
Stage II 5-year survival 80–90%
Stage III 5-year survival 56–77%
Stage IV 5-year survival 40–70%

In each case the lower figure applies to patients with systemic symptoms of fever, night sweats or more than 10% weight loss.
- Patients need to be warned against acquiring a gloomy outlook because of the experience of patients before new forms of treatment were introduced.

TREATMENT

1. Treatment is carried out at specialized centres and ranges from local deep X-ray (DXR) in clinical stage I to chemotherapy for stages II to IV.
2. Counselling to support patients and maintain morale throughout this period is essential. They must not believe that the condition is hereditary or hopeless.
3. Chemotherapy causes azoospermia and this must be discussed with young males. Use of a sperm bank is possible.

Follow-up is carried out in specialized centres but contact with the general practitioner is helpful and should be regular in order to answer queries and anticipate problems.

[1] Peckman MH, McElwain TJ (1977) *Recent Advances in Haematology*, **2**, 264–87. Edinburgh: Churchill Livingstone.

Haemophilia

Haemophilia is a bleeding disorder caused by an absence of factor VIII in the coagulation cascade. It is hereditary, confined to males and occurs with a prevalence of about 1 in 10 000 people. This possibility of AIDS developing in patients who have received infected blood products is an added tragedy.

PROGNOSIS

- Prognosis depends upon the severity of the condition. Half the patients with haemophilia are severely affected but with appropriate treatment should have a normal expectation of life. However catastrophic bleeding may occur and, at certain sites, such as the brain or the floor of the mouth, may be lethal.
- Other patients can expect a normal length of life. Haemophilia does not affect the fetus or small infant because fetal haemoglobin does not carry the gene.
- The risk of the patient becoming human immunodeficiency virus (HIV)-positive was extremely high in the UK until October 1986 when blood products were screened for their antibodies.

TREATMENT

1. Replacement therapy with factor VIII is the mainstay. The patient or his or her parents can be taught to give intravenous injections of the blood product as soon as any signs of bleeding occurs and this can prevent hospital admission or absence from school.
2. For first aid treatment to a haemophiliac only very minor injuries should be dealt with outside hospital. Light pressure can be applied to an oozing surface. Suturing should be done in a special centre and all other problems such as epistaxis or haemarthrosis need immediate referral.

FOLLOW-UP

Whilst patients need to be seen regularly at a special haemophiliac centre the help and support of the doctor, parents and voluntary agencies[1] is vital both for the patient and for carriers of the gene (Haemophilia Society, PO Box 9, 16 Trinity Street, London SE1 1DE). Counselling from a geneticist is important.

[1] Jones PM (1974) *Living with Haemophilia*. Lancaster: MTP Press.

Haemoglobinopathies and Thalassaemia Syndromes

These are a group of genetically determined conditions with abnormalities of globin. The best known is sickle cell disease which occurs in Negroes, and is concentrated in certain practice areas in the UK. Thalassaemia occurs particularly commonly in people from around the Mediterranean and there are a number of varieties[1].

PROGNOSIS

- In thalassaemia major (the homozygous state) the prognosis is poor and many children fail to survive into adult life. With transfusion therapy some survive to the age of 20[2].
- Thalassaemia minor (the heterozygous state) is much more benign and may be so slight that diagnosis is extremely difficult and no treatment is indicated. In mild cases misdirected efforts to treat with iron therapy can cause iron overload.
- In established sickle cell disease the prognosis depends greatly on social and environmental factors and survival into middle age can be hoped for with good care. Pregnancy is rarely successful.

TREATMENT

1. Accurate diagnosis at a specialist clinic is required.
2. In thalassaemia major bone transplantation is feasible. Otherwise transfusion therapy in a specialized centre is required. Splenectomy is sometimes indicated.
3. In thalassaemia minor no treatment is usually required, but genetic counselling may be advisable.
4. In sickle cell disease good nutrition and a good standard of care are essential. The health visitor, nurse and social worker have very important roles.
5. Infections need treating promptly with appropriate antibiotics.
6. Deficiencies of iron, vitamin B_{12} or folic acid may need correction.
7. Infarctions or haemolytic crises will require hospital admission and transfusion therapy may be needed.

FOLLOW-UP

Lifelong and regular surveillance is required for thalassaemia major and sickle cell disease, preferably at a specialist clinic, but the general practitioner should see the family regularly to provide support.

---

[1] Sergeant GR (1985) *Sickle Cell Disease*. Oxford: Oxford University Press.
[2] Weatherall DJ (1981) *The Thalassaemia Syndromes*, 3rd edn. Oxford: Blackwell Scientific Publications.

Lymphomas

Lymphomas are neoplastic conditions of lymphoid tissue. The cause is unknown but it may be viral. Patients present in a similar fashion as in Hodgkin's disease. The lymphoma may be local and restricted or may manifest aggressive spread. Lymphomas involve a different type of lymph cell and tend to be low-grade in older people and more malignant in the young.

PROGNOSIS

- Low-grade lymphomas have a good prognosis and 60–70% survive more than 5 years.
- High-grade disease has a poor prognosis and the median survival is only 2–3 years[1].
- There is a subset within the group of large-cell lymphomas and these may be cured by aggressive chemotherapy.

TREATMENT

1. In low-grade disease in the elderly no treatment or only local radiotherapy may be required.

FOLLOW-UP

Follow-up is usually lifelong at specialized clinics but the general practitioner should keep contact with the patient.

---

[1] Stuart AE *et al.* (eds) (1981) *Lymphomas other than Hodgkin's Disease*. Oxford: Oxford University Press.

Myelomatosis

Myelomatosis is a malignant proliferation of plasma cells within the bone marrow. It is rare below the age of 30 and most common over 50. The clinical presentation is variable but may be skeletal, with renal failure or, rarely, neurological. Males are slightly more commonly affected than females.

PROGNOSIS

- The outlook is uncertain but early diagnosis and slow progression are the most favourable factors. Heavy Bence Jones proteinuria suggests likely renal failure.
- Untreated median survival is 7 months. Treated median survival is 28 months, with a few patients surviving many years[1].

TREATMENT

1. Treatment is chemotherapy carried out at a specialized centre with radiotherapy added for local painful lesions.

FOLLOW-UP

Follow-up is lifelong and should be 6-weekly visits to a specialist centre; however the general practitioner should also keep in touch with the patient and the family.

---

[1] Allan NC (1986) *Treatment and prognosis: Medicine* pp 166–7. (Hawkins R ed). Oxford: Heinemann

Polycythaemia

Polycythaemia is a chronic overproduction of red cells and is a neoplastic disorder. It occurs mainly in the 50–60-year age group and is slightly more common in men. Pruritus after a hot bath is a common feature but the condition should be borne in mind when thrombotic episodes occur or when unexplained symptoms arise such as headache, dizziness, tinnitus or angina.

PROGNOSIS

- Untreated, 50% of patients die within 18 months. Adequately treated, the mean survival is 12 years[1].
- Acute leukaemia may develop in some patients due to treatment with radioactive phosphorus. Myelofibrosis develops in about 25% of patients[1].

TREATMENT

1. Referral for specialist advice is required. Venesection is the treatment of choice for young people and some older patients can be treated with occasional venesection as well.
2. Other patients will be treated with busulphan orally or intravenous radioactive phosphorus.

FOLLOW-UP

Follow-up is carried out at a specialized clinic. The general practitioner should be alert to thrombotic disorders or, paradoxically, haemorrhagic complications.

---

[1] Gilbert HS (1975) *Clin. Haematol.*, **4**, 263.

Thrombocytopenic Purpura

Thrombocytopenic purpura may occur at any age but is most common in the children and young adults. It is more frequently acute and postinfectious in young people, where it can follow immunization, and chronic and idiopathic in older people. It is three times as common in females as in males. It is often due to the production of platelet antibodies. Accurate diagnosis is urgent and is preceded by blood and marrow examination.

PROGNOSIS

- Death due to intracranial bleeding can occur in cases following acute infection in children, although this happens in less than 1%. However recovery is usually complete and 90% of very young children remit without treatment[1].
- Haemorrhage may occur from respiratory or intestinal tract if the platelet count drops below 70×10^9 l but is rare after the first 4–6 weeks. The incidence is 6–11/100 000[2].
- Chronic cases in older children and adults may persist for many months and fluctuate.
- A total of 90% show a response to prednisolone but half relapse and require splenectomy.
- About a quarter of patients are left with long-standing disease.

TREATMENT

1. Under 5 years of age treatment is usually conservative, though some advocate corticosteroids for the first few days. Aggressive activities should be restricted until platelet count is normal.
2. Older patients who usually have a chronic condition and more severe cases require referral to hospital where treatment choices includes splenectomy, steroids and immunosuppressive therapy.

3. Steroids produce platelet increment in 75% of cases.
4. Of those who fail to respond, 60% will benefit from splenectomy and the remainder require immunosuppressive therapy using vincristine, cyclophosphamide or azathioprine.

FOLLOW-UP

Follow-up is not required in children who spont-aneously remit. Otherwise it should be carried out in a specialized clinic.

[1] Newland AC (1987) *Infect.*, **15** (Suppl 1), 41–9.
[2] Davies JA, Tuddenham EGD (1968) Haemostasis and thrombosis. In *Oxford Textbook of Medicine*, 2nd edn. (Weatherall DJ *et al.* eds). Oxford: OUP.

The Leukaemias

The leukaemias are characterized by uncontrolled proliferation of malignant cells arising from haemopoietic precursors.

Acute leukaemia

There is now strong evidence that many acute leukaemias are caused by viruses. In young children lymphoblastic leukaemia is most common but from about 7 years of age the incidence of granulocytic leukaemia begins to supersede. Acute leukaemia can occur at any age but peaks in the 5–14-year age group and again between 55 and 70 years, and usually presents as bruising and pallor associated with oral or chest infections.

PROGNOSIS

- In acute lymphoblastic leukaemia, prognosis is best in female children aged between 2 and 5 years with a low total white cell count. The majority of these cases are probably cured[1].
- In adults the prognosis is less good but lasting remission is obtained in 30% of patients.
- In acute myeloblastic leukaemia 50% of patients die within 5 weeks and 99% within 1 year[2].

TREATMENT

Immediate referral to a specialist centre is necessary. Treatment involves cytotoxic drugs and bone marrow transplantation.

FOLLOW-UP

Follow-up in a specialist clinic is necessary but regular support for the family by the general practitioner is required.

Chronic leukaemia

Chronic lymphocytic leukaemia is most common in males and the incidence increases steeply after the age of 50. The onset is insidious with fatigue, lymphadenopathy and liver spleen enlargement. Chronic myeloid leukaemia occurs almost equally in males and females. It is rare before the age of 30 and most common between 50 and 60 years. Splenomegaly is a common feature.

PROGNOSIS

- Chronic lymphocytic leukaemia has a variable prognosis according to type. The cases with the best prognosis may survive for more than 10 years but cases with worse prognostic features have a mean survival rate of 2 years.
- Chronic myeloid leukaemia cannot be cured without bone marrow transplant. In these up to 60% may be cured if an identical twin is available. In other cases the results are less

certain but the rest of patients usually die between 1 and 5 years after diagnosis.

TREATMENT

1. Early referral is required.
2. In some chronic lymphocytic leukaemias no treatment is needed; in others, chemotherapy and/or radiotherapy is prescribed.
3. In chronic myeloid leukaemia bone marrow transplant is offered to patients under 40 with a comparable sibling donor; otherwise chemotherapy is used.

FOLLOW-UP

Follow-up in a specialist clinic is necessary but regular support for the family by the general practitioner is very important.

---

[1] Mauer AM (1986) New directions in the treatment of acute lymphoblastic leukaemia of childhood. *N. Engl. J. Med.*, **315,** 316–17.
[2] Whitaker JA *et al.* (1981) Survival in acute myelogenous leukaemia. *Br. Med. J.*, **282,** 692–5.

16

Sexually Transmitted Diseases and HIV

F. M. Hull

Chlamydial Infection

The *Chlamydia* are a genus of coccoid Gram-negative micro-organisms that for a long time were classified with viruses because of their inability to replicate outside host cells. They are now regarded as obligate intracellular bacteria. Two species are pathogenic to man: *Chlamydia psittaci* and *C. trachomatis*. The former causes psittacosis in man and many animals, and the latter is responsible for many diseases in man especially trachoma, inclusion conjunctivitis, pneumonitis and a wide variety of genital diseases including urethritis, cervicitis, salpingitis and lymphogranuloma venereum. *C. trachomatis* is probably the commonest cause of sexually transmitted disease (STD) in the world and is an important cause of female infertility.

Chlamydial STD – in the male

Non-gonococcal urethritis with or without symptoms is a common STD in men (see p. 319). It may be caused by a number of organisms, including *Mycoplasma* and *Gardnerella* species. In about 30–50% of cases *C. trachomatis* serotypes D–K can be isolated. Uncommonly in some males there may be associated epididymitis or prostatitis and, in homosexuals, proctitis.

Chlamydial STD – female

Chlamydia transmitted to women by men with urethritis may give rise to asymptomatic (in up to 60%) or symptomatic infection of the genital tract, especially cervicitis, salpingitis and pelvic inflammatory disease. In Sweden[1] pelvic inflammatory disease was caused by *Mycoplasma hominis*, in 10–15% women by *C. Trachomatis* in 60% and by the gonococcus in 10–15% of women. In another series[2] of 248 women whose cervical organisms were cultured during speculum examination regardless of symptoms in a British inner city general practice, 4 were found to have gonorrhoea and 19 showed definite and a further 4 presumptive evidence of chlamydial infection. Infection at birth may give rise to neonatal inclusion conjunctivitis or pneumonitis in 30–50% of infants born to infected mothers. *Chlamydia* is the commonest cause of pneumonia among neonates (5 per 1000)[3].

PROGNOSIS

- Uncommonly in some males there may be associated epididymitis or prostatitis and, in homosexuals, proctitis.
- Untreated, the infection may persist for years and may cause female infertility.
- Eye involvement may occur through auto-inoculation but blindness does not occur (as it does with the serotypes A–C which cause trachoma).
- Perihepatitis may occur as a rare complication.
- Reiter's syndrome may follow chlamydial infection.

TREATMENT

1. Chlamydiae are sensitive to sulphonamides and many broad spectrum antibiotics. The treatment of choice is tetracycline (500 mg 2–4 times daily for 2 weeks) or, in pregnancy, erythromycin (500 mg 2–3 times daily for 2 weeks).
2. When the disease is suspected in males it is important to treat female sexual partners with tetracycline since undetected female genital chlamydial infections may lead to later sterility.
3. In lymphogranuloma venereum treatment should be prolonged e.g. doxycycline 100 mg for a minimum of 21 days.
4. Neonatal infections should be treated with erythromycin (50 mg/(kg·day)) for 14–21 days with topical tetracycline into the conjunctiva.

[1] Mardh PA (1984) Microbial etiology of pelvic inflammatory disease. *Sex. Transm. Dis.*, **II** (suppl 4), 428–9.
[2] Southgate LJ *et al.* (1983) *Br. Med. J.*, **287**, 879–81.
[3] Gilbert GL (1986) *Aust. Paediatr. J.*, **22**, 13–17.

Lymphogranuloma Venereum

This rare disease, endemic in many tropical areas, is caused by *C. trachomatis* serotypes L1–L3. It is an acute and chronic STD affecting both sexes. It has an incubation period of 5–21 days followed by a transient genital lesion associated with inguinal lymphadenopathy. Later the infection may spread to produce chronic ulcerative lesions involving the genitals and rectum, leading to rectal stricture. Rarely the hip joint may be involved and there may be associated meningoencephalitis. An intradermal test (Frei) is available[1].

PROGNOSIS

- Untreated the infection may persist for years and may cause female infertility.
- Eye involvement may occur through autoinoculation but blindness does not occur (as it does with the serotypes A–C which cause trachoma).
- Perihepatitis may occur as a rare complication.
- Reiter's syndrome may follow chlamydial infection[2].

TREATMENT

1. In asymptomatic carriers eradication can be obtained in 95% of men with tetracycline (500 mg q.i.d. for 10 days) or, in pregnant women, erythromycin (500 mg t.i.d. for 10 days).
2. In pelvic inflammatory disease treatment consists of bedrest, analgesia and a full blood count followed by lower genital tract swabs. Combined treatment with metronidazole 400 mg b.d. and tetracycline 500 mg q.i.d. for 10 days should be instituted. If the diagnosis is in doubt laparoscopy should be considered.
3. When the disease is suspected in males it is important to treat their female sexual partners with tetracycline since undetected female genital chlamydial infections may later lead to sterility[3,4].
4. Treatment should be prolonged, e.g. doxycycline 100 mg for a minimum of 21 days.
5. Neonatal infections should be treated with erythromycin (50 mg/kg/day) for 14–21 days with topical tetracycline into the conjunctiva.

FOLLOW-UP

No routine follow-up is necessary.

[1] Hull R (1986) *Infective Diseases in Primary Care*. London: Chapman and Hall.
[2] Harris JRW, Forster GE (1986) Genito-urinary diseases. In: *Treatment and Prognosis, Medicine* (Hawkins RL ed), p. 276. Oxford: Heinemann.
[3] Schachter J (1980) *N. Eng. J. Med.*, **298,** 428, 490, 540.
[4] Southgate LJ *et al.* (1983) *Br. Med. J.*, **287,** 879–81.

Candidiasis

Infections with the yeast-like organism *Candida albicans*, which causes thrush, are common. Thrush is not entirely STD. The disease is particularly common among sexually active people – and is transmitted sexually – but the organism also occurs commensally (candidosis). *Candida albicans* can be cultured from the mouth or vagina of 30% of healthy women.

Candidiasis should prompt a search for the contributory cause. The progression from candidosis to candidiasis may be triggered by drugs, debilitation, immunosuppression or underlying disease. Drugs such as broad-spectrum antibiotics, steroids (including inhaled betamethasone which may give rise to candida stomatitis), and oral contraceptives predispose to the condition. Candidiasis is also seen in patients with debilitating disease such as metastatic carcinoma. *Candida* is particularly important in therapeutic or acquired immunosuppression, when it is a common opportunistic infection. Candidiasis may be the presenting symptom of diabetes, particularly occurring as vulvovaginitis or balanitis.

In sexually active women thrush can be a major cause of vaginal discharge and pruritus vulvae. Men are usually without symptoms but may carry the organism, usually in the penile coronal sulcus, and reinfect their partners. Recurrence may also occur from the rectum but less than half of patients with recurrent thrush have positive rectal cultures for *Candida*. Reports from STD clinics in England and Wales show a rise in incidence of new cases of candidiasis from 85.6 in 1979 to 123.6 cases per 100 000 in 1983.

Fungaemia due to *Candida* species and similar organisms (such as *Cryptococcus*) may occur in the immunocompromised host, in AIDS or following cancer chemotherapy, or when hyperalimentation is used in the treatment of alcoholism. Fungaemia carries a very bad prognosis, especially when it occurs in patients undergoing intensive care with intravenous lines. Candidaemia may be diagnosed by the ophthalmological appearances – raised white cotton wool spots extending into the vitreous humour – due to retinal candidiasis.

PROGNOSIS

- Except when candidiasis occurs in AIDS or other serious underlying disease the prognosis is good with rapid response to treatment in 75% of cases.
- Where the infection persists, an adequate search should be made for predisposing factors, such as poorly ventilated clothing, concurrent drugs (steroids or antibiotics) or diabetes[4,5].

TREATMENT

1. Only symptomatic cases need treatment.
2. Mild cases of vaginitis may respond to increasing the acidity of the vagina with local applications such as natural yoghurt or weak organic acids.
3. In all 90% of cases respond to imidazoles such as clotrimazole or isoconazole as cream and pessary (500 mg single dose or 200 mg daily for 3 days). Imidazoles may be given orally but there is little advantage over the topical application, they are expensive and may very rarely cause hepatotoxicity (1 in 15 000 treated patients).
4. It is important to treat all male sexual partners with topical imidazole cream to prevent reinfection.
5. Treatment of systemic candidiasis is described under opportunistic infection in AIDS (see p. 000).
6. Recurrent episodes may be treated with prolonged (6-week) courses of imidazoles.

FOLLOW-UP

The avoidance of *Candida* depends upon careful use of broad-spectrum antibiotics. Since transmission to newborn infants occurs at birth, care should be taken to treat *Candida* in pregnancy. There should be careful supervision of patients at risk because of immunodeficiency.

[1] Hull R (1986) *Infective Disease in Primary Care* p. 174. (From data published by Chief Medical Officer DHSS, London HMSO) London: Chapman and Hall.
[2] Henderson DK *et al.* (1981) *J. Inf. Dis.*, **143**, 655–61.

[3] Meunier-Carpenter F *et al.* (1981) *Am. J. Med.*, **71**, 363–70.
[4] Davidson F, Mould RF (1978) *Br. J. Ven. Dis.*, **54**, 176–83.
[5] Hay RJ (1985) *Br. Med. J.*, **290**, 260–1.

Trichomoniasis

Trichomoniasis is caused by infection with one of the flagellated protozoa belonging to the genus *Trichomonas*. *Trichomonas vaginalis* occurs in the male urethra where it is usually symptomless, and the vagina where it may cause symptoms varying from little to severe discharge and irritation. Though transmission is usually sexual it is not necessarily so. The protozoan has been shown to survive on moist lavatory seats or towels for 24 hours. Reports of trichomonas vaginitis at STD clinics in England showed a fall in incidence between 1979 and 1983 from 42.1 to 39.0 cases per 100 000[1]. Whilst this represents an overall fall in the condition it does not reflect the true prevalence since this condition is commonly treated in general practice[2].

PROGNOSIS

- Prognosis is good but reinfection commonly occurs, often due to poor compliance.
- As with all diseases which may be transmitted sexually, it is essential to be aware of the possibility of other venereal infections.

TREATMENT

1. Trichomonads are sensitive to the nitroimidazole derivatives such as metronidazole or nimorazole, which may be given as a single dose of 2 g or a 5-day course of 400 mg twice daily. It is important to treat both sexual partners simultaneously. Note that metronidazole has an Antabuse-like effect if taken with alcohol. The nitroimidazoles are not recommended in the first trimester of pregnancy.
2. Vaginal and rectal creams, pessaries and suppositories of nitroimidazoles are available for local treatment.

FOLLOW-UP

Follow-up is not necessary, provided coexisting STD is excluded.

[1] Hull R (1986) *Infective Disease in Primary Care*. p. 174. (From data published by Chief Medical Officer DHSS, London, HMSO) London: Chapman and Hall.
[2] Mindel A (1985) *Eur. J. Sex. Trans. Dis.*, **2**, 91.

Gonorrhoea

Gonorrhoea is caused by infection with *Neisseria gonorrhoeae*, a Gram-negative intracellular diplococcus. Though there has been a fall in the proportion of cases of gonorrhoea reporting to STD clinics in England and Wales from 24.6% in 1945 to 13.1% in 1979, absolute figures rose during this time from 33 000 to 56 000 per year (in 1982 this rose to nearly 59 000)[1]. Gonorrhoea is almost invariably sexually transmitted but changing patterns of sexual behaviour have led to increased incidence of rectal (of unknown incidence in male homosexuals; in 40% of women with gonorrhoea) and pharyngeal gonorrhoea (in 25% of homosexual males and 5% of heterosexuals with gonorrhoea). The disease is asymptomatic in over 70% of infected women and in as many as 10% of infected men[2,3].

PROGNOSIS

- Correct treatment will cure 95% of diagnosed acute gonococcal infections, though the incidence of penicillin resistance is increasing.
- Untreated urethritis in the male may lead to urethral stricture.
- Rarely local complications such as epididymitis or bartholinitis may occur.
- In 10–15% of females there may be ascending genital infection giving rise to pelvic inflammatory disease which may lead to chronic salpingitis or infertility.
- Disseminated gonococcal disease may occur as a result of bacteraemia leading to arthritis, skin rashes, endocarditis or meningitis.
- Neonates may be infected at birth from the maternal birth canal, giving rise to ophthalmia neonatorum.

TREATMENT

1. Most gonococci are sensitive to penicillin (spectinomycin is effective against resistant organisms) and repond quickly to relatively small dosages. However it is important to be aware of the possibility of other concurrent STDs, especially syphilis. It is important therefore to give an adequate dose of penicillin to kill treponemes as well.
2. Penicillin should be combined with probenecid in one of the following regimes: aqueous procaine penicillin 2.4 Mu preceded by 1 g probenecid orally, or 5 Mu benzylpenicillin in 8 ml 0.5% lignocaine with 1 g probebecid, or ampicillin 2–3 g in a single dose with 1 g probenecid.
3. Where the patient is allergic to penicillin alternative therapies include kanamycin 2 g intramuscularly, or 500 mg tetracycline 6–hourly for 5 days, or co-trimoxazole 2g twice daily for 2 days (NB tetracycline and co-trimoxazole are not treponemacidal).

FOLLOW-UP

Where treatment fails this may be due to reinfection, when treatment should be repeated. If there is no evidence of reinfection then the organism may be resistant to penicillin, in which case either spectinomycin 2 g intramuscularly or probenecid 1 g orally should be combined with cefuroxime 1.5 g intramuscularly. Postgonococcal urethritis may follow the acute infection in as many as 50% of men, due to chlamydial infection which responds to tetracycline.

All sexual contacts of patients should be traced and treated, particularly because so many patients are asymptomatic.

[1] Hull R (1986) *Infective Disease in Primary Care*. London: Chapman and Hall.
[2] Adler MW (1983) *Br. Med. J.*, **287**, 1360–2.
[3] Harris JRW, Forster GE (1986) Genito-urinary diseases. In *Treatment and Prognosis, Medicine* (Hawkins RL ed), pp. 269-70. Oxford: Heinemann.

Non-gonococcal urethritis

Non-gonococcal urethritis (NGU) is a loose term referring to any urethritis in which no gonococci can be cultured. In some cases urethral discharge may be physiological, as in spermatorrhoea, prostatorrhoea or in sexual stimulation. NGU may have no demonstrable cause in about 25% of cases. Specific NGU may be caused by *Chlamydia trachomatis* (see p. 314) in 30–50% of cases, by *Ureaplasma urealyticum* (a mycoplasma) in 10–40% of cases, and by other organisms such as *Trichomonas vaginalis, Candida albicans,* and by miscellaneous bacteria including *Escherichia coli* and *Proteus* spp[1].

NGU may also occur as a result of trauma or allergy, or secondary to other urethral or genitourinary pathology such as herpes, chancre or chronic kidney disease. Distinction between these causes may be made by careful history-taking but is largely dependent on laboratory investigation. A medium to isolate *Chlamydia* as well as other pathogens is required to enable a satisfactory NGU diagnosis in general practice[2].

PROGNOSIS

- NGU is frequently self-limiting and responds to treatment without complications.
- Rarely (in 1% of cases), sexually acquired reactive arthritis may develop.

TREATMENT

1. Treatment of NGU depends largely on tetracyclines, 500 mg q.d.s. for 7 days, or if this fails, erythromycin 500 mg for 7–14 days[3,4].

FOLLOW-UP

The sexual partners of known cases should be followed up and women should be treated with tetracycline to prevent possible infertility due to undetected chlamydial infection.

[1] Adler MW (1983) *Br. Med. J.,* **287,** 1360–2.
[2] Harris JRW, Forster GE (1986) Genito-urinary diseases, In *Treatment and Prognosis, Medicine,* (Hawkins RL ed), pp. 269–70. Oxford: Heinemann.
[3] McCutchan JA (1984) *Rev. Infect. Dis.,* **6,** 669–88.
[4] Fitzgerald MR (1984) *Br. J. Vener. Dis.,* **60,** 312–15.

Syphilis

Syphilis is caused by the spirochaete *Treponema pallidum*. In most European countries the disease is increasing but there has been a decrease in the UK during the late 1970s, especially among homosexuals. Syphilis is classically described as having primary, secondary and tertiary stages but from the point of view of treatment it is convenient to divide the history of the disease into 'early infectious' and 'late syphilis'. The early disease manifests itself from 10 to 90 days after exposure as an often painless genital, anal or oral ulcer. At this stage exudate from the lesion contains abundant spirochaetes and is highly infectious. After spontaneous healing of the primary sore the disease becomes latent and may reappear as a secondary skin rash which may involve mucous membranes and be highly infectious or may remain dormant for many years before producing late manifestations of gummata involving viscera, skin and bones or as cardiovascular or central nervous system disease[1].

PROGNOSIS

- In untreated syphilis a third of patients will undergo spontanous cure, in a third the disease will remain latent and in a further third it will progress to tertiary manifestations in the cardiovascular or central nervous system or as gummata.
- Treatment with antibiotics will cure early syphilis and arrest the progress of late disease.
- Immunosuppression may reactivate quiescent disease. Since syphilis may coexist with HIV infection, florid syphilitic disease may sometimes be seen in AIDS patients.

TREATMENT[2]

1. All patients in whom syphilis is suspected should be referred to a specialist in genito-urinary medicine.
2. Penicillin is the antibiotic of choice in the treatment of syphilis[1] In early infection procaine penicillin G should be given i.m. as 0.6 Mu daily for 10 days or benzathine penicillin 2.4 Mu as a single dose.
3. In later stages the duration of procaine penicillin G therapy should be increased to 15–20 days to give a total dose of 9–12 Mu or when benzathine penicillin is used 2.4 Mu weekly for 3 weeks.
4. Late infection involving the central nervous system (confirmed by cerebrospinal fluid examination), cardiovascular system or viscera should be treated with procaine penicillin as in point 3 above, to a total of 12 Mu.
5. Where the patient is allergic to penicillin, tetracycline (40–60 g over 14–20 days) or erythromycin (30–50 g for a similar period) may be used.
6. Herxheimer reactions, though usually mild, may cause fever and generalized aches and pains within 24 hours of starting any treponemacidal therapy.
7. Syphilis in pregnancy must be treated to protect the fetus and mother. Penicillin in dosage appropriate to the stage of the disease (see points 2–4 above) should be administered. When the diagnosis is not made until the third trimester larger doses should be used. If the patient is allergic to penicillin erythromycin should be used, but since this drug has poor placental penetration the infant should also be treated with penicillin after delivery – 50 000 units/kg as a single dose[2].
8. Where congenital syphilis is proven by positive cerebrospinal fluid tests or rising titres of blood (Venereal Disease Research Laboratories (VDRL)) the infant should be given procaine penicillin 50 000 units kg for 10 days.

FOLLOW-UP

Sexual contacts of all patients with syphilis and those who receive treatment for early syphilis should be followed clinically and serologically for at least a year. Patients with other forms of the disease should be observed for at least 2 year.

[1] Harris JRW, Forster GE (1986) *Treatment and Prognosis, Medicine*. Oxford: Heinemann.
[2] McCormach WM (1983) *Diagnosis and Treatment of Sexually Transmitted Diseases*. Bristol: John Wright.

Viral Genital Infections

Condylomata acuminata are anogenital warts caused by human papillomavirus (HPV). They are quite common, accounting for 4.3 and 3% of male and female attendances at clinics for STD[1]. Although they were formerly regarded as not very serious, association observed between HPV and cervical cancer has increased interest in condylomata acuminata[2]. The picture is confused since there is a huge number of HPV types and the precise relationship between them and cervical cancer is far from clear. The overwhelming majority of individuals with warts never experience any significant complication as a result of their HPV infections but fragments of HPV DNA are detectable in some genital malignancies, suggesting an aetiological relationship. Which of the many strains of virus is implicated is not clear and some authorities question whether the apparent relationship is any more than the commonly observed association between all STDs and cervical cancer.

Herpes genitalis

Herpes genitalis caused by the herpes simplex virus (HSV) II, has been described as the most important STD because it is common and because it produces severe neonatal infection[3]. In the USA the incidence of herpes genitalis rose from 50 to 130 cases per 100 000 between 1965 and 1979. Similarly, neonatal infection has risen 10-fold to about 28 per 100 000 livebirths over a similar period. In Britain between 1979 and 1983 rates of new cases of herpes reporting to STD clinics in England and Wales rose[4] from 19.1 to 35.3 per 100 000. In the adult the disease may be asymptomatic but is commonly characterized by a vesicular – later ulcerated – extremely painful genital rash. The infection may involve the vagina and cervix, and may give rise to ulceration on the cervix that may be mistaken for carcinoma. Rarely there may be generalized infection with symptoms of viraemia and meningism.

PROGNOSIS

- The importance of condylomata acuminata lies in the association with genital malignancy. While this possibility exists, yearly cervical smears should be taken from women known to be at risk of infection with HPV.
- HSV infections undergo spontaneous remission after 2–6 weeks. Recurrence is common but less severe than in the first episode.
- Neonatal herpes is a devastating central nervous system infection with a mortality of around 50% and survivors may have neurological complications. The majority of babies developing HSV infections are born to mothers without signs of the disease at delivery.
- Herpes central nervous system infection limited to the meninges has a good prognosis but mortality with encephalitis may be as high as 70%.
- Herpes infections are very severe in immunocompromised individuals.

TREATMENT

1. Classically condylomata acuminata were treated by local application of podophyllin (25% in spirit). This may be painful, has a cure rate of only 30% and is contraindicated in pregnancy. Cryotherapy with liquid nitrogen and vaporization treatments with carbon dioxide laser are becoming available and are less uncomfortable. They have a better cure rate of 90%.

2. Herpes genitalis may be treated with topical acyclovir 5% cream. Severe infection may require oral or even intravenous acyclovir but for maximum effect the drug should be given as soon as possible in the disease. Oral use, 200 mg q.i.d. for 12 weeks, can reduce the recurrence rate but is very expensive.

[1] Centres for Disease Control (1979) *Morbidity and Mortality Weekly Report*, **28,** 61–3.

[2] Lynch PJ (1985) *Clin. Obstet. Gynaecol.*, **28,** 142–8.

[3] Kaufman RH et al. (1985) *Clin. Obstet. Gynaecol.*, **28,** 152–61.

[4] Hull R (1986) *Infective Disease in Primary Care*, p. 174. (From data published by Chief Medical Officer, DHSS, London). London: Chapman and Hall.

Pediculosis pubis

Pubic lice are usually transmitted during sexual intercourse and their presence should alert the clinician to the possibility of other STDs. The pubic louse *Pthirus pubis* is rather smaller than head and body lice but like them reproduces by eggs which are cemented on to hair by a chitinous tube. Although infestation of the pubic hair is most common, any hairy part of the body such as the scalp and eyelashes may be affected.

PROGNOSIS

- Prognosis is good apart from secondary infection of abrasions or the possibility of louse-borne rickettsial disease.
- Beware of other coexisting STD: 15% of women and 7% of men attending a skin clinic in Denmark with pediculosis pubis were found to have gonorrhoea and 1.5% of men had syphilis[1].

TREATMENT

1. Treatment consists of local application of gamma benzene hexachloride or preparations containing carbaryl or malathion.

[1] Munkvad IM, Klemp P (1982) *Acta. Derm. Venereol.* (Stockholm) **62,** 366–7.

AIDS and other HIV-related Conditions

Acquired immune deficiency syndrome (AIDS) is one of the manifestations of infection with the human immunodeficiency virus (HIV). This virus is a retrovirus with special affinity for human T4 lymphocytes. Cell nuclei into which the viral RNA has become incorporated become factories for the production of the new viruses. Once infected the host cannot lose the infection, though it does not follow that any of the HIV-related conditions will develop[1].

The virus has been isolated from blood, semen, vaginal secretions, saliva, tears, breast milk, cerebrospinal fluid, amniotic fluid and urine. However only with blood, semen, vaginal secretions and, rarely, breast milk is there epidemiological evidence of transmission between individuals. The virus is usually transmitted sexually, particularly under circumstances which permit blood-to-blood or semen-to-blood contact; the commonest route is penetrative anal sexual intercourse. Other sexual contact may also transmit the virus, as may blood contact through shared needles and syringes among drug addicts. Infection can occur – and still does in undeveloped countries – through blood transfusion and blood products such as factor VIII. Vertical transmission from mother to fetus occurs and there are several documented cases where mothers who were uninfected at delivery but who subsequently received infected blood transfusions conveyed the infection to their breastfed neonates[2].

Following infection with HIV there is often an acute influenzal or glandular fever-like illness and seroconversion usually occurs within 8 weeks but may occasionally be longer. The acute infection is followed by a chronic phase of indeterminate length which may be asymptomatic or associated with varying degrees of illness. A number of clinical pictures in this chronic phase have been described as persistent generalized lymphadenopathy (PGL), AIDS-related complex (ARC) or frank AIDS[1,2].

The fullblown syndrome is characterized by the presence of opportunistic infections, particularly *Pneumocystsis carinii* pneumonia (PCP), and bizarre infections of the skin[3], gastrointestinal tract or central nervous system (due to protozoan, bacterial, fungal and viral organisms) or unusual forms of neoplasia[4].

Yet another manifestation of HIV infection produces neurological involvement[5]. HIV attacks glial cells, giving rise to symptoms of depression, seizures and progressive dementia in as many as one-third of AIDS patients and there is post-mortem evidence of brain damage in as many as 80% of patients with AIDS. HIV neuropathy may develop independently of AIDS and the occurrence of a subacute encephalitis leading to dementia in otherwise fit young individuals has led to the view that the neurological features of the disease may well come to dominate HIV disease.

PROGNOSIS

- The epidemiological pattern of epidemics varies between localities (e.g. it is largely associated with drug abuse in Edinburgh, with blood products in Birmingham and with homosexuality in Amsterdam). The epidemiological pattern influences the clinical manifestations with different distribution of opportunistic infections and neoplasia in different populations. For example, Kaposi's sarcoma is more common among homosexual than drug-abusing AIDS sufferers. The median survival time in patients presenting with Kaposi's sarcoma is 18 months, while that of AIDS patients with PCP is 7–8 months. Where the two diseases coexist median survival is only 6.6 months[6].
- An individual who has seroconverted may be well; may progress through PGL and ARC to AIDS itself; may bypass PGL and ARC or may remain chronically sick with glandular enlargement similar to mild mononucleosis. ARC is a debilitating condition with fever, might sweats, malaise, diarrhoea and weight loss. Many patients with PGL remain well and relatively few progress to more severe disease, but those with ARC have a high risk of progressing to AIDS[1,2].
- The proportion of antibody-positive subjects progressing to fullblown AIDS appears, at present, to lie between 20 and 30%[6,7].
- About 10–15% of infected individuals develop AIDS within 3 years of acquiring the virus.
- Overall mortality is close to 100%; 92% of those who developed AIDS by 1982 had died by October 1985[8].

TREATMENT

1. In a double-blind placebo-controlled trial[9] patients receiving AZT (Retrovir) had less mortality, fewer episodes of opportunistic infection and improved T4 lymphocyte counts compared to controls. It remains to be seen how effective prolonged AZT therapy is, but it appears to prolong mean survival time by postponing death.

2. Patients with severe opportunistic infections tend to be treated in hospital and only an outline of therapy for commoner opportunistic infections is mentioned here.

   Protozoan infections

   a. PCP can be treated with high-dose co-trimoxazole. The first episode responds well but second or subsequent episodes are often unresponsive.

   b. *Toxoplasma gondii* infection may respond to pyrimethamine and sulfadoxine.

   c. Intestinal infections with *Isospora* or *Cryptosporidium* give rise to intractable diarrhoea. The former may respond to treatment with co-trimoxazole but the latter is usually resistant to treatment.

Viral infections

Infection with herpes simplex or cytomegalovirus may respond to acyclovir.

Candidal infection

Systemic fungal infections are common in AIDS, leading to severe gastrointestinal involvement or fungaemia, at which time retinal candidiasis may be observed ophthalmologically. This fungaemia may require systemic ketoconazole or amphotericin B. Note that ketoconazole may be hepatotoxic and may reduce the white cell count in patients who are already lymphopenic. Amphotericin may be nephrotoxic.

Bacterial infection

Numerous Gram-negative organisms, such as *Escherichia coli*, *Shigella* or *Salmonella* species, may give rise to serious infection in AIDS patients and can be very difficult to manage. A typical tuberculous bacilli may also cause opportunistic infection and is often resistant to conventional antituberculous therapy.

FOLLOW-UP

Much support should be offered to HIV-positive patients. This will be both personal and family counselling about the prognosis for the patient and the risk to the family. The general practitioner should encourage the patient to contact voluntary support groups as well (e.g. Terence Higgins Trust, 52-4 Grays Inn Rd, London, WC1X 8JU. Tel 071 831 0330). If AIDS develops the general practitioner may need to involve a hospice in terminal care. The most difficult complication to manage may prove to be the early dementia.

[1] Adler MW (1987) ABC of AIDS *Br. Med. J.*, **294**, 1083–5.

[2] Adler MW (1987) ABC of AIDS *Br. Med. J.*, **294**, 1145–7.

[3] Kaplan MH *et al.* (1986) *J. Am. Acad. Dermatol.*, **16**, 485–505.

[4] Smith N, Spittle M (1987) ABC of AIDS *Br. Med. J.*, **294**, 1274–7.

[5] Pinching AJ (1986) AIDS and the AIDS virus (HIV). *The Magistrate*, 192–8.

[6] Harris JRW, Forster GE (1986) *Treatment and Prognosis – Medicine* (Hawkins RL ed). London: Heinemann.

[7] Wells N (1987) *The AIDS Virus, Forecasting its Impact.* London: Office of Health Economics.

[8] Morbidity and Mortality Weekly Reports: Centers for Disease Control, Atlanta (1987) *J.A.M.A.*, **258**, 1293–305.

[9] Fischl MA *et al.* (1987) *N. Engl. J. Med.*, **317**, 185–91.

17

The Urinary Tract

A. J. B. Carson

Urinary Tract Infections in Adults

Urinary tract infections are the commonest form of urological disorder and account for almost 6%[1] of all consultations in general practice in the UK, although the true incidence is not known. Infection reaches the bladder by the ascending route and females are three times more commonly affected than males. Sexually active or pregnant females are particularly at risk. Other important risk factors include increasing age, underlying defects causing a disturbance of flow of urine (hydronephrosis, diverticulae, calculi and neurogenic bladder), and instrumentation of the urinary tract, including the presence of an indwelling catheter. The commonest infecting organisms are the gut flora. Infection with other more unusual organisms, such as *Pseudomonas* species, is suggestive of an underlying lesion such as neurogenic bladder[2]. Common presenting symptoms include urinary frequency, dysuria, fever and, occasionally, macroscopic haematuria.

PROGNOSIS

- Bacterial cystitis responds readily to antibiotic treatment and does not cause long-term sequelae.
- In adults, acute pyelonephritis in the absence of obstruction does not cause renal scarring or hypertension.
- Some 20% of adults and 30% of children in end-stage renal failure have suffered from chronic pyelonephritis.
- Bacteriuria in pregnancy results in pyelonephritis in 25% of cases[3].
- Pyelonephritis and instrumentation of the urinary tract are important causes of Gram-negative septicaemia which may be fatal if prompt treatment is not undertaken.

TREATMENT

General measures

1. A high fluid intake is recommended.
2. The bladder should be voided regularly, including after sexual intercourse if appropriate.
3. Alkalinization of the urine with subsequent control of symptoms may be achieved using potassium citrate mixture 3 g 3 times daily, diluted with water.
4. Local hygiene is of the utmost importance, particularly in cases of recurrent cystitis in females. A urine specimen should be obtained and sent for microscopy, culture and sensitivity.
5. An appropriate antibiotic may be started (e.g. co-trimoxazole 2 tablets twice daily; trimethoprim 200 mg twice daily, ampicillin 250 mg 4 times daily, nitrofurantoin 50 mg 3 times daily). Treatment need not exceed 1 week.
6. Alternatively, single-dose therapy with co-trimoxazole 1.92 g (4 times normal-strength tablets) or amoxycillin 3 g may be used.
7. Recurrence of symptoms of cystitis within 1 week of treatment suggests infection higher in the urinary tract (pyelonephritis). Antibiotics should be used for 4–8 weeks and any relapse requires referral for further investigation. Some patients will be acutely ill and will need hospitalization for parenteral antibiotic therapy.

FOLLOW-UP

Some experts advocate that urine should be cultured 1 and 6 weeks after treatment of proven infections to exclude relapse or reinfection.

Recurrence of symptoms within 1 week is suggestive of either pyelonephritis or abnormal pooling of urine and requires referral for further investigation. Bacteriuria in children, or in adult males, is frequently associated with urinary tract abnormalities and further investigation is mandatory. Whether symptomatic or not, bacteriuria in pregnancy requires treatment to avoid complications of ascending infection. In males, bacteriuria not associated with instrumentation is nearly always indicative of an anatomical abnormality and further investigation is required.

[1] Catto RD, Powler DA (1986) *Nephrology in Clinical Practice*. London: Edward Arnold.
[2] Stanney TA (1980) *Pathogenesis and Treatment of Urinary Tract Infections*. Baltimore: Williams & Wilkins.
[3] Barton I (1986) In *Treatment and Prognosis, Medicine*. Oxford: Heinemann.

Urinary Calculi

The incidence of urinary calculi in the UK is approximately 70 per 100 000 population per year; about 50 new cases per 100 000 population presenting annually. This figure is gradually increasing and currently 2% of the population of the UK will develop a stone at some time in their lives. Most patients present with renal colic. There may be associated sweating, shock, haematuria, symptoms of urinary tract infection and occasionally, a palpable kidney. Stones form in the urine when the concentration of various substances exceeds their saturation point. In all, 70% of calculi are composed of calcium oxalate, usually caused by a low urine volume, increased urinary calcium and oxalate concentrations and an increased urinary pH. Infection or struvite stones (triple phosphate) constitute a further 20% of all calculi and are caused by underlying infections. They are typically staghorn calculi and are more common in women of childbearing age. Uric acid stones and cystine stones make up the remaining 10%.

The peak incidence of urinary calculi presentation occurs between 30 and 60 years of age. The male to female ratio is approximately 3 : 1. A total of 96% of stones are radiopaque. Some 50% of patients presenting with renal colic require hospital admission.

PROGNOSIS

- Most calculi under 5 mm diameter will be passed spontaneously[3].
- Some 30% of all calculi do not pass spontaneously and require surgical removal to prevent complications.
- Half of all patients with urinary calculi will have a recurrence within 10 years and two-thirds within 15 years.
- Underlying infection may cause renal parenchymal damage and impaired renal function.
- Uric acid calculi may be the initial presentation of an underlying metabolic disorder.

TREATMENT

1. Ureteric colic can be treated with 75 mg diclofenac i.m., or 200 mg by suppository, which gives more effective relief than 50 mg pethidine. Diclofenac suppositories may be given to patients for self-administration if they are subject to renal colic and are away from medical care.
2. An adequate fluid intake should be maintained and the urine strained in an attempt to recover any stones passed.
3. Most patients will require referral for screening of the urinary tract for residual calculi.
4. Residual ureteric calculi may be removed by a variety of techniques including extracorporeal shock-wave lithotripsy, ureteroscopic extraction and ureterolithotomy.
5. Staghorn calculi and other large stones may require open surgical removal.

FOLLOW-UP

Any patients who have required surgical intervention will need specialist follow-up. Those who have passed a small isolated calculus are recommended to have an annual x-ray for 2 years. No further long-term follow-up is required in this group.

[1] Catto GRD, Power DA (1988) *Nephrology in Clinical Practice*. London: Edward Arnold.
[2] Drach GW (1986) In *Campbell's Urology*, 5th ed. Philadelphia: WB Saunders.
[3] Blandy JP (1986) In *Treatment and Prognosis; Surgery*. Oxford: Heinemann.

Acute Nephritic Syndrome

This condition presents with acute microscopic or macroscopic haematuria associated with a variable combination of proteinuria, oedema, oliguria and impaired renal function. The syndrome usually follows an episode of infection although other primary causes of glomerulonephritis such as membranoproliferative glomerulonephritis or immunoglobulin *gamma* A nephropathy may give rise to the same clinical picture. Several multisystem disorders such as systemic lupus erythematosus, Wegener's granulomatosis and polyarteritis nodosa can also cause acute nephritic syndrome. The disease predominantly affects children and young adults, although it can occur at any age.

Postinfectious glomerulonephritis remains the most common cause, particularly in developing countries, accounting for up to 30% of hospital admissions in areas of Africa and South America[1]. In adults, the male to female ratio is 2 : 1. Group A streptococci causing cutaneous or pharyngeal infections are the most commonly implicated organisms but the syndrome is also seen following infection with group C streptococci. The usual time between infection and onset of symptoms is approximately 20 days, although it can be as long as 60 days. There may be an inherited susceptibility to the disease. Acute nephritic syndrome frequently occurs in small epidemics.

PROGNOSIS

- Most symptoms settle without treatment over a 2–3-week period[2].
- Proteinuria may persist for several years.
- Some 20% of patients develop a nephrotic syndrome at some time during their illness[1].
- Encephalopathy and pulmonary oedema are fatal complications in less than 1% of cases[2].
- A small group of sufferers—less than 1%—develop a rapid decline in renal function. Of these cases, 25% are idiopathic and most of the remaining 75% are found to have an underlying acute vasculitis.

TREATMENT

1. All cases require specialist referral for assessment and regular monitoring of renal function.
2. Treatment is mainly supportive.
3. Salt and water restriction are usually all that is needed to control oedema and hypertension, although these problems may occasionally require drug treatment.
4. Short-term dialysis is occasionally required to control fluid overload, uraemia or electrolyte disturbances.

FOLLOW-UP

These patients should have their renal function assessed every 1 or 2 years.

---

[1] Catto GRD, Power DA (1988) *Nephrology in Clinical Practice*. London: Edward Arnold.
[2] Barton I (1986) In *Treatment and Prognosis, Medicine*. Oxford: Heinemann.

Nephrotic Syndrome

Patients with this illness have heavy proteinuria, hypoalbuminaemia and oedema. The proteinuria is usually 5 g or more in 24 hours and the serum albumin falls to below 30 g/l[1]. Once the serum albumin falls below 20 g/l, peripheral oedema will develop in dependent areas and often also periorbitally. In severe cases pleural effusions and ascites may be found. Almost any cause of primary or secondary glomerular pathology can give rise to a nephrotic syndrome.

In children under 15 years of age 83% of cases of nephrotic syndrome are due to minimal change disease; in adults membranous glomerulonephritis constitutes over 50% of cases. In children the male to female ratio is 2 : 1, whereas in adults the sex ratio is equal[2].

Nephrotic syndrome usually follows a viral illness in children whereas in adults there is rarely a history of preceding infection. Hyperlipidaemia is nearly always present although the underlying mechanism involved in its production remains obscure.

PROGNOSIS

- The ultimate prognosis is largely dependent upon the underlying cause of the glomerular pathology.
- Patients with nephrotic syndrome are particularly prone to infection, probably due to reduced levels of immunoglobulin gamma G. Primary pneumococcal peritonitis is a well recognized complication in children.
- Most nephrotic patients have reduced levels of low molecular weight inhibitors of coagulation and increased levels of several clotting factors. Some 35% develop arterial or venous thrombi.
- Renal vein thrombosis is a common complication and may result in pulmonary embolism.
- Renal impairment results from the underlying glomerular damage or from hypovolaemia, causing acute renal failure. Hypovolaemia may be exacerbated by diuretic therapy.
- Azoospermia may follow treatment with cyclophosphamide for minimal change disease in boys.

TREATMENT

1. All cases of nephrotic syndrome will require specialist referral for a full assessment, monitoring of renal function and treatment. Specific therapy will depend largely upon the underlying cause.
2. Most children who have minimal change disease will respond to treatment with steroids. Half of these children will relapse.
3. In adults treatment is directed towards minimizing oedema and preventing complications.
4. In adults salt intake should be restricted to 40 mmol/day.
5. Protein intake in adults should be above 60 g/day unless the patient is uraemic, in which case protein intake should be lowered.
6. Loop diuretics may be used to encourage a diuresis but the risk of hypovolaemia and subsequent renal failure should be borne in mind.
7. Hyperlipidaemia does not appear to lead to an increase in atheroma formation and does not require treatment.

FOLLOW-UP

These patients require regular specialist review.

---

[1] Glassock RJ et al. (1986) The Kidney. Philadelphia: WB Saunders.
[2] Wach F et al. (1981) Am. J. Med., **69**, 819.

Acute Renal Failure

Acute renal failure may be defined as the rapid deterioration of renal function over a period of a few days with an associated accumulation of nitrogenous wastes in the body. The impaired renal function is frequently reversible, although temporary dialysis may be required. Clinically, acute renal failure can be divided into the more common oliguric form, with a urine output of less than 15 ml/h, and a non-oliguric form which appears to carry a better prognosis.

Acute renal failure is generally classified as being prerenal, renal or postrenal. Prerenal failure mainly follows acute circulatory failure, resulting in a reduced glomerular filtration rate. There is no structural damage and the ability to concentrate urine is retained. The situation is rapidly reversible if the circulation is restored to normal.

Postrenal failure is caused by a mechanical or functional obstruction within the urinary tract and again is reversible following removal of the obstruction.

Intrinsic renal failure may be classified according to the nephron segment involved: acute glomerulonephritis (glomerulus), acute tubular necrosis (tubule) or acute interstitial nephritis (surrounding interstitium).

The incidence of acute renal failure is uncertain but some 1500 new cases are treated annually in the UK[1]. Usual causes are ischaemia, such as after major trauma; nephrotoxins such as carbon tetrachloride or phenylbutazone, and diseases such as systemic lupus erythematosus or streptococcal infection.

Complications include biochemical derangement, fluid overload, arrhythmias, anaemia, thrombocytopenia, confusion, gastrointestinal bleeding (20–30%) and infections.

PROGNOSIS

- The eventual outcome depends largely on the underlying cause.
- Older patients have a worse prognosis than younger patients.
- Patients in a catabolic state are likely to accumulate nitrogenous wastes faster and are therefore likely to require dialysis earlier.
- Acute prerenal and postrenal failure can cause intrinsic renal failure if not treated promptly.
- Non-oliguric acute renal failure has a mortality rate of 10–40% and thus carries a better prognosis than oliguric renal failure[2,3].
- Acute tubular necrosis is associated with a 50% mortality rate.
- Acute renal failure associated with severe burns, severe pancreatitis, hepatorenal syndrome, intra-abdominal sepsis, pre-existing cardiovascular disease, gastrointestinal haemorrhage and pulmonary infection carries a mortality rate of 80–90%.
- Hyperkalaemia may be life-threatening and if the serum potassium exceeds 7.0 mmol/l, urgent treatment is required.
- The average duration of non-oliguric renal failure is approximately 7 days.
- The average duration of oliguric renal failure is approximately 2 weeks.

TREATMENT

1. Prevention of acute renal failure is of the utmost importance. Patients with acute pre- or postrenal failure should receive prompt treatment of the underlying cause.
2. In some cases, the conversion of oliguric to non-oliguric renal failure is possible with the use of plasma-expanding diuretics (such as mannitol), thereby improving the prognosis.
3. Early treatment should be aimed at restoring fluid and electrolyte balance.
4. Some centres routinely use H_2 antagonists in order to reduce the incidence of gastrointestinal haemorrhage.
5. Hyperphosphataemia can be corrected using aluminium-containing antacids with meals and at bedtime. These antacids bind phosphate within the gastrointestinal tract.
6. Magnesium-containing antacids should be avoided as renal magnesium clearance will be reduced and magnesium intoxication can ensue.

7. A low protein diet with an adequate calorie intake of 110–130 kJ/kg body weight will reduce protein breakdown, reduce mortality and enhance the rate of recovery. Parenteral nutrition may be required, although this is associated with a risk of catheter-induced sepsis.
8. Some 50% of patients require dialysis as a temporary measure while renal function improves.
9. Sepsis requires prompt treatment with an appropriate antibiotic.

FOLLOW-UP

Patients who survive will require regular review until renal function returns to normal. Some patients may be left with a significant impairment of renal function; these individuals require long-term monitoring of renal function.

[1] Catto GRD, Parks DA (1988) *Nephrology in Clinical Practice*. London: Edward Arnold.
[2] Dawborn KC (1986) *Med Int.*, **2**, 1309–16.
[3] Molitoris BA, Schrier RW (1986) *Campbell's Urology*, 8th ed. Philadelphia: WB Saunders.

Chronic Renal Failure

Chronic renal failure is characterized by irreversible loss of renal function over a period of months or years, usually secondary to chronic, progressive renal parenchymal disease. There may be considerable variation in the causes of chronic renal failure between different countries. In Switzerland and Australia, for example, 20–25% of patients have suffered analgesic nephropathy. Malaria, schistosomiasis and sickle cell disease are significant causes of chronic renal failure in tropical countries. In most developed countries glomerulonephritis accounts for 30% of cases of chronic end-stage renal disease, with pyelonephritis and interstitial nephritis contributing a further 20% of cases. Other common causes include diabetes, amyloidosis, hypertension, obstructive nephropathy and hereditary renal disease.

Accurate information on the incidence of chronic renal failure is not available but in the USA approximately 100 patients per million population per year present in end-stage renal failure, requiring long-term dialysis or renal transplantation. In the UK, 40 patients per million population per year present with end-stage renal disease in the under-50 years age group. Taking all ages into account, the total figure for the UK is approximately 80 patients per million population per year.

The onset of chronic renal failure is frequently insidious and many patients present with a variety of vague symptoms such as general malaise, fatigue, anorexia, dyspnoea and nocturia. Physical examination may reveal the characteristic 'muddy' skin complexion, signs of cardiac failure (secondary to hypertension and fluid imbalance), and occasionally peripheral neuropathy. The rise in serum urea is not proportional to the fall in glomerular filtration rate and the urea may not begin to increase until the glomerular filtration rate has fallen to at least 50% of normal. The serum creatinine level is a more reliable indicator of renal function, although it may also fail to detect early changes in the glomerular filtration rate. Many patients remain asymptomatic until the glomerular filtration rate falls to 15 ml/min and some patients do not develop symptoms with even lower glomerular filtration rates. Chronic renal failure results in various metabolic disturbances including hypernatraemia, hyperkalaemia and acidosis.

PROGNOSIS

- A total of 75% of patients with chronic renal failure (almost 100% by end-stage renal failure) have associated hypertension. Hypertension accelerates the decline of renal function and requires treatment.
- Chronic renal failure will usually produce a normochromic, normocytic anaemia, probably due to reduced erythropoietin production.

- Patients with chronic renal failure are prone to developing various forms of bone disease including osteoporosis, rickets and osteomalacia.
- End-stage renal failure produces immunosuppression.
- Once the glomerular filtration rate has deteriorated to about 30 ml/min, continuing decline in renal function to end-stage renal failure is inevitable in most patients.
- Serial plotting of reciprocal creatinine clearance will usually reveal a linear relationship with time. This enables planning for renal replacement therapy to take place.
- Once the glomerular filtration rate has fallen to around 5 ml/min some form of renal replacement therapy is likely to be required.
- Peritonitis is a recognized complication of peritoneal dialysis. Current improvements in catheter design and techniques of bag exchange are reducing the rates of peritonitis.
- Many renal transplantation units are now achieving 1-year kidney graft survival rates of over 80%, and 1-year patient survival rates of 90–95%[3].
- In patients aged under 55 years a 10-year survival rate of 50% can be expected.

TREATMENT

1. All patients require referral to a specialist centre for a full assessment and follow-up.
2. The primary disease process should be treated where possible. Thus, treating the cause of an obstructive or hypertensive nephropathy and some types of glomerulonephritis or discontinuing nephrotoxic agents may lead to a significant increase in glomerular filtration rate.
3. The hypertension of chronic renal failure is usually unresponsive to treatment with thiazide diuretics. First-line treatment is usually with salt restriction and a loop diuretic (such as frusemide) in combination with a beta-blocker[4]. Calcium antagonists are an alternative to beta-blockers. Second-line therapies include vasodilators (such as hydralazine or minoxidil) or angiotensin I converting enzyme inhibitors (such as captopril or enalapril).

4. The hypertension seen in most patients with end-stage renal disease will be controlled by dialysis.
5. Dietary manoeuvres include lowering protein intake to reduce nitrogenous waste production and supplying approximately 2500 calories per day, mainly in the form of carbohydrates. Some patients develop hyperlipidaemia on this regime and in these cases the amount of carbohydrate can be reduced and the balance made up with polyunsaturated fats.
6. Salt restriction is contraindicated in salt-losing nephropathy but in most cases patients should avoid added salt or salty foods.
7. Treatment of the anaemia is aimed at correcting any underlying iron and folate deficiency and controlling bleeding and haemolysis. Blood transfusion is not used routinely and is mainly reserved for preoperative use before transplantation.
8. Patients in end-stage renal disease with uraemia, hyperkalaemia, acidosis, peripheral neuropathy, central nervous system disturbances or whose disease is poorly controlled with conservative measures will require peritoneal or intravenous dialysis.
9. Once the glomerular filtration rate has fallen to around 5 ml/min some form of renal replacement therapy is required.
10. Renal transplantation remains the treatment of choice in end-stage renal disease as it allows patients to return to a near normal lifestyle.

FOLLOW-UP

Patients with chronic renal failure require regular follow-up in specialist centres. The general practitioner has an important role to play in the support of patient and family, particularly once the need for renal replacement therapy arises.

[1] Catto GRD, Power DA (1988) Nephrology in Clinical Practice. London: Edward Arnold.
[2] Walls J (1986) Med. Int., 2, 1317–21.
[3] Michael J (1986) Med. Int., 2, 1321–8.
[4] Molitoris BA, Schiner RW (1986) In Campbell's Urology, 5th ed. Philadelphia: WB Saunders.

Catheter Problems and Care

Long-term indwelling catheters are predominantly indicated for use in patients with neurogenic bladders. Other less well accepted indications include chronic urinary incontinence and obstruction of the urethra. Counselling of the patient and relatives about long-term catheterization is extremely important. Catheter problems can be kept to a minimum if care is taken initially to choose a catheter of the correct size and material. Continence advisers are now available in most areas and they can provide a valuable source of information on the management of long-term indwelling catheters in the home.

PROGNOSIS

- Some 20–40% of deaths occurring in patients with neurogenic bladders treated with indwelling catheters are attributable to renal causes, secondary to infection of the upper urinary tract[1].
- Unnecessary treatment of asymptomatic urinary infection with antimicrobial agents may lead to the development of resistant organisms or infection with far more pathological organisms[2].
- Leakage occurs in 40% of patients with a catheter. This is usually due to an unstable bladder.
- If the catheter size is too large or if it is allowed to bend near the urethral meatus then urethral meatal ulceration can occur.

TREATMENT

1. Infection should only be treated if the patient is systemically ill. A catheter specimen of urine should always be sent for microscopy, culture and sensitivity before treatment with an antimicrobial agent, such as trimethoprim 200 mg twice daily for 5 days, is commenced. The antimicrobial agent may need to be changed once the results of culture and sensitivity are available.

2. Leakage due to an unstable bladder may often be remedied either by using a smaller diameter catheter or by using less water in the balloon and thereby reducing the residual volume of urine[3].
3. Haematuria does not require treatment unless it is heavy or persistent, in which case a urological opinion should be sought.
4. Urethritis can usually be resolved by using a smaller diameter catheter.
5. Blocked catheters may be flushed with 50 ml sterile water.
6. Maintenance of a regular high fluid intake may help to prevent blockage due to urinary debris.

FOLLOW-UP

Patients with long-term indwelling catheters will require regular catheter changes, usually every 2 or 3 weeks. The frequency with which these changes are required will be dictated by the rate of encrustation.

[1] Warren JW et al. (1981) J. Urol., **125,** 1–8.
[2] Brocklehurst JC, Brocklehurst S (1987) Br. J. Urol., **50,** 102–5.
[3] Norton C (1986) Nursing for Continence. Beaconsfield: Beaconsfield Publishers.

Carcinoma of the Bladder

Carcinoma of the bladder accounts for approximately 3% of all deaths from malignancies[1]. The incidence in both males and females increases at a constant rate with age and the overall incidence in populations over 40 years of age is 20 per 100 000[2]. The male to female ratio is approximately 3 : 1. Aetiological factors include exposure to industrial carcinogens, cigarette smoking, schistosomiasis and use of artificial sweeteners such as sodium saccharine and sodium cyclamate. Coffee drinking has also been implicated, although the results of studies are inconclusive. Exposure to Cyclophosphamide and pelvic irradiation are also associated with an increased risk of development of bladder cancer. A genetic predisposition for the development of bladder cancer has not been proven. Haematuria, either microscopic or macroscopic, is the most common presenting symptom[3] although urgency or frequency of micturition may also be present.

PROGNOSIS

- The overall 5-year survival rate for males and females is 60%[4].
- The prognosis is dependent upon the stage and grade of the tumour.
  1. Well differentiated tumours without invasion have a 90% 5-year survival rate.
  2. Invasion of the bladder muscle carries a 35% 5-year survival rate.
  3. Once surrounding structures have been invaded the 5-year survival rate falls to almost 0%.
- Most bladder tumours recur in other parts of the bladder, thus becoming multiple.

TREATMENT

1. Carcinoma *in situ* usually responds to intravesical or systemic chemotherapy.
2. Papillary tumours without invasion are usually treated by transurethral resection.
3. Invasive tumours may be treated with a combination of radiotherapy and cystectomy.
4. Chemotherapy may also be required.

FOLLOW-UP

All patients require regular specialist follow-up for life.

[1] Blandy JP (1986) In *Treatment and Prognosis; Surgery.* Oxford: Heinemann.
[2] Droller MJ (1986) In *Campbell's Urology*, 5th edn. Philadelphia: WB Saunders.
[3] Varkarakis MJ et al. (1974) *Urology*, **R,** 414.
[4] Burbank F, Fraumeini JF (1970) *Nature*, **227,** 296.

Renal Cell Carcinoma

Renal cell carcinoma is relatively rare, accounting for only 3% of all adult malignancies, but 75% of all renal malignancies[1]. There is a male to female ratio of 2:1. The peak incidence occurs in the fifth to seventh decades of life, although the tumour may be seen in younger patients. The condition is occasionally found to run in families and polycystic kidney disease appears to be a predisposing factor, although this has not been firmly established. Tobacco smoking, especially of pipes or cigars, also appears to be a significant aetiological factor[2]. No other specific aetiological factors have been identified.

Presenting signs and symptoms may include haematuria or pain due to primary disease, but weight loss, night sweats or a varicocoele of recent onset are more common presentations due to metastatic spread. The triad of haematuria, pain and a mass in the loin usually indicates advanced disease and a poor prognosis.

PROGNOSIS

- Although the prognosis is influenced by the stage and grade of the tumour, these are not totally reliable predictors of outcome.
- Tumours less than 3 cm in diameter have a cure rate of almost 100%[3].
- In the absence of local or distant spread of the tumour there is an 80% 5-year survival rate following nephrectomy.
- Local extension of tumour into the perinephric fat reduces the 5-year survival rate to 45% even after radical nephrectomy[4].
- Involvement of lymph nodes draining the renal parenchyma is associated with a 5-year survival rate of 0–30%[5].

TREATMENT

1. All patients require referral to a urologist for specialist treatment.

2. Radical nephrectomy is performed for all patients except those presenting with inoperable disease.
3. Some distant metastases may regress spontaneously, although this does not appear to be influenced by nephrectomy.
4. Neither chemotherapy nor radiotherapy improve survival but local metastases may be controlled by radiotherapy.

FOLLOW-UP

All patients require indefinite specialist follow-up.

---

[1] de Kernion JB (1986) In *Campbell's Urology*, 5th edn. Philadelphia: WB Saunders.
[2] Kantor AF (1977) *J. Urol.*, **117**, 415.
[3] Kirchner FK *et al.* (1976) *J. Urol.*, **115**, 643.
[4] Simonistch JM *et al.* (1983) *J. Urol.*, **130**, 20.
[5] de Kernion JB (1980) *Urol. Clin. North Am.*, **7**, 697.

18

The Male Genitourinary Tract

A. J. B. Carson

Carcinoma of the Prostate

Carcinoma of the prostate is one of the most common cancers occurring in developed countries. The reported incidence in the USA between 1973 and 1977 was 69/100 000 males per year[1], accounting for approximately 10% of all cancer deaths[2]. The prevalence of prostatic carcinoma is variably reported as being between 5 and 40% in males over 50 years of age. One-third of cases of carcinoma of the prostate manifest themselves clinically during a patient's lifetime. Two-thirds are discovered at post-mortem as an incidental finding.

Genetic, hormonal and environmental factors probably all contribute to the aetiology of prostatic cancer[3]. The role of infection is unclear. There may be local, vascular or lymphatic spread of the tumour. Presentation is usually with symptoms of urinary outflow obstruction such as hesitancy, poor urinary stream, nocturia and, occasionally, signs of urinary tract infection. Rarely there may be associated hydronephrosis or uraemia.

PROGNOSIS

- The natural history of the disease is extremely variable. The prognosis is dependent upon the grade and stage of the tumour.
- Well differentiated carcinoma of the prostate without local or distant spread is associated with a normal life expectancy.
- Patients with evidence of metastatic spread at their initial presentation have a 2-year survival rate of 50% and a 5-year survival rate of 20%.

TREATMENT

1. Any suspected case of carcinoma of the prostate should be referred for specialist investigation and treatment.
2. Transurethral resection is the treatment of choice for urinary outflow obstruction.
3. Total prostatectomy is not advocated in the UK as there is no evidence that survival is improved and the risk of incontinence combined with the certainty of impotence cannot be justified[4].
4. Radiotherapy may be used both to prevent local regrowth of tumour and to treat painful metastases.
5. A total of 75% of cases of carcinoma of the prostate respond to some form of hormone manipulation including orchidectomy or oestrogen therapy, such as diethylstilboestrol 1 mg 3 times daily.

FOLLOW-UP

All patients require specialist follow-up for life.

[1] Young JD et al. (1981) Natl. Cancer Inst. Monogr., 57, 1.
[2] Silverberg E, Lubera JA (1983) C.A. 33, 2.
[3] Catalona WJ, Scott WW (1986) Campbell's Urology, (Walsh PC, Gitters RF, Perlmutter AD et al. eds.) 5th edn. Philadelphia: WB Saunders.
[4] Blandy JP (1986) In Treatment and Prognosis; Surgery (Hawkins ed). Oxford: Heinemann.

Testicular Tumours

Testicular neoplasms are the most common solid tumours occurring in males between 20 and 34 years of age. Seminoma is the most common tumour although it is rarely seen below 10 or over 60 years of age. Yolk sac tumours are the most common tumours in infancy and testicular lymphomas in men over 50 years of age. Approximately 2–3% of testicular tumours are bilateral.

Important aetiological factors include cryptorchidism, hormonal factors such as inutero exposure to diethylstilboestrol[1] and testicular atrophy due to mumps or other non-specific causes. Approximately 10% of males with testicular tumours have a history of cryptorchidism[2] and 5% of unilaterally cryptorchid males will develop a tumour in the contralateral, normally descended testis. The most common presentation is as a painless enlargement of the testis, although 10% of patients present with acute pain and symptoms similar to epididymo-orchitis. A further 10% of patients present with symptoms due to metastatic spread such as lymphadenopathy, or shortness of breath.

The average annual age-adjusted incidence is approximately 4 per 100 000 adult males[3]. The peak incidence occurs between 20 and 40 years of age although there are smaller peaks in infancy and in males over 60 years of age.

PROGNOSIS

- The management of these tumours has been revolutionized in recent years with a significant improvement in overall cure rate.
- The prognosis is dependent upon the histology of the tumour, including the proportion of yolk sac and choriocarcinoma cells present, and the stage.
- In patients with stage I seminoma – i.e. when the tumour is confined to the testicle – the overall 5-year survival rate is 90%[4].
- If there is involvement of retroperitoneal nodes (stage II), the 5-year survival rate is 70%.
- Spread to mediastinal nodes (stage III) or other distant sites (stage IV) reduced the 5-year survival rate to 22%.
- Stage I non-seminomatous tumours carry a 3-year survival rate of 80% and stage II tumours a 50% 3-year survival rate[4].
- One-quarter of stage I tumours relapse in the first year.

TREATMENT

1. Early diagnosis of the tumour is critical. All adult males, especially those with a past history of cryptorchidism, in-utero exposure to diethylstilboestrol or with testicular atrophy, should be taught the principles of testicular self-examination. All patients with painless testicular enlargement should be referred for specialist assessment.
2. Orchidectomy is the initial treatment of choice for all testicular tumours.
3. Subsequent treatment with chemotherapy or radiotherapy will depend upon the histology of the tumour and the stage.

FOLLOW-UP

All patients will require regular specialist follow-up for life.

[1] Cosgrove MD et al. (1977) J. Urol., **117**, 220.
[2] Whitaker RH (1970) Br. J. Hosp. Med., **4**, 25.
[3] Morse MJ, Whitmore WF (1986) Campbell's Urology, 5th edn. Philadelphia: WB Saunders.
[4] Blandy JP (1986) In Treatment and Prognosis; Surgery (Hawkins ed). Oxford: Heinemann

Benign Prostatic Hyperplasia

Benign prostatic hyperplasia is probably the most common neoplastic growth in men. The prostate gland increases slowly in size from birth to puberty. Following puberty there is a more rapid increase in size until the end of the third decade. Prostatic size then remains constant until approximately 45 years at which time benign prostatic hyperplasia may develop, causing a rapid increase in volume, continuing until death. Histological evidence of benign prostatic hyperplasia is found in approximately 23% of men by the ninth decade. At present, a 50-year-old man has a 20% chance of requiring a prostatectomy.

The aetiology of the condition is unclear, but ageing and the presence of testes appear to be the two most important factors. Benign prostatic hyperplasia is not seen in men who have been castrated before puberty. The precise role of the testis remains unclear. Carcinoma of the prostate, urethral stricture, carcinoma of the bladder and neurogenic bladder should all be considered in the differential diagnosis.

PROGNOSIS

- Approximately 10% of patients with urinary outflow obstruction will require prostatectomy.
- Prostatectomy has a mortality rate of less than 0.5% and provides effective relief of symptoms in the majority of cases.
- Postoperative recurrence of outflow obstruction occurs in 3% of cases[2].
- Urethral stricture develops postoperatively in 2% of cases[2].
- If the patient with prostatic hypertrophy is left until complications such as infection, urinary retention, hydronephrosis, uraemia, bladder diverticula or detrusor instability have developed, there is an increased operative mortality rate.
- One-quarter of patients who have symptoms of bladder instability associated with outflow obstruction will not be helped by prostatectomy.
- Retrograde ejaculation occurs in the majority of men who have undergone any operative procedure to the prostate or bladder neck.
- Impotence is a rare complication of transurethral resection of the prostate but is seen more commonly in men who have undergone open prostatectomy.
- There is no evidence that benign prostatic hyperplasia is a precursor of prostatic carcinoma but carcinoma of the prostate is found in approximately 10% of all patients with benign prostatic hyperplasia.

TREATMENT

1. Not all patients with benign prostatic hyperplasia require treatment. Indications for the relief of urinary outflow obstruction include acute urinary retention, recurrent urinary tract infection, hydronephrosis, uraemia, haematuria, obstruction symptoms associated with bladder instability or symptoms which are troublesome enough to cause the patient to desire treatment.
2. Referral to a urologist for transurethral resection is the treatment of choice. Occasionally open prostatectomy may be required if the prostate is too large for transurethral prostatectomy to be performed safely.
3. Research is currently underway to develop a medical treatment for benign prostatic hyperplasia but a reliable and safe medical treatment is unlikely to be available for many years.

FOLLOW-UP

It is probably wise to review patients with evidence of benign prostatic hyperplasia periodically so that treatment can be offered at an early stage, before the onset of complications. Postoperatively, once a patient has been discharged from follow-up by the urologist, he should be advised to return if symptoms of urinary outflow obstruction recur.

[1] Walsh PC (1986) Benign prostatic hyperplasia In *Campbell's Urology*, 5th edn. Philadelphia: WB Saunders.
[2] Blandy JP (1986) In *Treatment and Prognosis, Surgery*. (Hawkins ed) Oxford: Heinemann.

Undescended testis

If a testis is not found in the scrotum it may be retractile, ectopic or undescended. A retractile testis can normally be encouraged down into the scrotum once the cremaster muscle has relaxed. An ectopic testis may be found either at the base of the penis, in the inguinal area but not within the canal itself, or in the femoral area of the thigh. Among undescended testes, 15% are intra-abdominal. The remainder are found either at the external ring of the inguinal canal or within the canal itself. Unilateral cryptorchidism is found in 1% of male infants at 1 year of age. The incidence of unilateral cryptorchidism in adult males is 0.8%.

PROGNOSIS

- A single scrotal testis should be adequate for normal fertility.
- Bilateral cryptochidism is associated with poor-quality semen; infertility is common in this group.
- Cryptorchidism may be associated with dysgenesis of both testes and this is borne out by the finding that the contralateral testis normally atrophies (although approximately 5% undergo compensatory hypertrophy).
- The risk of tumour formation in an undescended testis is 30–35 times greater than in a properly descended testis[3,4]. The actual risk in intra-abdominal testes is 5% and is reduced to 1% in the case of testes within the inguinal canal.
- One-tenth of all germinal tumours of the testis develop in undescended testes.
- The site of the testis is important. The 15% of undescended testes that are intra-abdominal are responsible for 50% of the germinal tumours that develop in cryptorchid testes.
- Unilateral cryptorchidism is associated with an increased risk of tumour formation in the contralateral testis.
- In infants, testes that have not descended into the scrotum spontaneously by 12–18 months of age will require orchidopexy. Current evidence suggests that early orchidopexy may improve subsequent fertility and reduce the risk of tumour formation.
- If orchidopexy is performed after 3 years of age the risk of tumour formation begins to rise.
- Currently, tumour development is seen only rarely in boys who underwent orchidopexy before 5 years of age but, since the average age of tumour formation in a previously undescended testis is 40 years, the period of follow-up is not sufficient at present to establish the effect of orchidopexy with certainty.
- Orchidopexy performed after puberty does not reduce the risk of tumour formation and so orchidectomy is the treatment of choice in this group.

TREATMENT

1. Orchidopexy is currently the treatment of choice. The optimal time is between 18 and 30 months of age. Some workers have suggested that the cryptorchid testis interferes with spermatogenesis in the contralateral testis in spite of orchidopexy, and advocate orchidectomy at all ages. This issue is presently under debate.
2. Orchidectomy is the treatment of choice in postpubertal undescended testes.
3. Approximately 9% of males with hypospadias also have undescended testes. This group should be referred for screening of the whole urinary tract as other developmental abnormalities may be discovered.

FOLLOW-UP

All cryptorchid males should be encouraged to examine their own testes regularly for life in order to detect tumour formation as early as possible. Subsequent follow-up and referral will be required if patients present with subfertility or tumour formation.

[1] Rajfer S (1986) Congenital anomalies of the testis. In *Campbell's Urology*, 5th edn. Philadelphia: WB Saunders.
[2] Sherins RS, Howards SS (1986) Male infertility. In

Campbell's Urology, 5th edn. Philadelphia: WB Saunders.
[3] Snyder HM *et al.* (1986) Pediatric oncology. In *Campbell's Urology*, 5th edn. Philadelphia: WB Saunders.
[4] Blandy JP (1986) In *Treatment and Prognosis, Surgery*

(Hawkins ed). London: William Heinemann Medical Books.
[5] Khun FJ *et al.* (1981) Urologic anomalies associated with hypospadias. *Urol. Clinics, North Am.*, **8**, 565.

Varicocele

Varicocele is caused by dilatation of the veins draining the testis. The overall incidence is unknown but varicocele is found in 30–50% of infertile males and is thus the most common cause of male infertility. A varicocele may cause pain which can be relieved by the use of a scrotal support or by lying down. In all, 90% of varicoceles are left-sided. Infertility or severe pain are indications for referral for treatment. Some varicoceles may be subclinical and may then only be detected by ultrasound or thermography.

PROGNOSIS

- A number of recent studies[1,2] have demonstrated that varicocelectomy, with or without medical treatment, improves the sperm count and the quality of the sperms in a significant number of cases.
- Pregnancy rates following varicocelectomy have also been shown to be significantly better when compared with a group of patients who did not undergo surgical treatment[1].
- Testicular infarction is a rare but serious complication of varicocelectomy.

TREATMENT

1. If there is no pain and the patient is not concerned about fertility, then no treatment is required.
2. Scrotal support may relieve any discomfort[3].
3. If definitive treatment is required, the patient should be referred for surgical varicocelectomy.

4. A few centres can now offer varicocele embolization, an outpatient procedure performed under local anaesthesia[4].
5. Medical treatment for varicocele-induced infertility with agents such as clomiphene or human chorionic gonadotrophin has been tried, both alone and in combination with surgery – with limited success.

FOLLOW-UP

If the patient is being treated for infertility then the normal follow-up for infertility should continue. In other cases follow-up is not required.

[1] Sherins RJ, Howards SS (1986) Male infertility. In *Campbell's Urology*, 5th edn. Philadelphia: WB Saunders.
[2] Netto NR *et al.* (1987) *Int. J. Fertil.*, **32**, 432–5.
[3] Blandy JP (1986) In *Treatment and Prognosis, Surgery*. (Hawkins ed), Oxford: Heinemann.
[4] Reidy JF (1987) *Br. J. Hosp. Med.*, **38**, 484.

Hydrocele

A hydrocele is a collection of fluid between the parietal and visceral layers of the tunica vaginalis. Hydroceles present most commonly in middle-aged men and in about 6% of all full-term male infants. It is believed that, in infancy, a hydrocele may be due to a patent processus vaginalis which allows peritoneal fluid to collect in the tunica vaginalis. In adulthood it is possible that changes in the secretory and absorptive capacities of the parietal and visceral layers of the tunica vaginalis lead to a build-up of fluid. Inflammatory or neoplastic diseases of the testis can also give rise to hydrocele formation.

PROGNOSIS

- Primary hydroceles, if left untreated, will continue to enlarge slowly[2].
- Mesenteric adenitis may accentuate the size of a hydrocele.
- Aspiration of the fluid should be avoided if possible in infancy as there is a risk of infection which may lead to peritonitis.
- Hydroceles presenting in adolescence and early adulthood are frequently the first presenting sign of an underlying tumour and require urgent referral for specialist assessment. In the case of secondary hydroceles, the prognosis depends upon the underlying cause.

TREATMENT

1. In infancy hydroceles should be observed for the first 12–18 months of life. Those that persist beyond this stage will require surgical intervention by ligation of the processus vaginalis.
2. The treatment of hydroceles in young males will clearly depend upon the underlying cause.
3. Aspiration is an appropriate treatment in many cases, depending upon the length of time that it takes for fluid to re-accumulate. Prevention of sepsis is of paramount importance.

4. Various sclerosing agents may be injected into the hydrocele in adults following aspiration in an attempt to get adhesions to form between the parietal and visceral layers of the tunica vaginalis. Sclerosing agents frequently cause pain and may give rise to further hydrocele formation. Their use should be avoided in infants as the agent can pass into the peritoneum and cause intra-abdominal adhesions.
5. Several surgical procedures exist to effect a more radical cure of hydrocele.

FOLLOW-UP

A successfully cured primary hydrocele requires no follow-up. Hydroceles treated with regular aspiration will require follow-up at intervals dictated by the rate of accumulation of fluid. Follow-up of secondary hydroceles will depend upon the underlying cause.

[1] Rajfer J (1986) Congenital anomalies of the testis. In *Campbell's Urology*, 5th edn. Philadelphia: WB Saunders.
[2] Blandy JP (1986) In *Treatment and Prognosis, Surgery* (Hawkins ed). Oxford: Heinemann.

Epididymo-orchitis

Acute epididymitis is the most common intrascrotal infection. Patients with clinical evidence usually have simultaneous involvement of the testis. The true incidence is unknown but acute epididymo-orchitis accounts for 20 per cent of urological admissions in the American military population[1,2]. The peak incidence occurs between 20 and 29 years of age. The infection usually spreads from the urethra or bladder and the most common causative organisms vary according to the age of the subject. The most common organisms in children and older men are coliforms, in men under 35 years of age, C. trachomatis, N. gonorhoeae and coliforms[2]. In men aged over 35 years sexually transmitted organisms are uncommon. If it follows urethritis, sexual exposure to the causative organism can be up to 30 days prior to the onset of symptoms.

Testicular torsion and tumour formation should be considered in the differential diagnosis. Occasionally, systemic disease such as tuberculosis can present with acute epididymo-orchitis. Serial early morning urine specimens should be examined and cultured for M. tuberculosis.

PROGNOSIS

- The incidence of complications is unknown but epididymo-orchitis can lead to abscess formation, testicular infarction, development of chronic pain and infertility.
- Early treatment may reduce the incidence of oligospermia, azoospermia and other complications.

TREATMENT

1. Hospitalisation may need to be considered.
2. If the infection is the result of bacteriuria, urine should be sent for microscopy, culture and sensitivity and an appropriate antibiotic commenced promptly.
3. If the infection is secondary to a sexually transmitted urethritis, a urethral smear should be examined. Referral to a Sexually Transmitted Diseases Clinic may be required. An appropriate antimicrobial agent should be administered such as tetracycline 500 m.g. orally four times daily for 10 days, or doxycycline 100 m.g. orally twice daily for 10 days, or amoxycillin 500 m.g. orally three times daily for 10 days. Erythromycin should also be given at a dose of 500 m.g. four times daily for 10 days to treat non-gonococcal causes.
4. Scrotal support and bed-rest are advisable for the first few days.
5. Cases of epididymo-orchitis secondary to bacterinna will require investigation for any underlying urinary tract disease. This will include all children and most men over 35 years of age.
6. In cases of epididymo-orchitis secondary to a sexually transmitted urethritis, sexual partners should be examined and treated.

FOLLOW-UP

Epididymo-orchitis is prone to relapse. Cases should be followed-up for at least twelve months.

[1] Berger, RE, 1986 Sexually Transmitted Diseases. In Campbell's Urology, 5th edn. Philadelphia: WB Saunders.
[2] Krieger JN (1984), Sex. Transm. Dis., **11(3)**, 173–81.

Testicular Torsion

Testicular torsion is a surgical emergency which threatens the viability of the affected gonad. The incidence is unknown. It can occur at any age and is thought to be due to a short mesenteric attachment which allows the testis to fall forwards and rotate on its axis. Torsion is more common in pubertal testes, as the testes undergo a five- or sixfold increase in volume at puberty, making subsequent rotation more likely. Torsion usually presents with pain and swelling on the affected side, although in the neonate the only finding may be a firm scrotal swelling, sometimes associated with restlessness and poor feeding.

PROGNOSIS

- The prognosis is good if the testis is operated upon within 6 hours of onset.
- Approximately 30% of testes are necrotic at operation[2].
- In almost all cases of neonatal testicular torsion, the testes are found to be necrotic at operation.
- One-third of 'saved' testes atrophy within 2 years of operation.
- If a necrotic testis is left *in situ*, the sperm count in adulthood is found to be low, possibly due to an autoimmune reaction.
- If the contralateral testis is left unfixed, approximately 30% will develop torsion in that testis[3].
- Torsion in an undescended testis may be due to an increase in testicular volume and may thus herald the onset of a tumour.

TREATMENT

1. If possible the torsion should immediately be reduced manually, followed by bilateral orchidopexy.
2. If manual reduction is not possible, then urgent exploration of the scrotum is required.
3. The contralateral testis will require orchidopexy to avoid the 30% risk of torsion in that testis.
4. If a necrotic testis is removed, a prosthesis may be inserted.

FOLLOW-UP

No long-term follow-up is required.

[1] Rajfer J (1986) Congenital anomalies of the testis. In *Campbell's Urology*, 5th edn. Philadelphia: WB Saunders.
[2] Backhouse KM (1982) *Urol. Clin. North Am.*, **9**, 315.
[3] Krarup T (1978) *Br. J. Urol.*, **50**, 43–6.

Phimosis

Phimosis is a condition in which the foreskin cannot be retracted over the glans penis. It is normally caused by infection underneath the foreskin, often as a result of poor hygiene. The prepuce may become scarred and fibrotic leading to discomfort on micturition, occasionally associated with ballooning of the foreskin and a thick preputial ring.

The development of the foreskin takes place between the 8th and 16th weeks of gestation. At this stage the inner surface of the prepuce is adherent to the glans. At birth only 4% of foreskins are fully retractile. This figure increases to 20% by 6 months of age and to 50% by 1 year[1]. By 3 years, 90% of boys have a retractile foreskin but 10% still have a physiological phimosis[1]. Symptomatic phimosis occurs in 10% of uncircumsized males[1].

PROGNOSIS

- Left untreated, phimosis may interfere with micturition and sexual function.
- Rarely, stones may form in the preputial sac.
- Circumcision, which is ultimately the treatment of choice, is associated with a 0.2% complication rate.
- Recognized complications include denuded penis, deformities of the penis, buried penis, penile amputation and over-cauterization. In spite of this there are probably fewer complications from circumcision than from any other surgical procedure.
- Inability to clean under the foreskin has been implicated in subsequent development of cancer of the penis[1,2].

TREATMENT

1. A phimosis may be prevented as follows:
   a. A non-retractile foreskin should not be forcibly retracted as this may cause cracking of the prepuce leading to further fibrosis and infection.
   b. Local hygiene is of the utmost importance, especially during the non-retractile phase. Once retractile, the foreskin should be retracted and cleaned routinely.

2. Once a phimosis has occurred:
   a. If there is severe infection and difficulty with micturition, the patient may require a dorsal slit[3].
   b. Control of infection is required. This can be achieved with saline bathing 2 or 3 times daily.
   c. Occasionally an antimicrobial agent may be required if infection is marked. The choice of antimicrobial agent should be based upon results of swabs sent for microscopy, culture and sensitivity.
   d. Once local infection and inflammation are under control, circumcision will be required.

FOLLOW-UP

Once the circumcision is healed, no further follow-up is required.

---

[1] Duckett JW, Snow BW (1988) Disorder of the urethra and penis. In *Campbell's Urology*, 5th edn. Philadelphia: WB Saunders.

[2] Blandy JP (1986) In *Treatment and Prognosis, Surgery* (Hawkins ed). Oxford: Heinemann.

[3] Smith DR (1984) *General Urology*, 11th edn. Los Altos, California: Lange Medical Publications.

Balanitis

Balanitis is a common condition affecting males of all ages, involving inflammation of the glans penis and prepuce. It is almost always associated with the presence of a foreskin which is frequently phimotic. Poor local hygiene is an important predisposing factor. The commonest reported infecting agents include coliforms, staphylococci, streptococci and *Candida* species[1,2,3]. Balanitis is occasionally associated with systemic disorders such as diabetes.

PROGNOSIS

- Severe or persistent balanitis may result in narrowing of the urethral or preputial meatus.
- Chronic balanoposthitis may be superimposed upon more serious underlying conditions of the penile skin, such as malignancy.
- Balanitis can give rise to vulvovaginitis in the sexual partner and vice versa.

TREATMENT

1. Daily local hygiene is of the utmost importance.
2. A topical antifungal agent such as clotrimazole cream should be applied 3 times daily where balanitis is due to *Candida* species.
3. If persistent or severe, balanitis may require treatment with an appropriate antimicrobial agent based on culture and sensitivity results.

4. The sexual partner(s) may require treatment for vulvovaginitis.
5. If there is an associated phimosis, a dorsal slit or circumcision may be required to facilitate local hygiene.

FOLLOW-UP

No follow-up is required once the condition has settled.

[1] Nickel WR, Plumb RT (1986) Cutaneous diseases of external genitalia. In *Campbell's Urology*, 5th edn. Philadelphia: WB Saunders.
[2] Gikar PW (1976) Uropathology. In *Fundamentals of Urology*. Philadelphia: WB Saunders.
[3] Harvard BM (1961) *J. Urol.*, **85**, 374.

Male infertility

Male infertility may result from a wide variety of causes. Careful and thorough assessment of both the male and the female partner is of the utmost importance. The true incidence of male infertility is unknown. Infertility is associated with a number of inherited endocrine disorders and other congenital syndromes such as Klinefelter's syndrome. Cryptorchid males have a higher than expected incidence of infertility and varicocoele is a well recognised cause of male infertility. A number of drugs and other toxins including alcohol may also interfere with sperm production. Infections of the genital tract can lead to infertility. In the UK approximately 8% of marriages are childless although not all of these are because of problems with fertility[1]. Difficulties still exist in interpretation of seminal analysis and it is a dangerous assumption on the part of the clinician that an ejaculate is inadequate for impregnation[2].

PROGNOSIS

● The prognosis ultimately depends upon the underlying cause but in general few cases respond to treatment and the results from those that do are unpredictable.

TREATMENT

1. All infertile couples require referral for a detailed assessment and subsequent treatment.
2. Treatment will depend largely upon the underlying cause and thus precision in diagnosis is of paramount importance.
3. Depending upon the underlying cause, the treatment may involve surgery or hormonal therapy. Treatment of male infertility is generally disappointing.
4. Counselling and truthfulness are important aspects of treatment when adequate therapy is not available.

FOLLOW-UP

The general practitioner has an important role to play in counselling the infertile couple. Once assessment and treatment have been completed, long term follow-up is not required.

[1] Hargreave TB (1983) *Male Infertility*, Springer-Verlag, Berlin.
[2] Sherins RJ, Howards SS (1986) In *Campbell's Urology*, 5th edn. Philadelphia: WB Saunders.

19

Breast Disease

L. J. Southgate

Benign Breast Disease

Women present with breast symptoms relatively frequently in general practice; almost without exception extreme anxiety surrounds the consultation as all women fear breast cancer. The general practitioner's task is to begin the careful process of diagnosis so that cancer is dealt with urgently while sparing women with benign disease unnecessary anxiety. In one diagnostic breast clinic 55% of the women attending had a benign disorder and a further 30% had no abnormality[1]. Abnormalities of the ducts and lobules are the commonest benign breast lesions. Fibroadenomas and fibrocystic disease affect the terminal ducts and lobules whereas duct papillomas and duct ectasia occur within the large ducts close to the nipple.

The fibroadenoma is the commonest breast mass in young women under 35, and is well defined, painless and mobile. Fibrocystic disease, which is 10 times more common than breast cancer, affects late premenopausal and menopausal women and encompasses a range of pathological processes including cyst formation, adenosis, fibrosis and epitheliosis. Duct papillomas commonly occur just below the nipple and often present with a blood-stained or serous discharge. These benign papillomata occur 10 times less frequently than breast cancer; rarely they may be multiple. Duct ectasia is associated with chronic periductal inflammation and presents with discharge from the nipple, nipple inversion, painful breast mass and occasional abscess and fistula formation.

PROGNOSIS

Fibroadenoma

- Fibroadenoma is self-limiting and grows slowly, rarely exceeding 3 cm in size.
- Eventually the fibroadenoma forms a hard calcified mass if it is untreated.
- Fibroadenomas do not recur after excision.
- Rarely a giant fibroadenoma will occur in young adolescent women, growing rapidly to a large size.

Fibrocystic disease

- Some women experience cyclical symptoms of pain and nodularity, particularly in the upper outer quadrants, for many years. The situation resolves with the menopause.
- Epithelial hyperplasia and atypia are associated with a 2–3 times greater risk of cancer[2].
- Women who have had one breast cyst have a greater than 40% chance of having another one.

Duct ectasia

- There is a high rate of recurrence of fistulae after surgical excision.
- Some patients require multiple operations.
- Breastfeeding is not possible after total ductal excision.

Duct papilloma

- The tumour does not recur after excision.
- The rarer multiple duct papillomata may be associated with an increased risk of malignancy.

TREATMENT

Fibroadenoma

1. Some surgeons observe small fibroadenomas in young women providing the mammogram and cytology (obtained via fine needle aspiration) are negative. All women with fibroadenomata require these investigations.
2. Fibroadenomas should be treated by excision as it may be impossible to distinguish them clinically from carcinoma.

Fibrocystic disease

1. Breast cysts are diagnosed and treated by needle aspiration. Providing that the mammogram excludes carcinoma, there is no blood in the aspirate, there is no residual mass after aspiration and the cyst does not refill, the procedure is curative. If the above criteria are not met then breast cancer is still a possibility and must be excluded.
2. Cyclical breast pain associated with tender nodular breasts is a problem which is often brought to the general practitioner. If a careful

clinical examination of both breasts with the patient undressed, plus a mammogram in women over 35, does not reveal localized disease then the woman may be reassured. It is wise to examine the patient on at least two occasions, preferably before and after her period when a marked difference in symptoms and signs may be observed. Throughout these consultations the doctor should remember that the upmost thought in the patient's mind is likely to be 'Have I got breast cancer?' and the subject should be openly and sensitively discussed. If it is appropriate to reassure the patient it is important to ensure that she leaves feeling that she has not wasted the doctor's time, and that she is able to consult again with the same problem if she wishes. These patients should be taught breast self-examination during the consultation with a follow-up visit to the practice nurse to ensure good understanding and technique.

3. Some women experience extreme discomfort and require medication for cyclical breast pain due to fibroadenosis. The antioestrogen tamoxifen given 10 mg daily helps about two-thirds of sufferers; bromocriptine 2.5 mg is sometimes effective despite normal prolactin levels. Research using danazol given 200 mg daily suggests that the considerable beneficial effects persist long after the drug has been stopped[3].

Duct ectasia

1. Surgery is postponed in the acute inflammatory phase. Recent research has raised the possible role of aerobic and anaerobic bacteria in this condition and appropriate antibiotics such as tetracyclines appear to have a beneficial effect on the inflammatory component of the lesion[4].

2. Biopsy may be urgently required to differentiate the lesion from an inflammatory carcinoma.

3. Total ductal excision may be performed subsequently.

Duct papilloma

1. Excision of the duct (microdochectomy) is curative.

2. Multiple duct papillomata require a total ductal excision. Those showing a proliferative histological picture may be treated by simple mastectomy.

FOLLOW-UP

No follow-up is necessary for a simple fibroadenoma or a solitary duct papilloma. Women with multiple duct papillomata should be followed up at yearly intervals.

Patients with simple benign breast disease do not require planned follow-up, provided they report any unusual events. Women with epithelial hyperplasia and atypia on biopsy require annual examination and mammography.

No follow-up is necessary for duct ectasia once treatment is complete and successful.

[1] Chetty U (1980) *Br. J. Surg.*, **67**, 789–90.
[2] Dupont WD *et al.* (1985) *N. Engl. J. Med.*, **312**, 146.
[3] Panahy C *et al.* (1987) *Br. Med J.*, **295**, 464–6.
[4] Bundred NJ *et al.* (1985) *Br. J. Surg.*, **72**, 844.

Breast Cancer

Breast cancer is the commonest malignant disease in women, with 21 000 new cases reported annually in England and Wales. One in 14 women will develop the disease in her lifetime. The incidence rates vary greatly worldwide and are highest in northern Europe and the USA and lowest in Asia and parts of Africa.

Increased risk (threefold) is associated with having a first-degree relative with the disease and with a history of benign breast disease. Women having their first child over the age of 30 have three times the risk of those having their first child before 20. The overall incidence in the UK is rising, with an 11% increase in the years 1968–1978[2].

The relationship between breast cancer and oral contraceptive use has been widely studied. In general there appears to be no cause for concern, except in women under 45 years who have had 4 or more years of use before their first fullterm pregnancy and who may have a 2.5-fold increase in the risk of breast cancer. Many of these women were not, of course, taking modern low-dose pills[1]. There is also an association with dietary fat and obesity.

Most tumours present in general practice as a breast lump in women over 35, with 75% of cases occurring in women over 50. All breast lumps should be regarded as potentially malignant, although the majority are not. Associated symptoms include discharge or bleeding from the nipple, and pain. Signs include skin or deep tethering, axillary or supraclavicular nodes, and pain from distant metastases, notably backache. The diagnosis is confirmed by mammography, aspiration cytology, drill biopsy, and excision biopsy.

PROGNOSIS

- The vast majority of breast cancers are adenocarcinomata. The histology is of great importance as it reflects the power of the neoplastic process and is a predictor of outcome. The size of the primary tumour is correlated with the likelihood of spread to the axillary lymph nodes. Spread is local, lymphatic and bloodborne and many patients experience a particular pattern of spread (e.g. bone not soft tissue), for which the reasons are not known[2].

  The TNM staging notation for breast cancer is increasingly used and is shown below: it is more detailed than the Manchester staging which it is replacing and will allow greater precision in prospective evaluations of different therapies[2].

Table 1 TNM staging notation for breast cancer: International Union Against Cancer

Stage	Definition
T1	Tumour < 2 cm diameter
T2	Tumour 2–5 cm diameter
T3	Tumour > 5 cm diameter
T4	Tumour of any size with direct extension to the chest wall
N0	No palpable node involvement
N1	Mobile ipsilateral nodes
N2	Fixed ipsilateral nodes
N3	Supraclavicular or infraclavicular nodes or oedema of the arm
M0	No distant metastases
M1	Distant metastases

- The prognosis is very variable but overall about 50% of women with breast cancer are alive and well 10 years after treatment.
- In all, 75% of women presenting with tumours T1–2 N0 are alive at 10 years. Of those presenting with N1–3 M0, 35% are alive at 10 years.
- The 5- and 10-year survival rates do not give the real picture as women continue to die from breast cancer many years after initial diagnosis. The overall survival rate is about 20–25%.
- Postoperative radiotherapy in patients with positive axillary nodes does not appear to improve survival but has a notably beneficial effect on local recurrence.

Table 2 The 5-year survival rates for operable breast cancer: different therapies[6]

Therapy	5-year survival
Extended mastectomy	67%
Radical mastectomy	69%
Modified radical mastectomy (patey)	76%
Simple mastectomy and radiotherapy	66%
Radical radiotherapy and lumpectomy	74%

- One-quarter of women experience depression or psychosexual problems in the year following mastectomy[2].

TREATMENT

Early ('operable') breast cancer
1. A breast cancer is deemed 'operable' if there is no peau d'orange, no chest wall fixation, no fixed axillary nodes, no arm oedema and no supraclavicular nodes (T1–2 N0 M0).
2. The treatment of early breast cancer is controversial and comprises combinations of surgery and radiotherapy, as shown in Table 2. Now that the disease is recognized to be systemic in many cases, the more radical surgical approaches are performed less frequently[3].
3. Many British surgeons favour the modified radical mastectomy (Patey) which is a simple mastectomy with axillary dissection and the removal of pectoralis minor.
4. Even if a simple mastectomy or lumpectomy is preferred it is usual to examine at least one representative axillary node to exclude spread to the axilla.
5. Radical radiotherapy and lumpectomy gives excellent cosmetic results but the long-term survival rates are still under review.
6. Some centres recommend adjuvant therapy in the treatment of early disease. Postmenopausal women who are node-positive with oestrogen receptor-positive tumours (ER+) are given tamoxifen. Premenopausal node-positive women may be given chemotherapy orally for 1 year.

Locally advanced disease
1. Radiotherapy is the preferred treatment. The principal complications are swelling of the arm and a stiff shoulder. The disease is controlled locally in 90% of those patients still alive at 5 years.

Metastatic disease
1. For premenopausal women with ER+ tumours oophorectomy or radiation-induced menopause is the first line of treatment, followed by chemical adrenalectomy using aminoglutethamide. Postmenopausal women with ER+ disease are treated with tamoxifen.
2. Chemotherapy is of major importance in the management of advanced disease and gives the best response in fit women with soft tissue rather than bony disease. It is the first line of treatment in women with a short disease-free interval or in the management of ER− tumours.
3. In the UK hormone manipulaton is often used first because it has fewer side-effects than chemotherapy, although the response rate is lower (30% compared with 60%). Chemotherapy comprises multi-drug regimes and is usually supervised by the regional oncology service[2,4].

General
1. The family doctor has an important role in the management of breast cancer. Priority should be given to forming a close relationship with the woman to enable support throughout the illness. The doctor should be aware of the current research findings and of the way in which these findings are implemented by the local cancer care team. It is unhelpful to refer a patient who does not wish to consider mastectomy to a surgeon who always performs it. Combined clinics between surgeons and radiotherapists who plan treatment together with the patient are the ideal.
2. Patients with breast lumps referred for investigation always suffer great anxiety while waiting for appointments and results. The experience can be made less traumatic if a careful explanation of the process of investigation is given and an invitation to discuss the results and proposed treatment is offered. Many women are very upset at the thought of losing

a breast and fear loss of femininity and sexual difficulties. Partners often share these feelings and should be given the opportunity to express their worries and to participate in treatment decisions.

3. The provision of this level of support for patients is dependent on a good working relationship with the secondary care team and good practice organization. It is imperative that information about diagnosis, prognosis and proposed action should be promptly received; in particular, it is crucial to know what the patient has been told and by whom. A diary of referrals kept in the practice serves as a reminder to request information that has not been received after a suitable interval, and avoids consultations between a distressed patient and an ill informed general practitioner which can seriously harm future confidence.

4. All mastectomy patients should have the opportunity to discuss prosthetic implantation surgery versus external prosthesis. The mastectomy counsellor will explain the range of possibilities, and that the internal prosthesis will not restore the woman to a completely normal appearance.

5. Patients who have undergone mastectomy are often put in touch with self-help groups such as the Mastectomy Association (Breast Care and Mastectomy Association of Great Britain, 26A Harrison St, London WC1H 8JG) while in hospital. The family doctor should be aware of the service provided by the local team and ensure that the patient has been given the opportunity to contact the appropriate people. If a prosthesis is to be worn, the general practitioner should ensure that it satisfies the patient; if it does not then the patient should be referred back to the consultant for further discussion.

6. Women with locally advanced or metastatic disease require treatment for the side-effects of therapy and support in coming to terms with their illness and prognosis. Many women become depressed and need encouragement to persevere with unpleasant therapies such as chemotherapy which causes nausea, vomiting and hair loss. Premature menopause induced by treatment can lead to severe menopausal symptoms which must *not* be treated with hormone replacement[5].

FOLLOW-UP

All women with breast cancer will be followed up by the cancer care team which treated them. Women in remission need not be seen regularly in general practice provided they know that they are welcome to discuss any problems as they arise, and that they should report any new lumps or unusual symptoms immediately. The patient's records should be clearly marked and the problem entered on the summary of problems list at the front of the notes so that the fact that she has had breast cancer, however long ago, is not overlooked should she consult with possible signs of recurrence later on. Women with active disease should be followed up in conjunction with the specialist: the primary care team will provide support to the woman and her family and eventually terminal care for many patients. First-degree relatives are at increased risk of the disease and should be encouraged to seek regular screening.

[1] McPherson K *et al.* (1987) Early oral contraceptive use and breast cancer. Results of another case–control study. *Br. J. Cancer*, **56**, 653–60.
[2] Souhami R, Tobias J (1986) Cancer and its management. Oxford: Blackwell Scientific Publications.
[3] Spittle M (1985) Radiotherapy in the management of breast cancer. *Practitioner*, **229**, 247–53.
[4] Howell A, Ribeiro G (1985) Management of advanced carcinoma of the breast. *Practitioner*, **229**, 355–62.
[5] McPherson A (ed) (1988) *Women's Problems in General Practice.* Oxford: Oxford University Press.
[6] Pierquin B, Baillet F, Wilson JF (1976) Radiation therapy in the management of primary breast cancer, *Am. J. Roentgenology*, **127**, 645.

Abbreviations

AIDS	acquired immune deficiency syndrome	**iu**	international unit
ALS	amyotrophic lateral sclerosis	**IUCD**	intrauterine contraceptive device
ARC	AIDS-related complex	**i.v.**	intravenous
b.d	twice daily	**LEA**	local education authority
CIN	cervical intraepithelial neoplasia	**MS**	multiple sclerosis
CT	computerized tomography	**NGU**	non-gonococcal urethritis
		NIDDM	non-insulin-dependent diabetes mellitus
DHA	district health authority		
DVT	deep vein thrombosis	**NSAID**	Non-steroidal anti-inflammatory drugs
ECG	electrocardiogram		
ECT	electroconvulsive therapy	**ORT**	oral rehydration therapy
EEG	electroencephalogram		
ENT	ear, nose and throat	**PBP**	progressive bulbar palsy
ER⁺	oestrogen receptor–positive	**PCP**	*Pneumocystic carinii* pneumonia
ER⁻	oestrogen receptor–negative	**PGL**	persistent generalized lymphadenopathy
FEV₁	forced expiratory volume in 1 second	**PMA**	progressive muscular atrophy
		PMS	premenstrual syndrome
HDL	high density lipoproteins	**PUVA**	psoralen and ultraviolet A
HIV	human immunodeficiency virus	**q.i.d.**	four times a day
HLA	human leukocyte antigen		
HPV	human papillomavirus	**SAH**	subarachnoid haemorrhage
HRT	hormone replacement therapy	**SSPE**	subsclerosing panencephalitis
HSV	herpes simplex virus	**STD**	sexually transmitted disease
HTIG	human tetanus immunoglobulin		
		t.d.s	three times a day
ICP	intracranial pressure	**TIA**	transient ischaemic attacks
IDDM	insulin-dependent diabetes mellitus		
		VDRL	Venereal Disease Research Laboratories
i.m.	intramuscular		
IQ	intelligence quotient	**VPB**	ventricular premature beats

Index